Ancient Greek Medicine in Questions and Answers

Studies in Ancient Medicine

VOLUME 54

The titles published in this series are listed at *brill.com/sam*

Ancient Greek Medicine in Questions and Answers

Diagnostics, Didactics, Dialectics

Edited by

Michiel Meeusen

BRILL

LEIDEN | BOSTON

Cover illustration: central scene of a floor mosaic depicting a physician and his patient during a medical examination (?). Tomb of Cornelia Urbanilla, 3rd century CE, Lambaesis, Algeria. Source: Carcopino, J. 1922. 'Le tombeau de Lambiridi et l'hermétisme Africain', *Revue Archéologique, Cinquième Série*, 15: 211–301, 302, Table 1.

Library of Congress Cataloging-in-Publication Data

Names: Meeusen, Michiel, editor.
Title: Ancient Greek medicine in questions and answers : diagnostics, didactics, dialectics / edited by Michiel Meeusen.
Description: Leiden ; Boston : Brill, [2021] | Series: Studies in ancient medicine, 0925-1421 ; volume 54 | Includes bibliographical references and index.
Identifiers: LCCN 2020038335 (print) | LCCN 2020038336 (ebook) | ISBN 9789004437654 (hardback : acid-free paper) | ISBN 9789004442672 (ebook)
Subjects: LCSH: Medicine, Greek and Roman. | Medicine–Case studies.
Classification: LCC R135 .A58 2021 (print) | LCC R135 (ebook) | DDC 610.938–dc23
LC record available at https://lccn.loc.gov/2020038335
LC ebook record available at https://lccn.loc.gov/2020038336

Typeface for the Latin, Greek, and Cyrillic scripts: "Brill". See and download: brill.com/brill-typeface.

ISSN 0925-1421
ISBN 978-90-04-43765-4 (hardback)
ISBN 978-90-04-44267-2 (e-book)

This book is printed on acid-free paper and produced in a sustainable manner.

Contents

Acknowledgements

The volume at hand collects a series of 9 papers stemming from an international conference which aimed to study the use of questions and answers (Q&A) in ancient medical literature: *Where Does It Hurt? Ancient Medicine in Questions and Answers* (Leuven, August 30–31, 2016). Most of the papers read during this conference are published, after revision, in the present volume. I would like to record my sincere gratitude to the contributors for their pleasant cooperation and for their patience in the face of delay. Special thanks to Dr. Erika Gielen for co-organising the event in Leuven and to the KU Leuven Doctoral School for the Humanities and Social Sciences, the Department of Literary Studies, the De Wulf-Mansion Centre for Ancient, Medieval and Renaissance Philosophy, and the Leuven Centre for the Study of the Transmission of Texts and Ideas in Antiquity, the Middle Ages and the Renaissance (Lectio) for their financial and organisational support. The conference was organised in conclusion of my postdoctoral project "Between Tradition, Ingenuity and Innovation. Authorial Strategies in Ancient Greek Natural Problems" (funded by the Research Foundation Flanders—FWO).

Michiel Meeusen
Leuven, 1 May 2020

Figures

Notes on Contributors

Isabella Bonati

is a lecturer and Postdoctoral Fellow at the North-West University of Potchefstroom (South Africa). She was previously a Postdoctoral Fellow in Papyrology at the University of Parma (Italy), and holds a PhD in Papyrology from the same University, where she also completed both her BA and her MA in Classics. Her research interests range widely and include papyrology, classical philology, linguistics, material culture, history of medicine and science. She has several publications in Papyrology and Classics, among which a book entitled *Glosse esotiche nei frammenti di Ipponatte. Gli esotismi nella lingua del giambografo di Efeso* (EAI, Saarbrücken 2015), and the monograph *Il lessico dei vasi e dei contenitori greci nei papiri.* Specimina *per un repertorio lessicale degli angionimi greci* (APF-B 37, De Gruyter, Berlin-Boston 2016).

Luca Gili

(PhD KU Leuven, 2016) is an assistant professor of philosophy at the Université du Québec à Montréal. He wrote a dissertation on Thomas Aquinas' philosophy of change, a book on Alexander of Aphrodisias' logic (*La sillogistica di Alessandro di Afrodisia*, Olms 2011) and several articles on Aristotle's logic and metaphysics. He is currently working on a book project on the uses and the meanings of the copula from Parmenides to Epicurus. Recent publications include *Non-Existent but Potentially Actual. Aristotle on Plenitude* (Revue de philologie, 2016, with L. Ferroni) and the edited collection *Third Pisa Colloquium in Logic, Language and Epistemology* (Ets, 2019, with L. Bellotti, E. Moriconi and G. Turbanti).

Laura Mareri

completed her PhD in Classical Philology in 2016 at the University of Macerata. After an initial training on the subject of ancient medicine at the University of Siena, where she primarily focused on the study of Galen, she subsequently concentrated her main research efforts on Byzantine medicine, with particular regard to Alexander of Tralles, as well as on the ancient theories of mental disorders, especially melancholy.

Robert Mayhew

is Professor of Philosophy at Seton Hall University (New Jersey, USA). His publications in ancient philosophy include *Aristotle's Lost Homeric Problems* (Oxford UP), *Theophrastus: On Winds* (Brill), *Prodicus the Sophist* (Oxford UP),

Plato: Laws 10 (Oxford UP), and *The Female in Aristotle's Biology* (U. of Chicago Press). He is the editor of *Aristotle: Problems* in the Loeb Classical Library, and of *The Aristotelian Problemata Physica: Philosophical and Scientific Investigations* (Brill). He is currently in the early stages of work on the *De mirabilibus auscultationibus* (*On Marvelous Things Heard*) attributed to Aristotle.

Michiel Meeusen
(PhD KU Leuven, 2013) specialises in ancient science and medicine and the literature and culture of the High Roman Empire. Among his publications are a monograph on Plutarch's *Natural Questions* (Leuven 2016) and a co-authored edition of the same text in the *Collection des universités de France* (Paris 2018). He also published on the broader genre of natural-medical problems after the model of the Aristotelian *Natural Problems* with specific attention to the collection's circulation in the High Imperial era.

Katerina Oikonomopoulou
is Assistant Professor of Greek Literature at the University of Patras. Her research focuses on imperial Graeco-Roman encyclopaedic and compilatory writing, including the ancient literature of *problemata*. Her publications include book chapters on the pseudo-Aristotelian *Problemata Physica* ('The *Problemata*'s medical books: structural and methodological aspects', in: *The Aristotelian* Problemata Physica*: Philosophical and Scientific Investigations*, ed. Robert Mayhew, Brill 2015: 61–78), and on Plutarch's *Quaestiones*-collections ('Plutarch's corpus of *Quaestiones* in the tradition of imperial Greek encyclopaedism', in: *Encyclopaedism from Antiquity to the Renaissance*, eds. Jason König and Greg Woolf, Cambridge University Press 2013: 129–153). She has also co-edited a volume of essays on Plutarch's *Quaestiones Convivales* (*The Philosopher's Banquet: Plutarch's 'Table Talk' in the Intellectual Culture of the Roman Empire*, with Frieda Klotz, Oxford University Press 2011). She is currently preparing a monograph on Greek miscellanistic writing in the Second Sophistic.

Andrés Pelavski
is a medical doctor and works as a qualified anaesthetist. He is a final year PhD student at Cambridge University. His research focuses on disturbances of consciousness in ancient medical texts. His interest in the History of Medicine developed during his MPhil (also in Cambridge, Faculty of Classics). Prior to that, he studied Classics at the University of Barcelona.

Antonio Ricciardetto
est docteur en langues et lettres (2015) de l'Université de Liège. Sa thèse de doctorat a porté sur des papyrus documentaires grecs de médecine. Poursuivant des recherches dans les domaines de la papyrologie et de l'histoire de la médecine, il est membre statutaire de l'équipe « Monde byzantin » (UMR8167 Orient & Méditerranée), membre du CEDOPAL de l'Université de Liège, et secrétaire de la Société belge d'études byzantines. Il est l'auteur de *L'Anonyme de Londres* (P.Lit.Lond. *165*, Brit.Libr. *inv. 137*). *Édition et traduction d'un papyrus médical grec du Ier siècle apr. J.-C.* (2e éd. Paris, 2016), et coéditeur du volume *En marge du* Serment *hippocratique: contrats et serments dans le monde gréco-romain* (Liège, 2017).

Nicola Reggiani
is Researcher of Papyrology at the University of Parma. He continues Isabella Andorlini's work to build a Digital Corpus of the Greek Medical Papyri and is particularly interested in the material aspects of the ancient papyri of medical content and on their digital representation, on which he published several articles. His long-standing experience in Digital Papyrology led to the recent monographs *Digital Papyrology I—Tools, Methods and Trends* (De Gruyter 2017) and *La papirologia digitale* (Athenaeum 2019); he is also the editor of the volumes *Digital Papyrology II—Case Studies on the Digital Edition of Ancient Greek Papyri* (De Gruyter 2018) and *Greek Medical Papyri—Text, Context, Hypertext* (De Gruyter 2019).

Ancient Greek Medicine in Questions and Answers: A Short Introduction

Michiel Meeusen

> An ill-tempered doctor who only had one eye asked his patient how he was.
> "I am as you can see."
> "Well, as far as *I* can see, you are half dead!"[1]

∴

What makes this joke 'sick', apart from the fact that its two main protagonists suffer from a physical condition, is the total communicative breakdown taking place between a doctor and his patient at the outset of what would otherwise probably be just an everyday medical consultation. The question and answer that structure this amusing dialogue are formulated in such a way that they are open to interpretation, thus rendering the message that is being conveyed semantically ambiguous. The doctor's ordinary greeting, 'How are you?' (πῶς ἔχεις;), can be interpreted as a prompt attempt to diagnose his patient's physical condition; whereas the patient's rather insensitive reply that the doctor can see for himself, 'As you can see' (ὡς βλέπεις—a phrase equally common in ordinary conversation), has non-ordinary implications in this specific context, considering the doctor's visual impairment.[2] The doctor feels personally prompted—and, ill-tempered as he is, probably also offended—by his patient to examine him visually (rather than verbally), so reacts with agitation and declares him half-dead at a single glance. The pun is in the 'I' of the doctor's 'autopsy' (ὡς ἐγὼ βλέπω: 'as far as *I* can see').

All laughing aside, this joke has something important to say about the underlying rationale of the use of questions and answers in doctor-patient communication more generally but also about the potential problems and misun-

1 *Philogelos* 185a (57 Dawe); tr. Baldwin (1983: 35).
2 Baldwin (1983: 97) is right that "in the present context, the expression *hos blepeis* (as you can see) [...] makes the joke sicker." On morbid laughter, see Kazantzidis—Tsoumpra (2018). More one-eyed-jokes in Plutarch, *Quaest. conv.* 2.1.633C (130.10–16 Clement—Hoffleit).

 | DOI:10.1163/9789004442672_002

derstandings involved in this dialogical strand of communication (a genuine risk, considering the sheer number of doctor jokes in the *Philogelos*). Indeed, asking the right questions and obtaining the right answers is vital to medical healthcare today as much as it was in the past. It is essential for efficient doctor-patient interaction not in the least because it provides access to information not otherwise accessible via sensory observation or via logical reasoning, thus forming an important component of medical diagnosis and treatment, including patient anamnesis and physical examination.

Already the Hippocratic writings underline the great importance for doctors of asking questions to their patients, and they also give us a concrete idea of what kind of questions were asked and what answers were given in return (e.g., about the patients' lifestyle, the afflictions they were experiencing, or the progress/decline that they had made).[3] Centuries later, Rufus of Ephesus in his *Medical Questions* gives a useful set of guidelines on how a doctor can gain valuable information from his patients through questioning, thus offering a fascinating insight into the bedside manner of physicians in Antiquity.[4] And in Galen we find all the typologies for interviewing the sick; he criticises the Methodical school for not asking questions at all as they simply dictate their patients what they should do without further inquiry into the underlying causes of diseases (which they reduce to only two kinds, depending on flow and astringency).[5]

This is indeed very revealing of the sociology of ancient medical practice and of how physicians and patients interacted with each other. But it also tells us something about the therapeutic methods that doctors employed in their daily practice and how much of it was based on the patients' verbal input and cognitive abilities. The information thus obtained was not always unambiguous though. One can imagine that patients or their relatives were often incapable of providing an accurate answer (if, indeed, any answer at all) to some of the

3 That the Hippocratics were highly reliant on asking patients questions can be deduced, for instance, from the case histories recorded in the *Epidemics* (see Pelavski and Ricciardetto in this volume). The author of the Hippocratic *Prognostic* ascribes great importance to questioning patients in addition to autoptic examination. See Jouanna – Anastassiou – Magdelaine (2013: xxxvi–viii, at xxxviii): "L'interrogatoire du malade par le médecin soit sur ce qu'il éprouve dans le présent, soit sur ce qu'il a éprouvé et fait dans un passé proche est donc un complément nécessaire pour établir un pronostic correct." Cf. Debru (1991: 38): "La parole du malade entre donc dans la collection des signes cliniques". See also Cambiano (2006: 3–8).

4 It is a great loss for this volume not to have been able to publish a contribution concerning Rufus of Ephesus' *Medical Questions*. Melinda Letts gave a stimulating talk on this topic at the conference in Leuven; her work can be consulted in Thumiger – Petridou (2015: 81–103).

5 Gal., *Meth. Med.* 2.5.3 (10.105.13–106.1 Kühn). For further references, see Cambiano (2006: 10 n. 44).

doctor's questions. In the case of mental disorders, for instance, where the issue of trustworthiness comes into play, the answering itself often offered a useful tool for diagnosing the patient's mental condition.[6] In other cases, clear communication between patients and physicians was complicated not by some physical or mental impairment, but by a lack of accurate terminology. Galen, for instance, says that certain types of pain are actually felt by patients, but that they cannot always clearly describe them when asked to.[7] As such, a proficient doctor had to be able not only to ask the right questions but also to look for the right answers himself, if needed, and to interpret (or 'translate') the information thus obtained with an eye towards establishing a proper diagnosis and treatment plan.

Also in the reverse direction of the communicative spectrum, physicians had to be able to formulate suiting answers to the questions asked by their patients, thus demonstrating their reliability as medical experts whilst securing an informed clientele (bear in mind the absence of a formal *Lizenzsystem* in Antiquity). Galen wrote a treatise on this topic, *On Examining the Physician*, preserved in Arabic.[8] And we also have evidence that doctors were examined by official authorities in legal contexts; they could also take an official exam for 'public doctor' (δοκιμασία): critical situations in which their technical expertise was at stake and which also illustrate the broader political contexts in which medical experts were active in the ancient world.[9]

As this snapshot overview shows, the use of Q&A formulas is widely attested in ancient medical sources, casting an intriguing light on its relevance for medical practice at large. However, by employing specific interrogative turns in their discourses, medical authors not only sought to provide practical information for diagnosing and treating patients, but also to amass theoretical insights about the human body, its anatomy and its physiological and nosological processes, which could then serve for future reference (e.g., in the form of medical catechisms for students, or practical manuals for medical professionals). These texts deal with several types of questions, including questions that sought to locate, define and explain certain illnesses or disorders in the body and also how to treat them (e.g., 'Where does it hurt?', 'What is it that hurts?', 'Why does it hurt?', 'Which therapy helps?'). Questions of this sort can be found, for instance, in medical manuals, medical papyri and collections of problems.

---

6 See Pelavski and Mareri in this volume.

7 Gal., *Loc. Aff.* 2.7 (8.88.15–89.7 Kühn; 328.4–12 Gärtner). On this passage, see Meeusen in this volume. On Galen's method of questioning more generally, see Gili's contribution.

8 See Iskandar (1988), with the study of Nutton (1990: esp. 244–249).

9 See Ricciardetto and Reggiani in this volume.

The popularity of the Q&A genre, where questions are raised and answered in a tight repetitive sequence, is largely due to the fact that it provided a user-friendly matrix for storing vast amounts of practical and theoretical knowledge on specific medical topics. By making this information accessible in a systematic and bitesize fashion, the genre was particularly useful for medical practitioners (e.g., when dealing with a specific case which they could not immediately diagnose or for which they wanted to verify the proper treatment). But it became well-entrenched also in the ancient medical school curriculum (e.g., in the Preface to Ps.-Soranus' *Medical Questions* the author specifies that the Q&A format suits the work's educational aims as being intended for beginners).[10] Through its dialogical and interrogative structure, it provided students and professionals with an efficient method to consult and memorise all types of medical knowledge, both practical and theoretical. And by being condensed in a textual form, it was also useful for transferring this knowledge between authors and readers, to future generations.

Despite the recent revival of scholarly interest in the Q&A genre more broadly, as testified by a number of recent text editions and a proliferation of individual studies, a specific thematic focus on ancient Greek medical Q&A as such is, despite its socio-historical, intellectual and literary significance, up to now lacking.[11] By providing a set of in-depth studies (without any ambition towards exhaustiveness) the volume in hand is intended to bridge this gap and to progress and expand the existing scholarship in meaningful ways as well as to stimulate further research in the field. Although the volume's main focus is on the specific function of Q&A as a genre of ancient Greek medical writing, it also aims to usefully contribute to our better understanding of more general issues relating to the history and the sociology of ancient medicine, and to the organisation and communication of medical knowledge in Antiquity.

As to method, questions that are of central interest in the contributions include: How does the structural use of Q&A inform the social and intellectual relation between different medical stakeholders (doctor-patient, teacher-student, author-reader, among peers), and how is this manifested in the literature? What can we learn from this about the political, intellectual and cultural contexts of the medical art in Antiquity? What do the traditions and sources

10 Ps.-Sor., *Quaest. Med., Pref.* (247.5–8 Rose; cf. 243.5–6 Rose). The use of problem-based learning (PBL) in medical faculties—the 'Canadian method'—now introduced in many medical schools around the world shows that this approach is still very much alive. Many thanks to Marie-Hélène Marganne for this point.

11 Fundamental is Ieraci Bio (1995). For further literature, see the bibliographic sections in the individual contributions.

employed in the Q&A format reveal about the author's medical or philosophical allegiances? What does it tell us about the development from oral communication to written text? And what type of 'performance' contexts are implied, broadly defined (e.g., medical consultation, demonstration, school debate, contests, discussion at symposia, etc.)?

In dealing with such issues, the contributions gathered here cover a wide range of sources and employ a great variety of methodological perspectives, including insights from medical history, ancient philosophy, papyrology, literary studies, linguistics, cognitive studies, and digital humanities. Especially the latter—digital—perspective is of great importance; it is unique in the volume and its inclusion is believed to strengthen the volume's contribution to the field of ancient medicine studies in so far that it places digital methods as inherent to it (rather than as a part discussed and presented in publications dedicated to digital tools and methods). This is not, of course, to deny the innovativeness of the other contributions, which all offer fresh and fascinating perspectives into numerous hitherto unexplored facets pertaining to ancient medicine.

As to sources, 'medical literature' is broadly defined so as to embrace not only the highly specialised medical treatises as those collected in the Hippocratic and Galenic corpora, but also non-canonical authors and texts, including anonymous papyrus fragments and collections of problems. It also includes questions relating to material and visual culture (e.g., the materiality and visual lay-out of texts). The applied timeframe spans most of ancient Greek medical history, from the Hippocratic writings up to, and including, Late Antiquity (Alexander of Tralles). A specific emphasis is put on the Graeco-Roman period, when the Q&A genre became more and more common in medical treatises (cf., e.g., Soranus' *Gynaecology*, also most of the medical papyri in Q&A stem from this period).

For reasons of efficiency I have opted for a (roughly) diachronic, rather than thematic, ordering of the contributions, starting with the Hippocratics and ending with Alexander of Tralles. Other ordering principles have been considered but not eventually taken aboard considering the categorical restrictions that they inevitably would have imposed (e.g., contributions focusing on philosophical questions *vis-à-vis* those dealing with formal and literary aspects). This does not, of course, imply that there are no recurrent themes distinguishable throughout the volume (see further). Nor should it go unnoticed that some thematic clustering has emerged organically from the chosen approach (e.g., aligning the contributions on *problemata* collections, or the ones on medical papyri). But whereas this dynamic is not pervasive, the use of mechanical subdivisions seemed redundant.

As to the recurring themes in the contributions, the most clearly identifiable ones centre around the conceptual relevance of Q&A for medical diagnostics, didactics, and dialectics (and related to these, for medical practice, education, and research respectively). In different ways and to different degrees the contributions shed a light on these three aspects—which indeed need not necessarily be understood as strictly disconnected from one another (and hence do not require structural disentangling in the book). For instance, medical diagnosis commonly includes a dialectical process where doctors, in a logical way, question their patients in view of obtaining important (yet often indeed 'invisible') information about the malfunctioning of their body or mind, on which a proper treatment can then be based.[12] The genre of medical *problemata*, to give another example, comes in the form of concrete applications (or 'case-studies') of the dialectical processes of medical-scientific research and explanation, and more than once serves a concrete educational goal by contributing to the instruction of aspirant doctors.[13] And one may also wonder if the genre of medical Q&A more generally was perhaps inspired, at least in its beginnings, by the kind of questions raised during medical practice (e.g., by patients to their doctors as a way of informing themselves, or by doctors among themselves when confronted with enigmatic medical cases).

The attentive reader of this volume (likely to include medical historians, specialists of ancient philosophy, scholars of ancient Greek literature focusing on technical-scientific texts) will find concrete manifestations of these three central thematical lines (diagnostics, didactics, dialectics) interwoven throughout the nine contributions. Whereas previous studies have mainly focused on distinct aspects relating to ancient medical Q&A (e.g., by analysing its function as a literary genre or its use in doctor-patient interaction), this book aims to break new grounds by exploring, for the first time as far as I am aware, the wider complexity of this phenomenon and to suggest a more coherent approach. Further study into medical Q&A and its prevalence in other authors, texts, languages, times and cultures will show if this is a fair assessment or not, but this goes beyond the scope of the present volume.

---

12 See the contributions of Pelavski, Gili, Mareri; indirectly also Ricciardetto.

13 See the contributions of Mayhew, Oikonomopoulou, Meeusen; also prominent in medical ἐρωταποκρίσεις on papyrus: see Bonati and Reggiani.

Bibliography

Primary Sources

Clement, P.A.—Hoffleit, H.B. 1969. *Plutarch's Moralia 8. Table Talk 1–6*. Cambridge, Mass.—London: Harvard University Press—William Heinemann Ltd.

Dawe, R.D. 2000. *Philogelos*. Munich—Leipzig: K.G. Saur.

Gärtner, F. 2015. *Galeni De locis affectis I–II* [CMG V.6.1.1]. Berlin: De Gruyter.

Iskandar, A.Z. 1988. *Galeni De optimo medico cognoscendo libelli* [CMG Suppl. Or. IV]. Berlin: Akademie-Verlag.

Jouanna, J.—Anastassiou, A.—Magdelaine, C. 2013. *Hippocrate 3.1. Pronostic*. Paris: Les Belles Lettres.

Kühn, C.G. 1821–1833. *Claudii Galeni Opera Omnia*. Leipzig: Car. Cnoblochii.

Rose, V. 1870. *Anecdota Graeca et Graecolatina*, vol. 2. Berlin: Ferd. Duemmler.

Secondary Sources

Baldwin, B. 1983. *The Philogelos or Laughter-Lover*. Amsterdam: J.C. Gieben.

Ieraci Bio, A.M. 1995. 'L' *erōtapokrisis* nella letteratura medica', in C. Moreschini (ed.), *Esegesi, parafrasi e compilazioni in età tardoantica. Atti del terzo convegno dell'associazione di studi tardoantichi*. Naples: D'Auria, 187–207.

Cambiano, G. 2006. 'Funzioni del dialogo medico-paziente nella medicina antica', in A. Marcone (ed.), *Medicina e Società nel Mondo Antico. Atti del convegno di Udine (4–5 October 2005)*. Florence: Grassina, 1–15.

Debru, A. 1991. 'Médecin et malade dans la médecine hippocratique: interrogatoire ou dialogue?', in P. Demont (ed.), *Médecine antique: cinq études de Jacques Jouanna, Armelle Debru, Paul Demont, Michel Perrin*. Amiens: Université d'Amiens, 35–49.

Kazantzidis G.—Tsoumpra, N. 2018. 'Morbid Laughter: Exploring the Comic Dimensions of Disease in Classical Antiquity', *Illinois Classical Studies* 43.2: 273–297.

Nutton, V. 1990. 'The patient's choice: a new treatise by Galen', *Classical Quarterly* 40: 235–257.

CHAPTER 1

Questioning the Obvious: The Use of Questions and Answers in Assessing Consciousness in the Hippocratic Corpus

Andrés Pelavski

Abstract

Ancient medical texts offer many examples where patients act weirdly, speak nonsense, or simply are not their usual selves. Recent scholarship, in its attempt to better understand how the ancients conceived of mental illness, has generally regarded these conditions as signs of madness. But my aim here is to show that many of these cases rather describe diseases where the patient's consciousness is impaired. To this end, I will explore the ways in which Hippocratic doctors assessed such patients. Specifically, I look at certain questions to which the actual answers were not the real aim, since the doctors presumably already knew them beforehand. Instead, by asking such questions, the cognitive functioning required to answer them was under assessment. In other words, the questions were a 'metacognitive' device, whereby doctors attempted to understand the way in which their patients were thinking and making sense of the world that they were experiencing. In my analysis, I will frame these practices as examples of interpersonal communication and will relate them to contemporary questionnaires that are often used in current medical practice as tools to measure cognition and consciousness. By focusing on the communicational aspect of this question-and-answer-based interaction, the paper will shed light on the manner in which doctors related to deluded patients, and the rules and roles taken for granted in such interactions. On a more medical level, the analysis of these passages will reveal an embryonic notion of consciousness, which has not been explored before.

1 Introduction

[Medicus]	Menaechmus, why do you uncover your arm? Don't you know how bad this is for this illness that you currently have?
[Menaechmus I]	Why don't you hang yourself? […]

 | DOI:10.1163/9789004442672_003

[Med.] Tell me what I am asking you, do you drink white or red wine?
[Men.] Why don't you go to hell?
[Med.] By Hercules! Right now he is only just beginning to go mad.
[…]
Tell me, do you ever feel that your bowels rumble?
[Men.] When I'm full they don't make noises, when I'm hungry they rumble.
[Med.] He's giving me this reply, by Pollux, certainly not likely of a mad person.[1]

This passage presents a comic situation, where a doctor-patient interaction takes the form of questions and answers. Despite its parodic nature, and the centuries that separate Plautus from the Hippocratic doctors, the dialogue illustrates some important features about this type of verbal interchange, particularly about the different kinds of questions that doctors utilise in order to understand their patients' conditions.

The normal questions of a typical medical anamnesis can be schematically classified according to different criteria and levels of depth. On the first level, two kinds of questions can be singled out: those where the questioner does not know the answer, does not have access to the information asked for, and needs that information;[2] and those where the doctor is not specifically interested in the facts that he is inquiring about, because he already knows them, but wants to find out how the patient is reasoning. Examples of the former are: 'How are you?', 'What seems to be the problem?', 'Where does it hurt?'; whereas the latter include questions aimed at exploring the patient's orientation to time, place and person: 'Where are we?', 'What day is today?', 'What's your name?'. With the second group of questions the aim is not to find out the reply as such, but to test the patient's ability to reply. They act, therefore, as metacognitive devices aimed at assessing the patient's capacity to think properly.

At a deeper level, questions can be classified according to their neurophysiological implications. At this level, Hargie has described two types of useful questions to assess cognition: recall and process questions. The former type presupposes a low degree of cognitive demand, because the respondent only recalls basic facts: e.g., 'Where were you born?', or 'Where does it

1 Plautus, *Men.* 910–930; all translations are my own.
2 These questions correspond with the assumptions, presuppositions, and inferences that are taken for granted, as described by Hargie (2016: 124).

hurt?'. The latter type, by contrast, requires the use of higher mental functions of reasoning,[3] as is the case in the opening question of the Medicus in the passage from Plautus' *Menaechmi* quoted above: 'Why do you uncover your arm?'.[4] In the rest of the anamnesis the Medicus asks a number of recall questions, presumably because the answer will help him to understand the causes and nature of his patient's ailment.[5] The replies that he obtains do not, however, clarify any of the specific information that he was inquiring about, but they do allow him to figure out the way in which Menaechmus is thinking. In other words, these recall questions are also functioning as metacognitive devices.

In order to assess a person's cognition or consciousness the doctor needs to read between the lines of the responses that he obtains. He needs to ask questions, the answers to which will not be relevant in terms of their content as such, but more so in terms of the information that they reveal about the working of the mind, as is manifested more precisely by the accuracy and the adequacy of the content of the answers (or the lack thereof).

This same principle applies to several tools that are in use today to quantify impaired consciousness or compromised cognition. Two popular examples are the Confusion Assessment Method for the Intensive Care Unit (CAM-ICU),[6] which is used to diagnose delirium, or the Mini Mental State Examination (MMSE)[7] by which the deterioration of cognitive skills in elderly patients is measured (See Figures 1.1–1.2). Both tools, as well as many others that contemporary medical professionals utilise in their daily practice, are comprised of several recall questions and process questions, in addition to practical tasks. The questioner already knows the answer to some of the questions beforehand, so he aims to read between the lines of the answers that he obtains, in order to evaluate the cognitive capacities of the individuals under assessment.

This paper will look at how similar questions were used already by the Hippocratic doctors to diagnose the mental conditions of their patients when they were acting strangely, speaking nonsense or simply not being their usual selves. My aim is to demonstrate that by means of such questions, these doc-

3 Hargie (2016: 124–125).

4 The uncovering of the arm is likely to be a reaction to Menaechmus' previous interaction with his parasite, see Baumbach (1983). By asking about its rationale the doctor is trying to assess the way in which his patient is thinking.

5 The issues about the wine and the bowel rumbling have a clear medical connotation. See Fitton-Brown (1967) and Baumbach (1983) respectively.

6 This score is one of the most frequently employed to assess delirium in the Intensive Care Unit. See Gusmao-Flores et al. (2012).

7 Folstein et al. (1975).

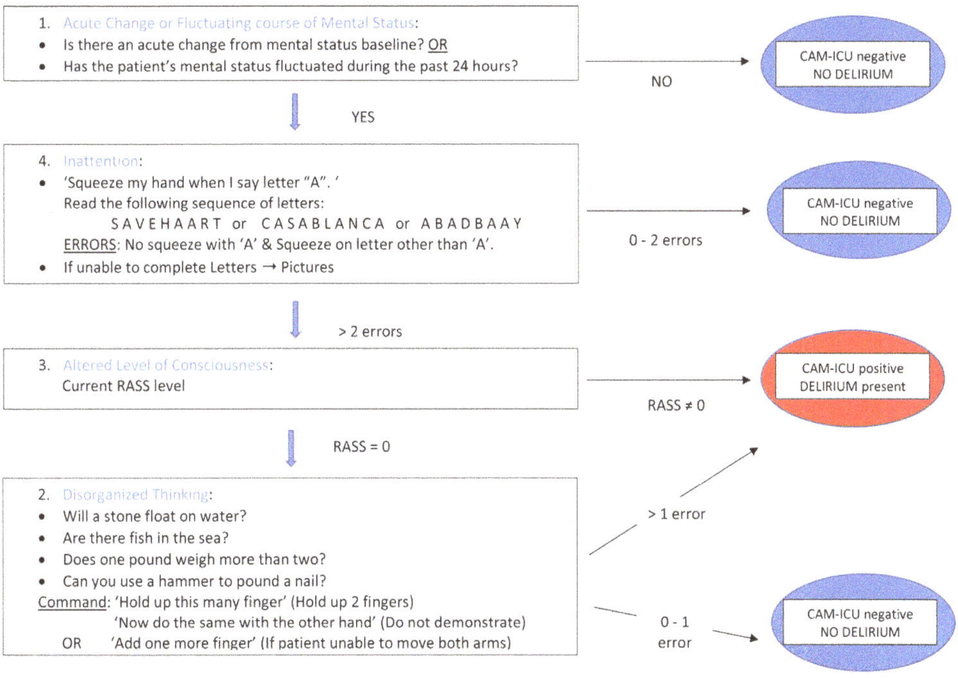

FIGURE 1.1 Confusion Assessment Method for the Intensive Care Unit. See Gusmao, Flores et al. (2012. R115). (RASS = Richmond Agitation-Sedation Scale)

tors were trying to assess cases of impaired consciousness rather than mental illness/madness/insanity (see below). Accordingly, the discussion will begin by distinguishing the notion of mental illness from impaired consciousness. Subsequently, I will draw a broad outline of the ways in which these texts have been recently interpreted by scholars in order to challenge them. I will then address a few passages from the Hippocratic corpus to support my claims; and finally, I will hypothesise that such descriptions reveal an embryonic or intuitive notion of consciousness amongst these early doctors.

2 Mental Illness/Madness/Insanity vs. Impaired Consciousness

Mental illness and its popular equivalents, madness and insanity, are used quasi interchangeably in every-day language and will be here. Their main difference is based on the slightly derogatory connotation of 'insane', and the colloquial nuance of 'madness'. Be that as it may, in order to set clear boundaries between what we consider within the sphere of mental illness/madness/insanity and what entails the notion of impaired consciousness, it is useful to take a look at their definitions.

Temporal orientation (5 points)	What is the approximate time? What day of the week is it? What is the date today? What is the month? What is the year?
Spatial orientation (5 points)	Where are we now? What is this place? In what district are we or what is the address here? In which town are we? In which state are we?
Registration (3 points)	Repeat the following words: CAR, VASE, BRICK
Attention and calculation (5 points)	Subtract: 100-7= (93)-7= (86)-7= (79)-7= (72)-7= (65)
Remote memory (3 points)	Can you remember the 3 words you have said?
Naming 2 objects (2 points)	Watch & Pen
REPEAT (1 point)	'NO IFS, ANDS OR BUTS'
Stage command (3 points)	'Take this piece of paper with your right hand, fold it in half and put it on the floor'
Writing a complete sentence (1 point)	Write a sentence that makes sense
Reading and obeying (1 point)	Close your eyes
Copy the diagram (1 point)	Copy 2 pentagons with an intersection

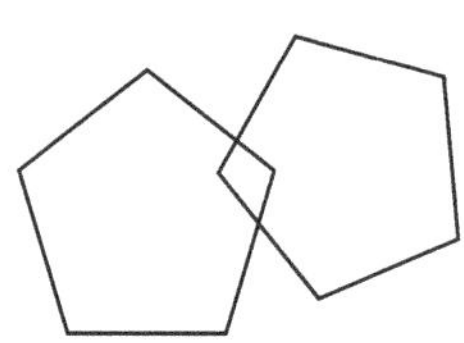

FIGURE 1.2 Mini Mental State Examination (MMSE). See Folstein et al. (1975).

Mental illness, according to the British Psychological Society, is a heterogeneous group of chronic conditions, where several or most of the following symptoms occur: extreme moods, hallucinations, delusions, thought disorders, and negative symptoms (such as apathy, inexpressiveness, lack of motivation, etc.).[8] It is important to highlight that this definition applies to a chronic condition, namely, one prolonged in time, as opposed to an acute one (whereas none of the Hippocratic descriptions below allude to a chronic affection).

Moreover, mental illness/madness/insanity should be clearly distinguished from acute psychosis or delirium,[9] which is one of the several possible manifestations of impaired consciousness (another heterogeneous nosologic entity). Indeed, acute psychosis, delirium or hyperactive impaired consciousness are different presentations of a similar syndrome characterised by a transient state of confusion, where patients seem to be temporarily out of touch with reality, and in which any of the above-mentioned symptoms can be present. In other words, hallucinations, mood swings, thought disorders can all be manifestations of impaired consciousness/delirium/acute psychosis, as long as they are short-lasting and in a permanent state of change or fluctuation.

Very schematically, medicine nowadays frames consciousness as a spectrum that goes from 'awake, alert and appropriate'[10] to deep coma or total loss of consciousness. In the middle, there are intermediate states or levels of consciousness, where individuals become confused, agitated, delirious (hyperactive impaired consciousness), or obtunded, drowsy, comatose (hypoactive impaired consciousness).[11] It should be noted that although delirium can occur during the course of a longer process such as mental illness, it is not specific to such psychiatric disorders. On the contrary, more often than not, impaired consciousness occurs in the context of severe systemic diseases such as serious infections, head trauma, intoxication, etc. Thus, the main distinction between madness and hyperactive impaired consciousness are the chronic and persistent course of the former as opposed to the acute, fluctuating and episodic character of the latter (the same can be said about the negative symptoms of mental illness and hypoactive impaired consciousness).

---

8 Cooke (2014). Each of these symptoms also has a specific definition. Extreme moods occur when patients are extremely aggressive, extremely sad, extremely happy, etc. Hallucinations refer to abnormal sensory perceptions (hearing voices, seeing, or smelling things that other people do not perceive). Delusions allude to situations where patients hold elaborated and complex beliefs that others do not share (mystic revelations, extreme suspiciousness, paranoia, persecution, conspiracy). Thought disorders are diagnosed in patients who experience difficulties in thinking, concentrating and speaking in a way that others can follow.

9 Acute psychosis, delirium and hyperactive impaired consciousness are often used interchangeably.

10 This is the usual medical jargon to describe the normal state of consciousness in a healthy wakeful individual.

11 Josephson—Miller (2011: 691–695).

Apart from exploring the medical phenomenon under study (viz. impaired consciousness) in the Hippocratic writings, this paper is aimed at examining a specific way of medical diagnosis, namely one that is based on a question-and-answer interchange between doctors and patients. Consequently, it is important to consider the specific nature of this type of communication more closely. We are dealing here with a dynamic communicative process,[12] where each reply modifies subsequent actions in light of the new information revealed by it. Plautus' passage illustrates very well the way in which the doctor is constantly gauging Menaechmus by his answers and modifying his questions accordingly. Also, within this interchange, the interactions are governed by implicit rules, which depend on the role of the actors, and their circumstances.[13] To be sure, an encounter between a doctor and a patient presupposes certain stereotyped sequences of acts and behaviours, where some implied communicative rules determine what is acceptable and what is not (Menaechmus' defiant attitude is clearly perceived as inappropriate by the Medicus). Thus, each actor plays his or her role, knowing and obeying social power relations that are taken for granted: one person asks the questions whereas the other replies to them. As stated, Plautus' scene illustrates both the 'acceptable' or 'natural' type of exchange (when Menaechmus answers soundly and reasonably regarding his bowels), and its unexpected—and therefore 'unacceptable' or 'unnatural'—disruption (when his reply is aggressive), which is interpreted by the doctor as the beginning of *insania*.

Furthermore, as is the case in any communicative situation such interactions are mostly goal oriented,[14] which means that every question has a purpose, and serves the doctor's medical agenda. The process is also multidimensional,[15] in the sense that non-verbal features such as body language, attitudes and behaviours convey implicit messages as well, even if the patient is not aware of it (i.e., unintentional communication). Finally, in order for the communication process to be successful, all participants need to have a notion of how the others are thinking and making sense of the world that they are experiencing, which can be defined as metacognitive processes.

It is worth bearing all these characteristics in mind when looking at the Hippocratic texts under scrutiny: there we will see that ancient authors also made certain assumptions and took certain rules for granted when communicating with their patients. It is my intention to make these more explicit. Like Plautus' Medicus, Hippocratic doctors also gave their own interpretation of those kinds

12 DeVito (2016: 47–49).

13 Argyle et al. (2011).

14 Westmyer et al. (1998: 9).

15 Adler—Elmhorst (2010: 77).

of situations and attitudes that did not comply with what they had expected. For the sake of my analysis, a 'question' will be defined as 'any statement or non-verbal act that invites an answer or a response in return'.[16] In other words, I will consider questions in their broader sense, and not only as verbal interrogative utterances.

3 Recent Scholarship

Before addressing the ancient texts, it is worthwhile to have a closer look at the ways in which they are currently being interpreted. Mental illness, madness and insanity have been the focus of interest among many scholars in the last two decades, whereas discussions on impaired consciousness in the Hippocratic corpus have generally been avoided. Two main reasons can explain this omission: a medical and a philosophical one. As stated above, from the medical standpoint, the boundaries between mental illness and impaired consciousness are sometimes difficult to draw. Therefore, umbrella terms such as madness or insanity are often used—without a clear definition—to talk about various conditions that are not always homogeneous. Furthermore, due to this vagueness, by extrapolating modern concepts into ancient texts—mental illness, madness, etc. are modern constructs—scholars end up assuming that certain similarities exist in descriptions by different authors, which lead them to group together conditions that were not necessarily considered to be connected.

Something similar occurs with the philosophical problem: because the idea of consciousness—as philosophers of mind currently conceive it—has clear Cartesian overtones, and according to Wilkes' influential paper "there is no [Greek] term that even roughly translates 'mind' or 'consciousness' ",[17] it is often assumed that little attention was paid in antiquity to this notion. This hypothesis might be tenable in purely philosophical texts, but it fails to realise that in order to describe and characterise clinical symptoms philosophical speculation is not strictly required (even if such descriptions often do trigger certain speculation).

As a result, the passages that describe deluded patients or report uncommon behaviours and attitudes have either been framed in terms of mental illness, madness, insanity, or as evidence of Hippocratic philosophical ideas about the soul, and the spirit, but not as cases of impaired consciousness. I aim to challenge this view and claim that these doctors were able to distinguish what

16 Stewart—Cash (2014: 57).
17 Wilkes (1988: 19).

we nowadays understand by mental illness from what we currently define as impaired consciousness. Moreover, I will posit that even if they did not have a coherent theory of mind, such conditions did prompt them to reflect about ideas that we do nowadays associate with the 'mind' and 'consciousness'.

Let us begin by taking a closer look at both scholarly approaches. To be sure, the first approach usually yields psychiatrically-informed analyses that attempt a general classification of mental illness. Benett[18] and Hugues,[19] for instance, draw parallels between the *DSM* (*Diagnostic and Statistic Manual*) of the American Psychiatric Association and ancient endeavours to classify mental disorders. Similarly, Matentzoglu[20] looks for 'psychopathologic symptoms' in some Hippocratic descriptions, and provides a systematic phenomenological classification by utilizing *the International Classification of Diseases* (ICD-10). Such an approach, however, demonstrates our own difficulty in categorizing mental diseases, rather than exploring the Hippocratics' views of such phenomena. Within this same group, Pigeaud tries to outline the notion of madness, *la folie*, and its later evolution in ancient texts of different periods,[21] whereas Thumiger[22] is specifically interested in the vocabulary of madness, exploring the composition of the specific terminology and trying to extract the exact meaning of each word by analyzing suffixes and lexemes.

As to the philosophical reading of the Hippocratic passages discussed below, on the other hand, Di Benedetto[23] argues in favour of a continuum between the physical and the psychic; Hankinson[24] questions the notion of soul, its location and its relation to the body; Gundert[25] explores how the ancients conceived the functioning and interaction between body, thought, and intelligence; and finally van der Eijk[26] reflects upon theories about their seat and the substances involved.

18 Benett (2013).
19 Hugues (2013).
20 Matentzoglu (2011).
21 Interestingly, Pigeaud (1987: 14–21) does mention that the ancient texts are not discussing psychopathologic conditions, but the loss and recovery of lucidity. Furthermore, his analysis looks at the vocabulary used by the Hippocratic authors to talk about both the loss and the recovery, and it even relates these conditions to the field of consciousness. However, in order to subsume these descriptions under a vaguely defined umbrella-notion of *folie*, he explicitly disregards this aspect (15). In my analysis below I will address the terminology utilised by the Hippocratic doctors to talk about delirium, and its recovery (*lucidité* according to Pigeaud).
22 Thumiger (2013: 63–81).
23 Di Benedetto (1986: 43–47).
24 Hankinson (1991).
25 Gundert (2000).
26 van der Eijk (2005).

Although allusions to consciousness arise in such discussions, the phenomenon is never looked at in depth. An exception to this is Boehm's analysis of insensitivity.[27] She describes the association of sensory perceptions with the spirit (*l'esprit*), and accurately identifies their impairment with a state of unconsciousness. However, her study is more concerned with insensitivity than with unconsciousness.

In summary, I will demonstrate that there are some descriptions in the Hippocratic corpus, which appear to be similar to conditions that we would nowadays associate with impaired consciousness and not madness. My approach does not take for granted that medical authors had an idea of consciousness. On the contrary, I use 'impaired consciousness' only to allude to the clinical symptoms that we nowadays understand by these terms, without making assumptions about abstract ideas regarding them. However, I will suggest in my analysis that in their attempt to understand the mechanisms underlying such conditions, these medical authors did manifest some interest and reflection on ideas akin to our notion of consciousness (for which they did have a specific—even if not well defined—terminology that I will discuss).

4 Q&A in the Hippocratic Corpus

I will now address some passages from the Hippocratic corpus, where the medical authors describe interactions in the form of Q&A between doctors and patients who are acting strangely or suffering unusual perceptions. Not surprisingly, such passages are found in treatises that describe case-records, such as the different books of *Epidemics*, or works that offer thorough characterisations of diseases. Among the latter, are some of the nosological treatises from the corpus, namely *On Internal Affections*, *On Diseases* 1 to 4, *On Regimen in Acute Diseases*, etc.

Let us begin with the case history of Hermoptolemos' wife described in *Epidemics* 7. After a period of symptoms that oscillated between irrational behaviour and coma, on the fifteenth day, the following happened:

> καὶ οἱ φόβοι καὶ ἡ βοὴ ἐγίνετο ἤπιος· παρηκολούθει δὲ τὸ ἀγριοῦσθαι καὶ τὸ θυμαίνειν καὶ κλαίειν εἰ μή οἱ ταχέως ὅ τι βούλοιτο ῥεχθείη· **καὶ ἐπεγίνωσκεν μὲν πάντας καὶ πάντα [...] εὐθὺς [...]**· ἡ δὲ μανίη καὶ τὸ παρὰ καιρὸν καὶ ἡ βοὴ καὶ ἡ μεταβολὴ ἡ εἰρημένη παρηκολούθει ἐς τὸ κῶμα.[28]

27 Boehm (2002).
28 *Epid.* 7.11 (5.384.16–22 Littré; 60.11–17 Jouanna—Grmek).

> Both the terrors and the shouts became mild, but she persisted in her wrath, her anger and her howling whenever what she wanted was not accomplished immediately. **She could recognise everybody, and every object straight away** [...]. Her rage, her lack of moderation, her shouting and the above-mentioned mood swings persisted until she became drowsy.

First of all, I would like to reflect on the underlined sentence: how can the doctor be sure that 'she could recognise everybody and everything at once'? It is very likely that he brought people to her with whom she was familiar, or that he showed her different objects for her to name. This is, indeed, not so different from the assessment recommended in point 2 of the CAM-ICU (Figure 1.1), where patients are asked to name letters or objects in pictures, or item 6 of the MMSE (Figure 1.2), where real objects, such as a pen and a watch are shown to the patient for him or her to name. We can posit, therefore, that in all these cases, the doctor is asking questions for which he knows the answers beforehand—hence, obvious questions. His interest is not focused on the reply itself, but on the information that such a reply can provide in terms of the patient's thinking capacities.

On the other hand, this case illustrates some of the unstated rules that govern doctor-patient encounters. The doctor probably felt that the anger and demands of his patient where abnormal because they evidenced a subversion in the normal social interactions, where individuals are expected to respect their doctor and be polite with those surrounding them. The clear breach in the implicit rules of communication is rightly attributed by the doctor to his patient's condition, rather than to her lack of social decorum.

Finally, considering our previous definitions of mental illness and impaired consciousness, the author is presenting us a case where a patient shows constant changes in her level of consciousness: first there are shouts and terrors (hyperactive impaired consciousness), then persistent extreme moods with rational intervals ('alert, awake, and appropriate'), followed by mood changes and drowsiness (hypoactive). This is clearly an acute situation that covers almost the whole spectrum of consciousness. Also of note is the fact that the medical author recognised all these rather different symptoms as part of the same problem. The polysyndetic use of καί and δέ suggests an accumulation of symptoms that are conceived as different stages within the same condition.

The author of *On Internal Affections* describes another interesting disease produced by bile, which he classifies among the 'thick diseases':

> [...] παραφρονέει· καὶ προφαίνεσθαί οἱ δοκέει πρὸ τῶν ὀφθαλμῶν ἑρπετὰ καὶ ἄλλα παντοδαπὰ θηρία καὶ ὁπλῖται μαχόμενοι, καὶ αὐτὸς ἐν αὐτοῖσι δοκέει

μάχεσθαι· τοιαῦτα λέγει ὡς ὁρῶν καὶ ἐπέρχεται [...]. ὅταν ἔννοος γένηται ἀφηγεῖται τὰ ἐνύπνια τοιαῦτα ὁρᾶν ὁποῖα καὶ τῷ σώματι ἐποίει καὶ τῇ γλώσσῃ ἔλεγε. [...] ἔστι δ' ὅτε καὶ κεῖται ἄφωνος ὅλην τὴν ἡμέρην καὶ τὴν νύκτα ἀναπνέων ἀθρόον πολὺ τὸ πνεῦμα. ὅταν δὲ παύσηται παραφρονέων, εὐθὺς ἔννοος γίνεται, **καὶ ἤν ἐρωτᾷ τις αὐτόν, ὀρθῶς ἀποκρίνεται, καὶ γινώσκει πάντα τὰ λεγόμενα.**[29]

[...] the patient becomes delirious: in front of his eyes there seem to appear reptiles, all other sorts of beasts, and fighting soldiers. He even thinks he is fighting amongst them, and speaks as though he could see such things [...]. When he regains consciousness,[30] he recounts what he saw in his dreams, which corresponds with what he did with his body, and said with his tongue. [...] There are also times when he lies speechless for the whole day and night taking frequent deep breaths. When delirium stops, he immediately regains consciousness and **if somebody asks him a question he answers accurately and is able to understand all that is said.**

This example again shows a rapidly changing situation that covers the whole spectrum of impaired consciousness: there is delirium with hallucinations or nightmares. It is, however, difficult to distinguish between the latter two in the passage at hand. Is the patient having nightmares in his sleep, or is he hallucinating while awake? Whatever may be the case, these blurred limits between states of wakefulness and sleep are typical of situations where the patient's consciousness is impaired. In this description there is yet another stage, which we would nowadays associate with 'vigil coma', where the patient looks awake, open-eyed, but he is not connecting with the environment, remains silent in his bed (negative symptoms) and therefore is considered to be unconscious.

It is interesting to highlight how the doctor perceives normality (ἔννοος γένηται/γίνεται) when communication takes place, and abnormality (παραφρονέει, κεῖται ἄφωνος) when it does not. This demonstrates the non-explicit assumptions of a doctor-patient encounter, as well as the metacognitive processes that are in place. As to the former, the patient should be able and willing to respond to the questions that are being asked, regardless of whether the doctor him-

29 *Int.* 48 (7.284.22–286.13 Littré; 232.15–234.9 Potter).

30 The adjective ἔννοος conveys the idea of 'becoming normal' again (it is the language of 'lucidity', as Pigeaud would call it). I have translated 'regains consciousness' because—to my mind—that is the clearest way to express it. However, it should be stressed that I am not necessarily presupposing an implicit idea of consciousness here, even if I will argue below that νοῦς is one of the terms used by several Hippocratic medical authors to allude to an embryonic idea of consciousness.

self or somebody else (τις) asked them. In either case, it is clear that the doctor was interested in the answer. Accordingly, since this basic rule of interaction is broken during the vigil coma, the situation is regarded as abnormal. Although the patient is awake and calm, he is not considered to be sound because neither does he reply to questions, nor does he obey requests, but remains speechless (ἄφωνος). Regarding metacognition, only when communication is possible can the patient explain the rationale for his actions and statements during the hallucinations/nightmares, thereby allowing the doctor to understand and make sense of his previous strange behaviour.

A final remark is in place here regarding the last sentence of the passage: 'if somebody asks him a question, he answers accurately'. How can the doctor know that the patient's reply is accurate? What kind of question should he or the present relatives have asked to be sure that he is being given the correct answer? Undoubtedly, a question for which he knew the answer beforehand; that is, an obvious question. Once again, the text suggests that this kind of questions was a common tool to assess consciousness in patients.

Very often modern scholars identify madness when descriptions allude to what we would nowadays define as delirium (hyperactive impaired consciousness). Hypoactive states, conversely, tend to go unnoticed. Consequently, it is useful to have a closer look at some other cases of negative symptoms or vigil coma (hypoactive), in order to show that they are presented with the same terminology, which suggests that they were conceived as related phenomena by ancient doctors.

The first extract is part of a description of φρενῖτις: patients suffering from this condition 'are delirious and stare fixedly' (ἔκφρονές εἰσι, καὶ ἀτενὲς βλέπουσι).[31] A condition with similar symptoms is experienced by Cydes in *Epidemics* 7, where we read that on the seventh day 'he was slightly delirious' and 'stared with his eyes into the void as if looking at something' (ὑποπαρέκρουε [...]. τὰ ὄμματα διὰ κενῆς ὡς εἴ τι βλέπων ξυνέστρεφε).[32] Even more explicit is the author of *Coan Prenotions* in his aphorismic sentence: 'silent deliriums in unsettled patients, with their eyes gazing around, and exhaling deep breaths are fatal [...]' (αἱ σιγῶσαι ἐκστάσιες, οὐχ ἡσυχάζουσαι, ὄμμασι περιβλέπουσαι, πνεῦμα ἔξω ἀναφέρουσαι, ὀλέθριαι [...]).[33]

Although there are no allusions in the passages to questions and answers, we can easily deduce that the doctors did try to interact with their patients

31 *Morb.* 3.9 (7.128.7 Littré; 76.21–22 Potter; 18.1–2 Potter).
32 *Epid.* 7.83 (5.440.4–6 Littré; 98.13–15 Jouanna—Grmek).
33 *Coac.* 476 (5.690.12–13 Littré; 222.8–10 Potter).

by asking questions. But even without these assumptions, the silence hints—once again—at an unusual breach in the natural doctor-patient interaction, if for no other reason than that patients are expected to talk to their doctor. Interestingly, in each of these descriptions doctors pay particular attention to the gaze of their patients. As such, these passages seem to suggest that whenever a patient could not express his thoughts and feelings through the spoken word, the doctor tried to make eye contact and determine whether the patient was able to fix the gaze. Managing to do so would be a form of non-verbal communication in itself. But in those cases where even that ability appeared compromised the doctor considered the patient to be delirious.

We have proof of successful non-verbal communication in another case, where the author describes how Polycrates' wife suffered from a disease that caused progressive shortness of breath. At the end of the disease, the symptoms were so serious that she had to remain sitting. It is well known that severe dyspnoea prevents patients from speaking. Hence, in order to explain that she remained conscious until the end, the doctor observes that 'her looks were particularly alert[34] until the very last moment' (ἐμβλέψιες ἐμφρονώδεις σφόδρα μέχρι τοῦ ἐσχάτου χρόνου).[35] In this case, unlike the previous ones, we can imagine a doctor asking questions and interacting with a patient who is unable to talk but is still able to communicate in a non-verbal way. Hence, the author highlights that although the patient's breathing was compromised so that she could not talk, her consciousness was still intact.

The opposite situation to these negative symptoms is what psychiatrists call thought and speech disorders, where the patients talk and interact, albeit in an utterly meaningless way. They seem to be replying to questions, but their speech makes no sense whatsoever. Such a condition is described regarding Philinus' wife after giving birth in *Epidemics* 1:

> ἑκταίῃ ἐς νύκτα παρέκρουσε πολλά, καὶ πάλιν κατενόει. [...] ὀγδόῃ [...] πολλὰ παρέλεγεν [...]. δεκάτῃ, σμικρὰ κατενόει. [...] περὶ δὲ τεσσαρεσκαιδεκάτην [...] λόγοι πολλοί· σμικρὰ κατενόει· διὰ ταχέων δὲ πάλιν παρέκρουσεν.[36]

---

34 Like ἔννοος above (n. 30), the adjective ἐμφρονώδης is part of the vocabulary of lucidity (to continue using Pigeaud's theorisation). I chose 'alert' instead of the translation offered in LSJ dictionary ('showing intelligence'), because these authors utilised different compounds of φρόνησις, νοῦς/νόος, etc. to allude to normal or abnormal consciousness, depending on the prefix they added (ἐν- and κατά- usually convey the idea of soundness, whereas ἐκ- and παρά- are used to describe derangement).

35 *Epid.* 7.7 (5.378.15–16 Littré; 56.15–16 Jouanna—Grmek).

36 *Epid.* 1.27.4 (2.692.3–10 Littré; 46.8–47.5 Jouanna—Guardasole—Anastassiou).

> On the sixth day, during the night, she was very delirious, then she was rational again. […] On the eighth she had wandering talk […]. On the tenth she was rational for short instants. […] Around the fourteenth day […] many (senseless) words, rational for short instants. Soon afterwards, again deluded.

Note how the author here uses three different concepts to allude to the same kind of chatty delirium: παρακρύω, παραλέγω, and λόγοι πολλοί. There is, again, no allusion to questions or answers, but we can easily suppose that the doctor tried to interrogate the patient and interact with her, thus delirium seems to be related in this case to disrupted speech. The link between lack of communication and delirium is so strong in this passage that specific terminology for speech disorders (παραλέγω and λόγοι πολλοί) is used interchangeably with a more general word to allude to delirium (παρακρύω).[37] The alternation between fits of delirium and moments when the patient is sound (κατενόει) points towards an impairment of the patient's consciousness rather than to a mental illness, where thought disorders do not occur in fits as described in this case, but are persistent and chronic.

Several other Hippocratic passages show that successful communication, by contrast, is related to lucidity. There are examples that illustrate how terms denoting normal speech were used to convey the idea of 'unimpaired consciousness'. For instance, in a passage from *On Diseases* 4, after a long description of dropsy, the author reports that his patient at the moment of his death was 'able to understand and to speak articulately' (ἐπαΐων τε καὶ διαλεγόμενος: *Morb.* 4.26 [7.614.2 Littré; 124.9–10 Joly; 184.20–21 Potter]), that is to say that the patient perished while fully conscious. For this medical author, then, the ability to communicate is a sign of being sound (despite the fact that the patient died not long after).

37 In the passage under discussion, the adverb πάλιν makes it clear that in this author's mind λόγοι πολλοί and παρέκρουσεν were probably used as synonyms: the sequence λόγοι πολλοί, κατενόει, πάλιν παρέκρουσεν leaves no doubt that the first and the last terms allude to similar symptoms. Rodríguez Alfageme in his descriptive analysis of speech pathology in the Hippocratic corpus (1999: 156–157) does remark that the loss of the ability to speak is often related to delirium, and its recovery to regaining consciousness. However, he fails to realise that often Hippocratic doctors use the terms as equivalent. Gourevitch (1983: 300–302), on the other hand, equated speechlessness with dumbness. Even though she rightly recognises that speech and its impairment are closely related to the level of consciousness, she did not consider *l'aphonie hippocratique* as a characteristic sign of impaired consciousness.

The final passage that I would like to discuss comes from *On Regimen in Acute Diseases* (*Appendix*). The author there offers an interesting description of patients whose abdomen is wet and whose mind (γνώμη)[38] disturbed:

> ὁπόσοισι δὲ [...] γνώμη τεταραγμένη, οἱ πολλοὶ τῶν τοιούτων τὰς κροκύδας ἀφαιρέουσι καὶ τὰς ῥῖνας σκάλλουσι καὶ κατὰ βραχὺ μὲν ἀποκρίνονται τὸ ἐρωτώμενον, αὐτοὶ δὲ ἀφ' ἑωυτῶν οὐδὲν λέγουσιν κατηρτημένον.[39]
>
> Most of those whose mind is disturbed pluck off bits of wool, and pick their noses, and although they can reply shortly to whatever they are asked, they cannot spontaneously say anything sensible.

In order to understand the implications of this account it is useful to try and visualise the real situation: it is not uncommon for doctors to treat patients who are confused, and speak diffusely without making sense, but when they try to connect with them, call them or stimulate them they do have short moments of lucidity. These patients are able to respond correctly to simple questions, but then continue in their delirium. Notably, the way chosen by the physician to connect with the patient is through a question. Probably an easy and obvious 'recall question' (as described earlier) the answer to which the doctor very likely knew beforehand. Again, checking the ability to communicate through questions is the chosen method to assess and report cognitive functioning.

Another important point is the kind of construction that the author is using to report this case. He describes it as γνώμη τεταραγμένη. This may well be a 'phrasal term', as defined by Langslow (in the context of Latin medical language), that is, a lexicalised phrase comprised of a 'determiner' and a 'noun head'.[40] The 'noun heads' (in this case γνώμη) tend to be abstract and can usually be assimilated to different mental functions, such as cognition, sense-perception, intelligence, etc.[41] The 'determiner', on the other hand, describes a

38 The concept of γνώμη, like νοῦς, φρόνησις, and σύνεσις, is a term that the Hippocratic medical authors used to allude to what I will later define as an embryonic idea of consciousness.

39 *Acut. Sp.* 16 (2.424.14–426.4 Littré; 75.20–24 Joly; 278.16–20 Potter).

40 Langslow (2000: 208–209).

41 A good testimony of the vagueness of these noun heads is the way in which different scholars have translated such terms: e.g., γνώμη is translated by Mann (2012: 62) as 'mind', by Gundert (2000: 26) as 'judgment', by Jones (1931: 251) as 'intelligence', and by Craik (2009: 77) as 'intellect', which, on a more abstract level, all allude to some mental capacities. If we interpret the use of γνώμη as part of a phrasal term that describes impaired consciousness, we are alluding to all of the above renderings in a comprehensive manner.

disturbance or dysfunction of the former. There are several examples of these constructions in the Hippocratic corpus, and most of them are used to illustrate cases where consciousness seems to be impaired. To name but a few: γνώμης παράφοροι ('deranged'),[42] τὴν γνώμην βλαβέντες ('distracted, mislead, hurt'),[43] τοῦ νοῦ παρακόπτει ('struck'),[44] ἡ διάνοια θρασυτέρη ('audacious, insolent'),[45] παραλλάξιες φρενῶν ('deviation, change').[46]

A common trait in these examples is that the abstract nouns are linked to a determiner that suggests the idea of deviation, alteration or blow. The relevance of these phrasal terms is that they hint at an underlying idea, namely, that the mental capability of the patient is damaged, which suggests an embryonic notion of consciousness. Furthermore, the doctors are exploring the impairment of these mental functions through obvious questions, as we have seen in the previous examples. Certainly, different authors from different treatises used diverse concepts like γνώμη, νοῦς, φρόνησις, σύνεσις, etc. to allude to these notions. For instance, the author of *On Diseases* 1 considers the σύνεσις to be affected during the delirium that characterises φρενῖτις,[47] whereas for the author of *On Affections* it is the νοῦς that becomes compromised.[48] Yet, as stated, these and other examples of compromised, deviated or struck mental capacities in the Hippocratic collection suggest an underlying embryonic idea of what we would nowadays associate with the sphere of consciousness.

5 Conclusions

What we learn from the above analysis is that by questioning the obvious, the Hippocratic doctors were able to gather much useful information about their patients' mental condition, very little of which derived from the actual

42 *Coac.* 31 (5.592.11 Littré; 112.25–114.1 Potter). Inserted in a miscellaneous description of symptoms, in which delirium is associated with pain.

43 *Acut.* 17 (2.260.6 Littré; 74.27 Jones; 43.2–3 Joly). The phrasal term alludes to a certain delirium associated with unstrained gruel.

44 *Aff.* 10 (6.216.24–25 Littré; 18.19 Potter). Used to characterise the kind of delirium that accompanies φρενῖτις.

45 *Epid.* 7.1 (5.364.17 Littré; 48.12 Jouanna—Grmek). This phrasal term has the same structure as the others but is used to convey the opposite situation. In this case Polycrates' διάνοια becomes more insolent, which suggests that although his consciousness was still affected, he became more alert.

46 *Acut. Sp.* 1 (2.396.1 Littré; 68.11–12 Joly; 262.12 Potter). Describes delirium in the context of ardent fever (καῦσος).

47 *Morb.* 1.30 (6.200.12 Littré; 176.24 Potter).

48 *Aff.* 10 (6.216.24 Littré; 18.19 Potter).

content of the answers they received. Indeed, by employing this simple tool doctors could test the ability of their patients to communicate properly, as well as their competence to respect the implicit rules of social interaction in a doctor-patient encounter, in short, their cognitive functioning. Accordingly, the impairment of any of these abilities was construed by the doctor as a symptom of mental disorder, which we would nowadays classify as impaired consciousness (but not madness). So much so, that some of our current tools to assess consciousness resemble certain strategies employed by Hippocratic medical authors (arguably, the recall and process questions from the CAM-ICU and the MMSE do not differ substantially from the ones that were used back then). Based on the examples discussed above, I have argued that these medical authors seem to have had a primitive intuition, or an embryonic notion of what we today call 'consciousness' (variably designated as γνώμη, φρόνησις, σύνεσις, or νοῦς). We can therefore posit that consciousness was an actual object of medical concern, observation and study, and that questioning the obvious was a useful diagnostic tool that doctors employed in assessing its (mal)functioning.

Bibliography

Primary Sources

Jones, W.H.S. 1923. *Hippocrates 2. Prognostic. Regimen in Acute Diseases. The Sacred Disease. The Art. Breaths. Law. Decorum. Physician (Ch. 1). Dentition*. Cambridge, Mass.—London: Harvard University Press.

Jones, W.H.S. 1931. *Hippocrates 4. Nature of Man. Regimen in Health. Humours. Aphorisms. Regimen 1–3. Dreams. Heracleitus: On the Universe*. Cambridge, Mass.—London: Harvard University Press.

Joly, R. 1970. *Hippocrate 11. De la génération. De la nature de l'enfant. Des maladies IV. Du foetus de huit mois*. Paris: Les Belles Lettres.

Joly, R. 1972. *Hippocrate 6.2. Du régime des maladies aiguës. Appendice. De l'aliment. De l'usage des liquides*. Paris: Les Belles Lettres

Jouanna, J.—Grmek, M.D. 2000. *Hippocrate 4.3. Épidémies V et VII*. Paris: Les Belles Lettres.

Jouanna, J.—Guardasole, A.—Anastassiou, A. 2016. *Hippocrate 4.1. Épidémies I et III*. Paris: Les Belles Lettres.

Littré, É. 1839–1861. *Oeuvres complètes d'Hippocrate: traduction nouvelle avec le texte grec en regard*. 10 vols. Paris: J.-B. Baillière.

Potter, P. 1980. *Hippocratis De Morbis* 3 [CMG 1.2.3]. Berlin: Akademie-Verlag.

Potter, P. 1988. *Hippocrates 5. Affections. Diseases 1. Diseases 2*. Cambridge, Mass.—London: Harvard University Press.

Potter, P. 1988. *Hippocrates 6. Diseases 3. Internal Affections. Regimen in Acute Diseases (Appendix)*. Cambridge, Mass.—London: Harvard University Press.

Potter, P. 2010. *Hippocrates 9. Coan Prenotions. Anatomical and Minor Clinical Writings*. Cambridge, Mass.—London: Harvard University Press.

Potter, P. 2012. *Hippocrates 10. Generation. Nature of the Child. Diseases 4. Nature of Women and Barrenness*. Cambridge, Mass.—London: Harvard University Press.

Secondary Sources

Adler, R.B.—Elmhorst, J.M. 2010. *Communicating at work: principles and practices for business and the professions*. New York: McGraw-Hill.

Argyle, M.—Furnham, A.—Graham, J.A. 2011. *Social Situations*. Cambridge: Cambridge University Press.

Baumbach, L. 1983. 'Quacks then as now? An examination of medical practice, theory and superstition in Plautus' *Menaechmi*', *Acta Classica* 26: 99–104.

Benett, S. 2013. ''Carving nature at the joints': the dream of a perfect classification of mental illness', in Harris (2013: 27–40).

Boehm, I. 2002. 'Inconscience et insensibilité dans la collection hippocratique', in A. Thivel—A. Zucker (eds.). *Le normal et le pathologique dans la Collection hippocratique. Actes du Xe colloque hippocratique, Nice, 6–8 octobre 1999*. Nice-Sophia Antipolis: Publications de la Faculté des Lettres, Arts et Sciences humaines, 257–270.

Cooke, A. (ed.). 2014. *Understanding Psychosis and Schizophrenia. A report by the division of Clinical psychology*. Leicester: The British Psychological Society.

Craik, E.M. 2009. *The Hippocratic treatise On glands*. Leiden: Brill.

DeVito, J.A. 2016. *The Interpersonal Communication Book*. Boston: Pearson.

Di Benedetto, V. 1986. *Il medico e la malattia: la scienza di Ippocrate*. Torino: Einaudi.

van der Eijk, P.J. 2005. 'The heart, the brain, the blood and the pneuma: Hippocrates, Diocles and Aristotle on the location of cognitive processes', in P.J. van der Eijk (ed.), *Medicine and Philosophy in Classical Antiquity Doctors and Philosophers on Nature, Soul, Health and Disease*. Cambridge: Cambridge University Press, 119–135.

Fitton-Brown, A.D. 1967. 'Black wine', *Classical Review* 12: 192–195.

Folstein, M.F.—Folstein, S.E.—McHugh, P.R. 1975. '"Mini-Mental State": a Practical Method for Grading the Cognitive State of Patients for the Clinician', *Journal of Psychiatric Research* 12: 189–198.

Gourevitch, D. 1983. 'L'aphonie hippocratique', in F. Lasserre—P. Mudry (eds.), *Formes de pensée dans la collection hippocratique. Actes du IVe colloque international hippocratique. Lausanne, 21–26 septembre 1981*. Genève: Librairie Droz, 297–305.

Gundert, B. 2000. 'Soma and Psyche in Hippocratic Medicine', in J.P. Wright—P. Potter (eds.), *Psyche and soma: physicians and metaphysicians on the mind-body problem from antiquity to enlightenment*. Oxford: Clarendon Press, 13–35.

Gusmao-Flores, D.—Salluh, J.I.—Chalhub, R.Á.—Quarantini, L.C. 2012. 'The confusion assessment method for the intensive care unit (CAM-ICU) and intensive care delirium screening checklist (ICDSC) for the diagnosis of delirium: a systematic review and meta-analysis of clinical studies', *Critical Care* 16: R115.
Hankinson, R.J. 1991. 'Greek medical models of mind', in S. Everson (ed.), *Psychology*. Cambridge: Cambridge University Press, 194–217.
Hargie, O. 2016. *Skilled Interpersonal Communication: Research, Theory and Practice*. London: Routledge.
Harris, W.V. (ed.). 2013. *Mental Disorders in the Classical World*. Leiden—Boston: Brill.
Hugues, J.C. 2013. 'If only the ancients had had the DSM, all would have been crystal clear: reflections on diagnosis', in Harris (2013: 41–58).
Josephson, S.A.—Miller, B.L. 2011. 'Confusion and delirium', in D.L. Longo—A.S. Fauci—D.L. Kasper—S.L. Hauser—J.L. Jameson—J. Loscalzo (eds.), *Harrison's Principles of Internal Medicine 18th Edition*. New York: McGraw Hill.
Langslow, D.R. 2000. *Medical Latin in the Roman Empire*. Oxford: Oxford University Press.
Mann, J.E. 2012. *Hippocrates, On the Art of Medicine*. Leiden—Boston: Brill.
Matentzoglu, S. 2011. *Zur Psychopathologie in den hippokratischen Schriften*. Diss. Erlangen-Nürnberg. Berlin: dissertation.de.
Pigeaud, J. 1987. *Folie et cures de la folie chez les médecins de l'Antiquité gréco-romaine. La manie*. Paris: Belles Lettres.
Rodríguez Alfageme, I. 1999. 'Patología del habla en el *Corpus Hippocraticum*', in A. Thivel—A. Zucker (eds.). *Le normal et le pathologique dans la Collection hippocratique. Actes du xe colloque hippocratique, Nice, 6–8 octobre 1999*. Nice-Sophia Antipolis: Publications de la Faculté des Lettres, Arts et Sciences humaines, 149–171.
Stewart, C.J.—Cash, W.B. 2014. *Interviewing: principles and practices*. New York: McGraw-Hill.
Thumiger, C. 2013. 'The early Greek medical vocabulary of insanity', in Harris (2013: 61–95).
Westmyer, S.—DiCioccio, R.—Rubin, R. 1998. 'Appropriateness and effectiveness of communication channels in competent interpersonal communication', *Journal of Communication* 48: 27–48.
Wilkes, K.V. 1988. '—, Yìshì, Duh, Um, and Consciousness', in A.J. Marcel—E. Bisiach (eds.), *Consciousness in Contemporary Science*. Oxford: Clarendon Press, 16–41.

CHAPTER 2

Peripatetic and Hippocratic Seeds in Pseudo-Aristotle, *Problemata* 4: Raising Questions about Aristotle's Rejection of the Pangenesis Theory of Generation

Robert Mayhew

Abstract

Although the *Problemata physica* attributed to Aristotle is beginning to receive more attention, Book 4 (περὶ ἀφροδίσια) has generally been neglected. This essay attempts to shed some light on *Pr.* 4 and to determine what it might tell us about the study of reproduction, and Aristotelian engagement with Hippocratic medicine, in the early Peripatos. After sketching the pangenesis theory (in the Hippocratic *On Seed*), and Aristotle's critique of that theory and his alternative account of generation (in the *Generation of Animals*), I examine three chapters of *Pr.* 4 (2, 15, and 21), each of which raises questions about Aristotle's rejection of the Hippocratic pangenesis theory. I argue that although there are no challenges to Aristotle's account of generation generally, doubts or concerns are being raised in connection with certain aspects of that account, including doubts about some of Aristotle's reasons for rejecting the pangenesis theory and about whether certain aspects of that theory might well be superior or in some way worth salvaging. I end by speculating—based on the available evidence—that the date of the three chapters I examine likely falls somewhere between the period in which Aristotle himself was active and the time when Strato was scholarch.

1 Introduction

The title of *Problemata physica* 4 is Ὅσα (sc. προβλήματα) περὶ ἀφροδίσια. The topics it deals with are by and large the biology or physiology of sexual intercourse and reproduction. In the present essay, I examine three chapters of *Pr.* 4 (2, 15, and 21) that raise questions about Aristotle's critique of the Hippocratic account of conception. So my interest in medical questions here is not of the sort that a physician asks a patient (e.g., Where does it hurt?), but rather the

 | DOI:10.1163/9789004442672_004

kind of question a physician-cum-philosopher asks about medical or physiological phenomena (e.g., *Why* does it hurt?—or rather, in the present context, Why is it so pleasant?).

Although the *Problemata physica* attributed to Aristotle is in general beginning to receive more attention, and scholarly attention is specifically being paid to the way in which the *Problemata* raises questions about medical phenomena, *Pr.* 4 continues to be neglected.[1]

I have more to say later, as a prelude to my examination of *Pr.* 4.2, 15, and 21, about how precisely the *Problemata* raises questions; but before I turn to these chapters, I need to set the Hippocratic and Peripatetic contexts by looking briefly at two texts: the Hippocratic *On Semen* or *On Seed* (Περὶ γονῆς),[2] which presents a version of the pangenesis theory of conception; and then parts of the *Generation of Animals* 1–2, wherein Aristotle (*inter alia*) criticises the pangenesis theory and presents an alternative account. At the end of the essay, I draw some conclusions—or perhaps more accurately, speculate—about what *Pr.* 4.2, 15, and 21 might tell us about Peripatetic biology and its engagement with Hippocratic medicine in the period during which Aristotle's biology seems to have disappeared.[3]

2 The Hippocratic *On Seed*

I have chosen the Hippocratic *On Seed* because it is arguably the best example (and perhaps a likely source) of the view criticised by Aristotle.[4] As Heinrich

1 See especially Oikonomopoulou (2015), Thomas (2015), and Ulacco (2011). I am referring not to the historical reception or influence of *Pr.* 4, which has been dealt with fairly often and quite well, but to the content of *Pr.* 4 itself, in its own intellectual context. On the former, see, e.g., Schleissner (1994), Cadden (1997), and Couke (2008). As for the latter, one older exception is the commentary on *Pr.* 4 in Flashar (1962: 456–469); and the only recent exception that I am aware of is Meeusen (2020). In addition, I should mention *Pr.* 4.26: this long and (in)famous *problema* (which begins: "Why do some men enjoy submitting to sex, and some at the same time enjoy being active, whereas others do not?") generally receives brief coverage in studies of homosexuality in the ancient Greek world: see, e.g., Dover (1989: 169–170) and Cantarella (1992: 68–69).

2 Traditionally rendered *De genitura* or *De semine* (or *On Generation* in English). The most accurate English translation of the title is arguably *On Semen* (but see note 9 below).

3 See Lennox (1994).

4 See Connell (2016: 96–98). Aristotle clearly also had in mind certain Presocratics—Democritus, Empedocles, and Anaxagoras—who defended some version of, or something akin to, this view. See Lonie (1981: 62–70). But I find unconvincing those attempts (e.g., De Ley [1980]) to show that Presocratics (*rather than* Hippocratic treatises) are the primary target of Aristotle's critique.

von Staden put it: "In general, [...] the pangenetic theory dominates the Hippocratic Corpus [...]."[5]

I cover just enough of the content of *On Seed* to provide the context necessary for understanding Aristotle's rejection of the pangenesis theory as well as the relevant chapters in *Pr.* 4.[6] Scholars tend to agree that the date of this work falls within the "End of the fifth century, beginning of the fourth".[7] But whatever its actual date, what is important for my purposes is that it was written long before Aristotle wrote on these topics, and so it is reasonable to think that he knew of this work and/or others like it (or at the very least of the ideas presented therein).[8]

In the opening chapter (*On Seed* 1 [7.470–472 Littré; 44–45 Joly; 6–8 Potter]), the author claims that "a man's [i.e., a male human's] seed[9] comes from all the moisture [or fluid] in his body (ἡ δὲ γονὴ τοῦ ἀνδρὸς ἔρχεται ἀπὸ παντὸς τοῦ ὑγροῦ τοῦ ἐν τῷ σώματι), and is the excretion of its most powerful part."[10] Proof of this is that what is emitted during sex, though small in quantity, causes us to become weak (ἀσθενέες). Further, "Vessels and nerves from the whole body extend to the penis (φλέβες καὶ νεῦρα ἀπὸ παντὸς τοῦ σώματος τείνουσιν ἐς τὸ αἰδοῖον), and

5 von Staden (1989: 290). He continues: "and it is represented both in the so-called 'Coan' treatises (e.g., *Airs, Waters, Places; On Sacred Diseases*) and in treatises traditionally known as 'Cnidian' (for example, the 'trilogy' *On Seed, On the Nature of the Child, On Diseases* iv)." See, e.g., *Airs, Waters, Places* 14 (2.60.1–2 Littré; 224.17–19 Jouanna): ὁ γὰρ γόνος πανταχόθεν ἔρχεται τοῦ σώματος, ἀπό τε τῶν ὑγιηρῶν ὑγιηρός, ἀπό τε τῶν νοσερῶν νοσερός, and *On the Sacred Disease* 2 (6.364.19–20 Littré; 10.16–18 Jouanna): ὡς ὁ γόνος ἔρχεται πάντοθεν τοῦ σώματος, ἀπό τε τῶν ὑγιηρῶν ὑγιηρὸς, ἀπό τε τῶν νοσερῶν νοσερός. See also Giorgianni (2006: 52–55).

6 For brief accounts of this Hippocratic work, see Lloyd (1983: 88–90), Jouanna (1999: 392), Craik (2015: 113–118), and Connell (2016: 97–98). For more detailed treatments, see the introductions in Lonie (1981) and Giorgianni (2006). See also Dean-Jones (1994: 153–176). On textual matters, see especially the commentary in Giorgianni (2006).

7 Jouanna (1999: 392). Cf. Lonie (1981: 71): "between 420–400"; Craik (2015: 118): "may be as early as around 430–420". See also Giorgianni (2006: 50).

8 For evidence of Aristotle's familiarity with the relevant Hippocratic texts, in the *Generation of Animals*, see Giorgianni (2006: 69–70) and van der Eijk (2007).

9 In Mayhew (2004: ch. 3), I am careful to distinguish in translation τὸ σπέρμα ('seed') and ἡ γονή ('semen'), for in his *Generation of Animals* Aristotle uses ἡ γονή for the male's contribution to generation, and τὸ σπέρμα either as a synonym for ἡ γονή or to refer to both the male's and the female's contributions to generation (the latter being τὰ καταμήνια, 'menses', in his view). But in the present context—comparing discussions in the Hippocratic *On Seed*, Aristotle's *Generation of Animals*, and *Pr.* 4—such a distinction can actually cause confusion, and so in translating the Hippocratic *On Seed*, I render both ἡ γονή and τὸ σπέρμα 'seed'.

10 I am using (with occasional variations) the text and translation of Potter (2012), though I have also consulted the text of Giorgianni (2006) and the translation of Lonie (1981).

these [vessels and nerves], as they are gently rubbed, warmed, and filled, are befallen by a titillation (κνησμός),[11] and from this, pleasure and warmth arise in the whole body." This rubbing, and the movement in general during sex, causes the moisture throughout the body to be heated, further liquefied or diffused, and agitated, and as a result it foams up, and from this foam the most powerful and richest part of this moisture is secreted. This is seed, and it moves from the whole body via the spinal marrow—and past the kidneys and through the middle of the testicles—to the penis.

As is made clear in ch. 2 (7.472–474 Littré; 45–46 Joly; 8–10 Potter), on this view the greatest part of the seed passes from the head and by the ears into the spinal marrow. (A disputed line in ch. 1 says that it passes particularly from the brain to the spinal marrow.[12]) That the author has the seed (or most of it, anyway) move to the spinal marrow via the brain has been thought to be odd. For instance, as Lonie puts it:

> This upsets the economy of the author's theory, and the easiest way to explain it is as an eclectic combination of two prevalent beliefs about the origin of [seed]: (i) the belief that it is derived from all the parts of the body, the pangenesis doctrine, and (ii) the belief that it is drawn from the brain to the spinal marrow.[13]

In ch. 3 (7.474 Littré; 46 Joly; 10–12 Potter), the author elaborates somewhat on what he means by seed coming from the whole body: he specifies the solid parts, the soft parts, and "all the moisture in the body." There are four kinds of moisture: blood, bile, water, and phlegm. These are the four kinds of substance

---

11 Lonie translates this 'irritation', Potter 'tickling sensation', Giorgianni *Kitzel*. LSJ s.v. has *itching, scratching*, "in a pleasurable sense, *titillation*," and "metaph., *irritation*." *The Brill Dictionary of Ancient Greek* (hereafter *BDAG*) s.v. has *scraping, scratching, itching, irritation*.

12 Most editors believe the relevant line ought to be obelised or bracketed (see, e.g., Lonie [1981: 107]): τείνουσι γὰρ ἐς τοῦτον ἐκ παντὸς τοῦ σώματος, καὶ διαχέει ἐκ τοῦ ἐγκεφάλου εἰς τὴν ὀσφὺν καὶ ἐς πᾶν τὸ σῶμα καὶ ἐς τὸν μυελὸν, καὶ ἐξ αὐτοῦ τείνουσιν ὁδοὶ, ὥστε καὶ ἐπιέναι τοῦ ὑγροῦ ἐς αὐτὸν καὶ ἀποχωρέειν. Potter translates it: "For they lead from the entire body to this part, and pass out of the brain to the loin, the whole body, and the marrow, and from it passageways lead such that moisture can both go to it and away from it." Cf. Giorgianni (2006: 146) for a different text, and (230–231) for commentary.

13 Lonie (1981: 101–102). See also von Staden (1989: 288–290), Dean-Jones (1994: 162–163), and Craik (2015: 115). Note however Jouanna (1999: 272): "neither of these two physicians [i.e., the author of *On Seed* and the author of *Airs, Waters, Places*] understood the distinction that modern scholars have sought to introduce between an 'encephalomyetic' theory and a 'pangenic' theory."

that exist naturally in a person.[14] There is no explanation of what these solid and soft parts are, nor of the relationship between the seed coming from the four kinds of moisture and from these solid and soft parts.

In ch. 4 (7.474–476 Littré; 46–47 Joly; 12–14 Potter), the author makes clear that what he's described so far, in the case of the male human, happens in essentially the same way—*mutatis mutandis*—in the case of the female as well. The rubbing and other motions that occur during intercourse cause pleasure and warmth to arise in the whole body, which leads in the same way to the emitting of seed (and the same kind of seed)—sometimes into the uterus, sometimes externally. Pleasure is a necessary part or by-product of the production of seed, on this view, and this explains the unusual claims the author makes about a woman's pleasure during sex—such pleasure, on this account, always accompanying conception.[15]

In ch. 5 (7.476 Littré; 48 Joly; 14 Potter), the author explains the purported fact that "When a woman has intercourse, if she is not going to conceive, generally the seed of both partners runs out of her, when this is what the woman intends."[16] In ch. 6 (7.478 Littré; 48 Joly; 14–16 Potter), both males and females are said to produce male and female seeds. Male seed is stronger, female seed weaker. Whichever kind of seed predominates (in quantity) in a particular mixture determines the gender of the child. In ch. 7 (7.478–480 Littré; 49 Joly; 16–18 Potter), evidence is provided for the claim that both males and females have male and female seed; and in ch. 8 (7.480–482 Littré; 49–50 Joly; 18–20 Potter), the author attempts to explain family resemblance. (I skip the details of these four chapters, as they are not part of the context necessary for understanding *Pr.* 4.)

The last three chapters (9–11 [7.482–484 Littré; 50–52 Joly; 20–22 Potter]) deal for the most part with offspring that are born weak, stunted, or deformed, and to some extent with parents that are such.[17] The author is arguably espe-

14 εἰσὶ δὲ τέσσαρες ἰδέαι τοῦ ὑγροῦ, αἷμα, χολή, ὕδωρ καὶ φλέγμα. τοσαύτας γὰρ ἰδέας ἔχει ξυμφυέας ὁ ἄνθρωπος ἐν ἑωυτῷ, καὶ ἀπὸ τουτέων αἱ νοῦσοι γίνονται [...]. See also ch. 11: ἐπὴν δέ τί οἱ νόσημα προσπέσῃ καὶ τοῦ ὑγροῦ αὐτοῦ, ἀφ' οὗ τὸ σπέρμα γίνεται, τέσσαρες ἰδέαι ἐοῦσαι, ὁκόσαι ἐν φύσει ὑπῆρξαν, τὴν γονὴν οὐχ ὅλην παρέχουσιν [...].

15 As Dean-Jones (1994: 157) comments: "The description of a woman's pleasure in [ch. 4] hardly shows an intimate knowledge of feminine experience."

16 ἐπὴν δὲ μιχθῇ ἡ γυνή, ἢν μὲν δὴ μὴ μέλλῃ λήψεσθαι πρὸς ἑωυτήν, πρὸς τῷ ἔθει χωρέει ἔξω ἡ γονὴ ἀπ' ἀμφοτέρων, ὁκόταν ἡ γυνὴ ἐθελήσῃ.

17 In chs. 10–11, the author often uses πήρωσις and its cognates (e.g., πηρωθέν at the opening of ch. 10, πεπηρωμένων at the opening of ch. 11). Lonie (1981: 145) notes correctly that "πήρωσις covers the notion both of mutilation and deformities" (cf. Mayhew [2004: 54 n. 1]). He goes on, however, to say that in ch. 11 the author has in mind deformities only; but I doubt

cially concerned with two kinds of cases that might prove difficult to account for according to the pangenesis theory: How it is that healthy and whole parents sometimes give birth to weak, stunted, or deformed offspring; and, how it is that a weak, stunted, or deformed parent sometimes contributes to the generation of healthy and whole offspring.[18]

As a last word on this view of conception, note that the same author says, in the first three chapters of *Nature of the Child* (7.486–492 Littré; 53–57 Joly; 30–38 Potter), which work is a continuation of *On Seed*,[19] that the seed from male and female mix in the uterus, and there the mixture is warmed, and it congeals and becomes thicker. It is formed and nourished by the blood and breath (*pneuma*) of the mother (the mother's breath entering via the umbilical cord).

3 Aristotle's *Generation of Animals*

The first book of the *Generation of Animals* provides a quick sketch of Aristotle's presentation of the evidence for, and his criticisms of, the pangenesis theory,

---

that. Perhaps like Aristotle after him, the author of *On Seed* is leaving open the possibility of the truth of the strange reports about children inheriting acquired characteristics. See Arist. *GA* 1.17.721b28–36 (and note 24 below).

18 In ch. 11, the author says that in some cases, when a parent is maimed or deformed, the child is not; in others, when the parent is maimed or deformed or diseased, so is the child. The difference is the following: In the case where a parent is maimed or deformed, the child may still be healthy (i.e., whole), "for the maimed/deformed (part) has the whole number (of seeds), as in the healthy one" (ἔχει γὰρ τὸν ἀριθμὸν πάντα τὸ πεπηρωμένον τῷ ὑγιεῖ). (Potter translates this: "for what is maimed still has everything equal in number to the whole." Cf. Lonie's: "This is because although an animal may be deformed, it still has exactly the same components as what is sound.") This is an important line (however obscure). For as Dean-Jones (1994: 165) comments, here the author has "made the first few stumbling steps towards the realization that seed carried information on how to structure the material rather than the material itself". It seems that if a man has a club foot, or loses a toe chopping wood, his children will or might still be born with two whole feet, not only because of the seed contributed by the mother, but also because the father's seed from this part of the body still has encoded in it (so to speak) the potential to form a complete foot. But this is all left to implication. Irrespective of their connection to the pangenesis theory, such questions concerning parent-child differences had a lasting appeal: see, e.g., Ps.-Alex., *Med. Puzz.* 1.28 (12.5–16 Ideler), which begins: "Why do many stupid people bear highly intelligent children, and many highly intelligent people very stupid ones?" (Διὰ τί πολλοὶ μωροὶ φρονίμους ἄγαν τίκτουσι, πολλοὶ δὲ ἄγαν φρόνιμοι μωροτέρους;)

19 There is a scholarly consensus that *On Seed* and *On the Nature of the Child* are two parts of one unified work (on conception and on embryology, respectively), and that *Diseases* 4 is a separate work by the same author. See: Lonie (1981: 49–51); Jouanna (1999: 384 & 392); Giorgianni (2006: 1–30); Craik (2015: 117).

followed by a brief summary of his own, alternative account of the contributions of the male and the female to generation.

In *GA* 1.17, Aristotle presents four pieces of evidence (τεκμηρίοις)[20] that one could use to support the view that "seed comes away from each of the parts"[21] (721b13–27):

1. The intensity of the pleasure (ἡ σφοδρότης τῆς ἡδονῆς). "For the same affection becomes more pleasant if there is more of it, and that which occurs in all the parts is more than that which occurs in one or a few." (This is implied in the Hippocratic *On Seed*, and it is also the topic of *Pr.* 4.15.)
2. The fact that incomplete/stunted offspring come from incomplete/stunted parents (τὸ ἐκ κολοβῶν κολοβὰ γίγνεσθαι).[22] This is because where a part is missing, no seed comes from that part. (The author of *On Seed* deals with this, as well as other, more difficult, cases.[23] But this is not an issue discussed in *Pr.* 4.)
3. Family resemblance: Offspring resemble parents not only in the body as a whole, but also (and especially) part for part (μόρια μορίοις). (This is implied in, and motivates, the discussion of family resemblance in *On Seed*. But this is not an issue discussed in *Pr.* 4.)
4. "It would also seem reasonable that just as there is some first thing in the whole out of which the whole develops, so there is in each part; hence if the whole has a seed, each part must have a seed of its own." (This general point is arguably implied in any version of the pangenesis theory—or at least Aristotle thought so. Once again, however, this is not an issue discussed in *Pr.* 4.)[24]

---

20 Connell (2016: 112) refers to *three* pieces of evidence, treating (3) and (4) together. The text, however, says τέτταρα, though the Greek at this point is arguably problematic: see 721b13–14, with Drossaart Lulofs's *apparatus ad loc.* (1965: 19). One could also argue, however, that Aristotle in fact presents *five* pieces of evidence, the four that τέτταρα refers to, plus the marvelous *endoxa* that directly follows them (721b28–36). See note 24 below.

21 Translations from *GA* 1 are from Balme (1972), in some cases modified. Translations from the rest of this work are my own. The text I am using is Drossaart Lulofs (1965).

22 LSJ s.v. κολοβός includes: 1. *docked, curtailed*. 2. *maimed, mutilated*; of trees, *stunted* (e.g., in Theophrastus); of persons, *undersized*: generally, *short*; of a cup, *broken, chipped*. *BDAG* s.v. has *mutilated, castrated, truncated, curtailed, incomplete, short, small, low*. See above note 17.

23 Cf. *On the Sacred Disease* 2 (the relevant part of which is quote in note 5 above).

24 After these four pieces of evidence, Aristotle refers to certain testimonies that plausibly support these opinions (πιθανὰ δὲ καὶ τὰ τοιαῦτα μαρτύρια ταύταις ταῖς δόξαις, see 1.17.721b28–722a1). He refers to two kinds of marvelous *endoxa*, of the sort that interested early Peripatetics—cases in which children were said to have inherited not only a parent's inborn characteristics, but also acquired ones (τὰ ἐπίκτητα): one account involves a scar,

Roughly the first half of the next chapter (*GA* 1.18)—a long one—is devoted to responding to this evidence, and to the pangenesis theory generally. I can be relatively brief—in fact, I skip Aristotle's replies to points (2) and (3)—as only one of these replies is dealt with directly in *Pr.* 4.[25]

Aristotle's set of replies to (4), and to any version of the theory generally (722a16–723b32), is quite long and sophisticated; but in brief, the main point is this: There is no clear or coherent account of whether the seeds that come from the whole body come from uniform parts (τὰ ὁμοιομερῆ: e.g., flesh, blood, bone) or non-uniform parts (τὰ ἀνομοιομερῆ: e.g., nose, face, arm).[26] And there are problems in either case: If the seed comes from the uniform parts, this cannot account for family resemblance nor—more importantly—does the theory account for how this mix of basic materials could produce such an incredibly complex entity as a human being. And if seed is said to come from the non-uniform parts, how can these bits of human being—little ears and noses etc.—stay alive during the process and then come together to form a unified whole living thing. That is the gist of the criticism.[27]

Next, here in full is Aristotle's reply to the first point (723b32–724a3):

> The reason that pleasure (ἡδονή) is intensified in sexual intercourse is not that something comes from the whole body, but that there is strong titillation (κνησμός);[28] and this is why if intercourse takes place often, the enjoyment (τὸ χαίρεν) becomes less for those who consort. Further, the joy (χαρά) is at the end; but it ought to be in each part, and not simultaneously, but earlier in some and later in others.

---

the other a tattoo. (Cf. Ps.-Arist./Alex., *Suppl. Pr.* 3.1 [256.2–4 Kapetanaki—Sharples].) I think it clear that Aristotle does not take these as seriously as he does the other four; but he does think they are worth mentioning, because they are *endoxa*, and they would support the pangenesis theory if they were true. And perhaps some defenders of this theory did make use of these stories. In any case, *On Seed* arguably leaves open the possibility of such cases.

25 As far as I can tell, these points are not dealt with elsewhere in the *Problemata*. Re. point 2 (on 'incomplete' offspring), see *Pr.* 10.41: "Why is a human much more likely to be born lame (χωλός) than any other animal?" Re. point 3 (on family resemblance), see *Pr.* 10.10: "Why in the other animals do the offspring resemble the natures (sc. of their parents) more than in humans?" But in neither case is the author's response concerned with the pangenesis theory.

26 But see above note 18.

27 There are other criticisms in this section as well, which I pass over: For instance, the pangenesis theory, Aristotle claims, cannot explain generation in those kinds of animals that come to be from larvae (723b3–9).

28 Peck translates this 'stimulation', Balme 'titillation'. See above note 11.

Aristotle seems to be claiming that if the cause of the intense pleasure experienced during intercourse were seed being drawn from the whole body, then that pleasure would never diminish, no matter how often one had sex; but the fact is, he claims, it does diminish with frequent intercourse. Whereas if the cause is titillation, then (like tickling) one would become sensitised to it. Further, if the pangenesis explanation is correct, we should expect the pleasure to occur all over the body, and at different stages, as the seed is being drawn from this or that part of the body; but the pleasure, he claims, does not occur this way.

It is perhaps surprising that Aristotle does not mention as a proof, and so does not reply to, the opening argument of *On Seed* 1: i.e., that the weakness following intercourse is evidence that seed is drawn from the whole body. Later in *GA* 1.18, however, while presenting his own account—and in particular, in defending his claim that seed is a residue (more on this shortly), in contrast to the view (attributed to the pangenesis theory) that it is a colliquation or liquefaction (σύντηγμα, σύντηξις)—he does say: "the exhaustion (ἔκλυσις)[29] produced by the smallest loss of seed is obvious, and suggests that the body is being deprived of the end product of the nourishment" (725b6–8). He then stresses that, with the exception of some people in their youth, most do not feel relief (κουφίζει) from sex but fatigue: "the result of sexual intercourse/indulgence[30] is rather exhaustion and incapacity (*συμβαίνει ἐκ τῶν ἀφροδισιασμῶν ἔκλυσις καὶ ἀδυναμία μᾶλλον*), and for the reasons stated" (725b9–19). I mention this, because although Aristotle seems not to have thought much of this argument from *On Seed* 1, he does agree with the author that sex produces weakness. Moreover, the author of *Pr.* 4.21 seemed to think this was a possible problem for Aristotle—that the pangenesis account may better explain this weakness.

I can be fairly brief in presenting Aristotle's alternative conception of generation (the basics of which are found for the most part in *GA* 1).[31] According to Aristotle, the male provides the form (semen, ἡ γονή), the female the matter (menses, τὰ καταμήνια). Both of these contributions are referred to as seed (τὸ σπέρμα) or sometimes as spermatic material.[32] And this is a residue of nourishment. Nourishment (food and drink) is concocted in the stomach, liver, and

29 The primary definition in LSJ s.v. is *release*, a secondary meaning is *feebleness* and *faintness*. *BDAG* s.v. has *release, liberation, slackening, weakening*.

30 LSJ s.v. ἀφροδισιασμός: *sexual intercourse, lustfulness*. *BDAG* s.v. *sexual intercourse, sensuality, lasciviousness*. Peck translates this 'sexual intercourse', Balme 'sexual indulgence'.

31 See Balme (1972: 127–165), Dean-Jones (1994: 184–193), and especially Connell (2016: chs. 3–6).

32 See Mayhew (2004: ch. 3) and above note 9.

heart (the heat from the heart is especially important), until (in the form of blood) it is sufficient to perform the nutritive functions of the soul: namely, growth and maintenance. After puberty, however, when growth stops, there is an excess of blood, and it is further concocted into seed—though the female's seed is not fully concocted, because she is not as warm as the male (which is why, Aristotle says, it still looks like blood): her contribution to generation is abundant enough to provide the material basis for the future embryo, and she has enough vital heat to form the nutritive part of the soul in her offspring (i.e., all the nutritive functions of the soul), but not enough to form a sentient being—nor a rational one, in the case of humans.[33] Formation of the rest of the soul (the sentient part, and in humans the rational part)[34] is the role of the male seed: it is fully concocted (which is why it looks different and is smaller in quantity), consisting of water and *pneuma*—a special kind of hot air (*GA* 2.2.736a1), which is or contains soul-heat (θερμότητα ψυχικήν, 3.11.762a20)—and it is "by means of *pneuma* that the parts of animals are differentiated" as the embryo develops (2.6.741b37).[35] I take this *pneuma* or soul-heat to be something akin to non-material D.N.A. that in conception and after forms or processes the material provided by the female.[36]

As the male's contribution to generation is more fully concocted than the female's, and must be emitted (whereas the female's is secreted), its production and passage through the body are more complicated (and in fact Aristotle's account is not entirely clear). I find Lesley Dean-Jones's summary (drawing especially on *GA* 1.4–6 and *HA* 3.1) quite useful:[37]

> Aristotle says that the two blood vessels leading to the head of each testicle from the kidneys are filled with blood, while two blood-vessel-like passages (φλεβικοὶ πόροι) leading to the head of each testicle from the

33 Contrary to the characterisations (or caricatures) of Aristotle's theory of generation by some of his feminist critics, the female seed on his view is not prime matter or any kind of inert matter; it is organic material possessing nutritive soul plus all the potentials for becoming a particular animal of a certain kind. See Mayhew (2004: ch. 3) and Connell (2016: chs. 3–4).

34 Apparently with the exception of intellect (*nous*), which enters from outside (*GA* 2.3.736b21–29). See Balme's long note on this passage (1972: 159–164).

35 I think it fairly certain that this is connate (σύμφυτον) *pneuma* and not external *pneuma*. See Meeusen (2020: 65 n. 4). (On this special heat in the *pneuma*, see *GA* 2.3.)

36 In this paragraph I have drawn on Dean-Jones (1994: 60–61 and 184–187), and Mayhew (2004: ch. 3). See also Peck (1942: lxiii–lxvii).

37 Dean-Jones (1994: 187). See especially *HA* 3.1.510a13–29.

> aorta are not. When the passages from the kidneys double back at the head of the testicles and converge in the penis they contain white liquid. At *GA* [1.5.]717b23–26[38] Aristotle says it is the heating of the penis during intercourse which causes the semen to collect together. It seems as if this heat causes the pneuma to rush to the testicles through the *phlebikoi poroi* leading directly from the aorta and to heat the bloodlike residue in the passages leading from the kidneys [...] to the penis.

So on this view, one could say (at most) that seed travels from the kidneys to the genitals, though it is perhaps more accurate to say that the seed itself (in contrast to the blood being concocted into seed) is formed in and around the genitals. The important point, in either case, is that on Aristotle's view, the seed does not travel through the length of the body, as it does according to the pangenesis theory. Nor of course is it drawn from the whole body. (The fact that blood—which is concocted into seed—courses through the entire body, is not a relevant part of Aristotle's conception of generation.)

Aristotle would claim that his account avoids the fundamental problem of the pangenesis theory: There are two different contributions to generation (male and female), and one works on or forms or processes the other. So there is no problem of explaining how the male and female contributions (of the same kind) mix together to form a unified whole living being.[39]

4 *Problemata Physica* 4

The most prevalent (and basic) format of the over 900 problems in the *Problemata physica* (though there are many exceptions) consists of three parts:

1. The statement of the problem, in the form of a question (beginning διὰ τί, 'Why [...]?').
2. The follow-up question (usually beginning ἢ ὅτι/διότι, sometimes πότερον διά, in any case translated 'Is it that/because [...]?'), which presents a tentative (or perhaps respected or widely held) solution to the problem (not necessarily or in every case the author's committed view).
3. Commentary on or discussion of that solution.

---

38 Balme (1972: 26 and 135) brackets this passage as irrelevant and Hippocratic—erroneously, in my view.

39 Aristotle later claims that his account is superior in another way as well, namely, in that it does not require the obviously false notion that conception is impossible without pleasure on the part of the female (*GA* 1.19.727b5–12).

There are more complex formats, involving more than one solution, and/or more than one follow-up question with discussion. Of the three *problemata* that concern me, *Pr.* 4.15 and 21 follow this basic format (except that the follow-up question in 4.15 begins with ἤ alone); and, 4.2 does so with respect to the first two points, though its commentary is lengthy and highly complex.[40]

István Bodnár writes that the question and answer format of the *Problemata* might give the impression that its chapters are part of a dialectical inquiry into matters that are open questions among Peripatetic thinkers, but this in fact is not the case generally.[41] He adds, however:

> But on some occasions—especially where there are several, alternative answers proposed—the indecisiveness is genuine, and the question and its answer may be the record of actual, tentative research, or of some school-discussion, where the answers of the pupils to the question of the teacher are recorded. Nevertheless, this is only so in the minority of cases.

I suspect I disagree with Bodnár about how rare or occasional this latter sort of *problema* is. In any case, I hope to show in what follows that the chapters from *Pr.* 4 that I examine in this essay fit his description of questions raised and answered as part of "actual, tentative research."

Book 4 of the *Problemata* is characterised by the lack of organisation typical of that work. The first three chapters are on the connection between sexual intercourse and the eyes (as is the last chapter). But after this initial grouping, there seems to be no method behind the ordering of chapters. For the most part, *Pr.* 4 focuses on sexual intercourse in humans (though they are sometimes compared to other animals). In some cases, the author is discussing humans generally, in others he seems to be or clearly is discussing males (or males compared to females). With two exceptions, the subject is heterosexual intercourse (and this is not surprising given the focus on generation). The longest and most famous chapter however, *Pr.* 4.26, is concerned with male homosexual intercourse or desire,[42] as is *Pr.* 4.27. On the whole, or for the most part, the chapters of *Pr.* 4 raise questions about the Aristotelian conception of generation and the mechanics of sexual intercourse.[43]

In *Pr.* 4, there are no questions raised of a global or fundamental nature, aimed directly at the heart of Aristotle's conception of generation itself, nor at

40 On its basic structure, see below note 62.
41 Bodnár (2015: 3).
42 See above note 1.
43 For much of this paragraph, I have drawn on my preface to *Pr.* 4 in Mayhew (2011: 141–143).

his main criticism of the pangenesis theory, namely, that there is no clear or coherent account of whether the seeds that come from the whole body come from uniform parts or non-uniform parts, and in either case, how they would do so. This absence is not, I think, insignificant. Of the three chapters that interest me here, one raises a question about the pleasure produced during intercourse, one raises a question about the exhaustion or weakness produced during intercourse, and one raises a question about a phenomenon or *endoxon* involving a purported effect of sex on a human's eyes, and implies or suggests that there is a tension between claims Aristotle makes in one section of *GA* 2.7 (which I have not yet discussed, but will shortly) and his basic theory as presented earlier in the *Generation of Animals*.

4.1 *Sex and Pleasure:* Pr. *4.15*[44]

The author begins by asking two questions (or one two-part question): "Why is having sex the most pleasant activity, and is it so for animals out of necessity or for the sake of something (ἐξ ἀνάγκης ἢ ἕνεκά τινος)?"[45] This latter is a rare instance in the *Problemata* of a concern for final causation.[46] To the question Why is sex the most pleasant activity? the tentative answer, in part in the form of a follow-up question, is:

> Is it pleasant because the seed (τὸ σπέρμα) comes from the entire body, as some claim, or indeed it does not come from the entire body (ἀπὸ παντὸς τοῦ σώματος), but through that region into which all the passages of the veins (οἱ πόροι τῶν φλεβῶν) extend?[47] Therefore, as the pleasure in the titillation (ἐν τῷ κνησμῷ)[48] is similar, this happens just as if it came from the entire body.

44 On *Pr.* 4.15, see Meeusen (2020: 82–84).

45 I use the text of Louis (1991), which is largely based on the four most important manuscripts: Ap[a] = *Parisinus gr.* 1865 (15th c.); C[a] = *Laurentianus gr.* 87,4 (13th c.); X[a] = *Vaticanus gr.* 1283 (15th c.); and especially Y[a] = *Parisinus gr.* 2036 (10th c.). But see Couke (2008, 1: lxviii–lxx) for corrections to Louis's reports on readings in Y[a] and especially C[a] (*Pr.* 4 only). I have read *Pr.* 4 in a copy of Y[a] available at: http://gallica.bnf.fr/ark:/12148/btv1b8470138s.r=Aristote+problemata.langEN. (*Pr.* 4 is on fols. 31r–38v.) The translations of *Pr.* 4 are from Mayhew (2011), in some cases revised.

46 But see Stoyles (2015).

47 I assume the author has in mind *something* like the Aristotelian view described above (pp. 37–38), so that the "region into which all the passages of the veins extend" likely refers to the testicles.

48 Forster (1927) translates this 'friction'; Flashar (1962), *Kitzeln*; and Louis (1991), *prurit*. The translation of Beets et al. (2010), *van het genitale contact*, is rather loose. See above notes 11 and 28.

We must first identify what the alternative to the pangenesis explanation is. David Balme takes it to be a variation on the account presented in the Hippocratic *On Seed*: "The pseudo-Aristotelian *Problems* has a version [of that account] in which seed comes only from the parts to which blood vessels extend (878b5)."[49] Now I cannot rule this out completely, given the brevity and ambiguity of the evidence; but I think it more likely that the author is contrasting the pangenesis explanation with his own understanding of Aristotle's account of generation. This may be why the author switches from using σπέρμα in the passage just quoted, to γονή in the passage I turn to next: because in the former case he has in mind the pangenesis theory, whereas in the latter he is discussing the emission of male seed, according to the Peripatetic theory.[50]

The author at first seems concerned to show *not* that the alternative explanation is superior to the one offered by the pangenesis theory, but that it too can explain the phenomenon just as well. That is, I take "as the pleasure in the titillation is similar, this happens just as if it came from the entire body" to mean: whichever view is correct, the pleasure would be the same, so the pleasure produced by the seed going through the region into which all the veins extend (Aristotle's view) is similar to what would be produced if the seed were drawn from the whole body. He next adds an explanation for sexual pleasure that better fits or supports the Aristotelian account. I think this is clear from the reference to pneumatic moisture, as *pneuma* plays a much more significant role in Aristotle's account than it does in the Hippocratic one. (On its role in the latter, see above p. 33.)

> Now the titillation (κνησμός) is pleasant, as is the exiting of pneumatic moisture that has been enclosed contrary to (its) nature (παρὰ φύσιν). But the (emission of) semen (γονή) is the exiting of such moisture in accordance with (its) nature (κατὰ φύσιν).

Recall Aristotle's critique of the pangenesis explanation of the intensity of sexual pleasure: (1) pleasure is strong because the κνησμός is strong (not really a critique but an alternative explanation), (2) sexual pleasure decreases with frequent intercourse, the implication being that this should not happen according to the pangenesis theory, (3) sexual pleasure is fairly localised and occurs at the end (the climax), which should not be the case (he claims) if the pangenesis theory is correct. The author of *Pr.* 4.15 seems to agree with this first point

49 Balme (1972: 141).
50 See above note 9.

("the titillation is pleasant"), but does not make use of or refer to the two other criticisms. Instead he offers an additional explanation: the natural release of built up pneumatic moisture is pleasant. This likely comes from *GA* 1.20, where Aristotle says: "the occurrence of pleasure in intercourse is due to the emitting not only of seed but also of *pneuma*, the constituting of which results in the emission" (τὸ δὲ συμβαίνειν ἡδονὴν ἐν τῇ συνουσίᾳ οὐ μόνον τοῦ σπέρματος προϊεμένου ἐστὶν ἀλλὰ καὶ πνεύματος ἐξ οὗ συνισταμένου ἀποσπερματίζει) (728a9–11).[51]

The author's answer to the second (part of the) question is that sex is pleasant for reasons of material necessity *and* final causality:

> It is pleasant both from necessity and for the sake of something (ἔστι δὲ καὶ ἐξ ἀνάγκης ἡδὺ καὶ ἕνεκά τινος): from necessity, because the path that is according to nature is pleasant, if it is perceived; for the sake of something, in order that there is generation of animals—for owing to this pleasure, animals are more roused to copulate.

The teleological explanation is pretty obvious and fits both the pangenesis theory and the Aristotelian alternative, but favors neither—except in that an Aristotelian would be more likely to offer this kind of explanation, than would a Hippocratic. The material explanation, however, once again better fits or supports the Aristotelian account, the pleasure in perceiving "the path that is according to nature" referring I take it to the aforementioned natural release of built up pneumatic moisture.

4.2 *Sex and Exhaustion:* Pr. *4.21*

Pr. 4.21 begins: "Why do those who have sex in most cases become exhausted and weaker?" (Διὰ τί οἱ ἀφροδισιάζοντες ἐκλύονται καὶ ἀσθενέστεροι γίνονται ὡς ἐπὶ τὸ πολύ;)[52] The reference to both exhaustion and weakness seems to indicate that the author wants to cover both the pangenesis and Aristotelian accounts.[53] This opening question is followed by a possible explanation in the form of a question:

---

51 The author may also be working with a Platonic conception of pleasure—though without Plato's moral evaluations. See especially *Phlb.* 31e–32b, 42c–d, and *Ti.* 64a–65b, 86b–e. My thanks to Gerd van Riel who, at the conference in Leuven, pointed me in this direction.

52 *Pr.* 4.6 deals with a related problem, but one unconnected to the pangenesis theory. It asks: "Why is a human especially of the animals exhausted from having sex?" (Διὰ τί ἐκλύεται μάλιστα τῶν ζῴων ἀφροδισιάσας ἄνθρωπος;)

53 Recall that in the Hippocratic *On Seed* 1, the author argued that the fact that what is emitted during intercourse is small in quantity and yet causes us to become weak is proof that

> Is it because (πότερον διά) the seed is an excretion from all (parts of the body) (ἀπὸ πάντων), such that, like the harmonies of a building, the composition of the body too is thus disturbed by losing something, for example if the blood or all of some other part were to escape?

This explanation takes seriously and in fact supports the pangenesis theory, but does so by offering support for it not found in *On Seed*: removing crucial material from all over the body would make it less stable (more feeble), just as would happen to a building.

If we accept the manuscript tradition—which of course we should, unless we have a good reason not to—then the author next seems to add a line of further support for the pangenesis explanation, and not, as we might expect, to present a balanced account by offering support for or an explanation of an Aristotelian alternative:

> What exits (the body during sex) is so very important, and (or 'i.e.'), what is little in quantity comes from a great deal of nourishment, like a small amount of starch from dough (or 'like a cookie from flour')[54] (οὕτω σφόδρα ἐπίκαιρον τὸ ἐξιόν ἐστι, καὶ ὃ ἐκ πολλῆς γίνεται τροφῆς ὀλίγον, οἷον τὸ ἀμύλιον ἐκ τοῦ σταιτός).

This is in line with *On Seed* 1 (the seed is small in quantity, and consists of the most powerful part of the moisture from which it comes), though the reference to nourishment sounds much more like an Aristotelian account.

Now *Pr.* 4.21 ends here. As there is no second answer or alternative explanation, the implication seems to be that according to the author, the pangenesis theory is superior to Aristotle's—at least with respect to explaining post-coital exhaustion. And that may well be the author's view. But I would like to offer the following conjecture: Could it be that an eta (i.e., ἤ) has dropped out of the text before οὕτω?[55] If we revise the text in this way, and change the final

---

seed comes from all the moisture in the body and contains its most powerful part; and in *GA* 1.18, Aristotle said that "the exhaustion produced by the smallest loss of seed is obvious, and suggests that the body is being deprived of the end product of the nourishment" (725b6–8).

54 These are the two approaches to rendering this last phrase (οἷον τὸ ἀμύλιον ἐκ τοῦ σταιτός): cf. the translations of Forster, Flashar, Louis, Ferrini, and Beets, and see Beets et al. (2010: 200–201 n. 47).

55 There are no (other) instances of ἢ οὕτω in the *Problemata*; but cf. Arist., *EN* 5.10.1134a17–19: ἐπεὶ δ' ἔστιν ἀδικοῦντα μήπω ἄδικον εἶναι, ὁ ποῖα ἀδικήματα ἀδικῶν ἤδη ἄδικός ἐστιν ἑκάστην ἀδικίαν, οἷον κλέπτης ἢ μοιχὸς ἢ λῃστής; ἢ οὕτω μὲν οὐδὲν διοίσει;

punctuation to a question mark, then the last line of *Pr.* 4.21 would be rendered something like: "⟨Or⟩ is what exits (the body during sex) so very important, and what is little in quantity comes from a great deal of nourishment, like starch from dough?" If this is correct, it is more natural to take it as an alternative to the first account. I think this conjecture gets some support from the fact that, of the nearly 120 occurrences of πότερον in the *Problemata*, all but four of them[56] are followed by a sentence or clause that begins ἤ (πότερον [...] ἤ [...]; meaning 'Is it [...], or is it [...]?').

If this is right (as I think it probably is), then the author would be doing precisely what he (if it is the same person) did in *Pr.* 4.15, namely, presenting (as a serious possibility) first a pangenesis explanation, and then (as he understands it) an alternative, Aristotelian account. In this case, however, the point would be not that the Aristotelian account is here superior to the pangenesis one, but that it can explain post-coital exhaustion or weakness just as well.[57]

4.3 *Sex and Sunken Eyes:* Pr. *4.2*

Just as there is arguably a tension in the Hippocratic *On Seed* between the idea that seed is drawn from the whole body, and that most of the seed moves to the spinal marrow via the brain, so there seems to be a tension between Aristotle's general account of generation, and certain claims he makes in *GA* 2.7 (among others, regarding the spermatic nature of the brain). And as it happens, this chapter is a crucially important part of the context necessary for understanding *Pr.* 4.2.

GA 2.7 is a lengthy chapter that covers a number of topics. The section that interests me is on infertility (746b12–747a22). Aristotle writes: "for what reason a male or female is infertile (ἄγονον) is a universal problem (πρόβλημα καθόλου)." He lists some causes of infertility (birth defects, advanced age, obesity, disease), and then turns his attention to fertility tests for both men and women. The tests for women are relevant here (747a7–22):

> They test women both with pessaries, (to see) if the odors penetrate from below upwards to the exhaled breath, and by colors rubbed on the eyes, (to see) if they color saliva in the mouth. For this not happening proves with respect to the body that the passages through which the residue is

---

56 Including the present case. The other three are in *Pr.* 16.9, 20.29 and 23.21.

57 Another Peripatetic text relevant to this discussion is *HA* 10.5.636b24–39. (The authenticity of *HA* 10 is disputed: see Balme [1985], van der Eijk [1999], and Dean-Jones [2011].) It is beyond the scope of this essay, however, to discuss its connections to the other texts covered in this section.

> secreted have been obstructed and fused. For the region around the eyes is the most spermatic (σπερματικώτατος) of those around the head. That this (region) alone is visibly transformed during sexual intercourse proves this, and (or 'that is', καί) the eyes clearly sink in in those who have sex too much. Now the reason is that the nature of semen (ἡ τῆς γονῆς φύσις)[58] is similar to that of the brain; for its matter is watery, though its heat is acquired. Moreover, the spermatic discharges (αἱ σπερματικαὶ καθάρσεις) are from the diaphragm; for the first principle of nature (ἡ […] ἀρχὴ τῆς φύσεως, i.e., 'of the natural organism') is there, so that the movements from the genitals (i.e., any changes occurring there) penetrate to the chest, and any odors from the chest become perceptible through respiration.

So Aristotle (or whoever is responsible for this passage, as I think it likely is or contains an interpolation) is saying that the explanation for sunken eyes that result from too much sex, and for the reliability of certain fertility tests,[59] is: the spermatic nature of the brain and the region around the eyes; that this material (in normal cases) passes through the length of the body, from those regions to the genitals; and, that there are in fact such passages between the head and the genitals. But what should we make of this, in light of his basic account of generation in the *Generation of Animals*?

Contemporary scholars of Aristotle's biology might well attempt to offer plausible explanations for how this text is consistent with what he says elsewhere in the *Generation of Animals* (though I have not seen such an explanation).[60] But I think one must at least admit that there is something unusual about it, in light of Aristotle's general account of generation: That is, the claim that spermatic material is prominent in the brain, and that it moves through passages from the region of the head to the genitals (in such a way that it affects how the eyes look, and can explain the passage of colored material from the eyes to the mouth, and of odors from the genitals to the mouth), is surprising. So too is the claim that spermatic discharges come from the diaphragm, and that certain changes occurring in the genitals can penetrate to the chest

58 Note the rare use (in Aristotle) of γονῆ to describe the *woman's* seed. See above note 9.

59 This is in agreement with certain Hippocratic treatises concerning these tests: On the eye test, see *Nature of Women* 99 (7.416 Littré; 83 Bourbon; 304 Potter). On the pessary test, see *Barrenness* 2 (8.414–416 Littré; 74–75 Bourbon; 338–340 Potter) and *Aphorisms* 5.59 (4.554 Littré; 174 Jones). Cf. Sor., *Gyn.* 1.35 (24–25 Ilberg; 32 Burguière—Gourevitch—Malinas).

60 The closest is Peck (1942: lxvii). There are brief discussions of aspects of *GA* 2.7.747a7–22 in Dean-Jones (1994: 201–202) and Connell (2016: 104–105), but neither mention its possibly problematic nature. See Connell (2016: ch. 2) on apparent contradictions in the *Generation of Animals* and how she believes scholars ought to approach them.

and then move on to the mouth (such that they can be detected in saliva or breath).[61] Such claims are more what one would expect from an advocate of, if not the pangenesis theory, then the aforementioned early prevalent belief that seed is drawn from the brain to the spinal marrow. In any case, at least one ancient Peripatetic had questions about this passage—as is clear from *Pr.* 4.2, which I turn to now.

For ease of reference, I have included the text and translation of *Pr.* 4.2 in an appendix, which I have divided into sections labeled with letters embedded in the text and translation.[62]

Pr. 4.2 begins (a): "Why do both the eyes and the haunches[63] of those who engage in sex a great deal sink in very noticeably, though the latter are near (sc. the sexual organs) and the former are far from them?" The author offers two alternative explanations:

> (b) Is it because even during intercourse itself these parts very noticeably cooperate in the act by contracting around the time of the emission of seed? Therefore, it is especially from here that any easily melted nourishment that is present is pressed out through pressure. (c) Or is it because things that are overheated melt most of all, and having sex produces heat, and those parts which are moved in the act are most heated?

So the alternatives are not (as we might have expected) a pangenesis explanation and an Aristotelian one; rather, there's one emphasizing pressure (θλῖψις) and the other melting (τῆξις). I shall focus on the eyes: One is suggesting that

61 Matters become even more mysterious or difficult when one compares *GA* 2.7.747a7–22 to *PA* 2.7, Aristotle's lengthiest discussion of the brain (and marrow). He begins the chapter by rejecting the view of many people that "the brain seems to be marrow, even the origin of the marrow" (Lennox [2001] translation here and in what follows)—it is not, as brain and marrow are opposite in nature (the former is cold, the latter hot)—and he goes on to say that the brain "is the most bloodless of all the moist parts in the body (indeed it has no blood at all in it)," and that it consists of water and earth (there is no mention of air or *pneuma*). And although blood vessels flow through the membrane around the brain—the purpose of the brain in fact is to temper the heat and boiling in the heart—there do not seem to be any passages from the brain to other parts of the body that could explain the fertility tests discussed in *GA* 2.7.

62 The section-divisions reflect what I take to be the structure of *Pr.* 4.2: (a) statement of the problem; (b) provisional solution no. 1; (c) provisional solution no. 2. (d)–(e) support for solution no. 1; (f)–(h) support for solution no. 2.

63 It is clear that by "the haunches" (τὰ ἰσχία) the author includes the buttocks, for he later refers to τὰ περὶ τὴν ἕδραν ("the buttocks"—lit. "the areas around the seat") and ἀρχός ("rectum").

pressure from the shutting of the eyes during sex pushes out material from the area around the eyes (which, owing to the heat generated during sex, has been melted) and this makes the area around the eyes leaner. The other explanation focuses exclusively on the heat generated, especially in the most active parts—the eyes (!) and the haunches—and the resultant melting of the material in those regions.

Section (d) supports the first (pressure) interpretation, by elaborating on the role of the pressure exerted by the buttocks and the eyes during sex. This section ends: "the closing of the eyes exerts pressure on the matter from the brain." Section (e) defends this statement: "And it is clear, from the experiment with ointments of both childless and fruitful women, that the eyes and the region around them have a great potential with a view to generation, *as potency must pass this way into the seed*" (ὡς δέον ταύτῃ διελθεῖν εἰς τὸ σπέρμα δύναμιν). Though one could give this an Aristotelian spin, I think it does sound closer to the Hippocratic account—especially if the potency is passing into the seed *in the region around the eyes*, which is a natural way of reading this. And of course, the account might also be a combination of Aristotelian and Hippocratic elements.

Sections (f) through (h) support the second (melting) interpretation. Basically, the claim is that because the buttocks and the region around the eyes both play a role in sex, produce a lot of heat, and contain fat, there is melting of the fat in these regions, which explains why the eyes and the haunches of those who engage in sex a great deal sink in very noticeably. As the author writes in section (f): "owing to their cooperation in sex they share in the heat (it produces), and for this reason they become leaner and much (of this melted material) is secreted into the seed" (συναποκρίνεται πολὺ εἰς τὸ σπέρμα). Again, I think such a statement could be incorporated into either a Hippocratic or an Aristotelian theory of generation—except that the author then refers, in section (h), to the "passage of the seed through these regions" (ἡ τοῦ σπέρματος πάροδος παρὰ τοὺς τόπους τούτους). Now "these regions" could refer to the regions around the kidneys and the genitals, mentioned in section (g), though I think it much more likely that they refer to the regions around the eyes and the buttocks, which are the focus of the entire chapter and which were most recently mentioned in section (f). And if that is the case, then the author is taking seriously the idea that seed travels through the body from as far away as the head—that is, he is taking the pangenesis[64] theory seriously—as a means

64 Or at least the encephalomyetic theory—assuming these were distinguished in antiquity. See the comment by Jouanna above in note 13.

of solving this problem, and perhaps (implicitly or in passing) as a means of explaining certain phenomena (or *endoxa*) referred to in *GA* 2.7.[65]

Two final comments on *Pr.* 4.2: (1) The reference to melting is much more Hippocratic than Aristotelian. Recall the contrast between Hippocratic colliquation or liquefaction, and Aristotle's view that seed is a residue, not the product of melting (though seed *is* a result of concoction, which is a kind of heating or cooking). (2) The reference to nourishment is much more in line with Aristotle's account than with the Hippocratic one. So the author seems to be accepting aspects of both accounts—or at least taking both accounts seriously in provisionally raising problems and offering solutions relevant to these issues.

5 Concluding Unsatisfactory Postscript

James Lennox has written of "The Disappearance of Aristotle's Biology: A Hellenistic Mystery."[66] In what follows I do not contribute to a solution to this mystery; rather, I raise two related questions, concerning the nature of Peripatetic biology during the period in which it disappeared: (1) What do my examinations of these three chapters in *Pr.* 4 suggest or imply about the study of biology (and particularly reproduction) in the Lyceum after Aristotle (if not during his lifetime)? (2) When should we suppose *Pr.* 4 (or at least the three chapters discussed in this essay) were written? I.e., where in the chronology of the Lyceum—or Peripatetic science more broadly—ought we to place them? My conclusion is an unsatisfactory postscript because I do little more than indicate what I think are the likely answers.

Re. (1): These chapters seem to be dealing with what are to some extent open issues. True, there are no challenges to or implied criticisms of or doubts

65 *Pr.* 4.3 and 32 both ask questions concerning the supposed connection between (too much) sex and deteriorating eyesight. This phenomenon or *endoxon* is not mentioned by Aristotle (so far as I know), though it seems clearly connected to the issue I am discussing here. I'll simply add that whereas the solution in *Pr.* 4.3 is at most arguably consistent with the pangenesis theory, the solution in *Pr.* 4.32 seems explicitly to rely on that account, as the author says that the semen "is spread throughout the person (or 'body') just like blood" (κέχυται γὰρ ἐν τῷ ἀνθρώπῳ [σώματι Ap[a]] ὥσπερ τὸ αἷμα). *Pr.* 4.1 also deals with sex and the eyes, beginning "Why do the one who is having sex and the one who is dying cast their eyes up, whereas the one who is sleeping casts them down?" (Διὰ τί ὁ ἀφροδισιάζων καὶ ὁ ἀποθνήσκων ἀναβάλλει τὰ ὄμματα, καθεύδων δὲ καταβάλλει;) But otherwise, so far as I can tell it does not involve the pangenesis theory.

66 Lennox (1994). See also Hellmann (2006).

concerning Aristotle's account of generation generally; but genuine doubts or concerns are being raised in connection with certain aspects of that theory, including questions about some of Aristotle's reasons for rejecting the pangenesis theory and about whether certain aspects of that theory might well be true or superior or in some way worth salvaging.[67] And I think this implies that according to the author of these chapters at least (or authors), Aristotle's own theory—including his criticisms of the pangenesis theory—was not entirely settled or established in the Lyceum.

Re. (2): Not only do these chapters from *Pr.* 4 give us some impression of Peripatetic natural philosophy after Aristotle, I think they also allow us to speculate with some reasonableness about when these discussions or debates or inquiries may have taken place. The *Problemata physica* is usually taken to be an accumulation of problems from Aristotle's own day till as late as (according to some scholars) the 6th c. AD. But I think we have good reason to think that *Pr.* 4 (or the bulk of it anyway, and my chapters certainly) are much closer to Aristotle's own time, if not initiated during his lifetime. Here's why: (a) As I have said, there are no questions (or doubts) raised about the Aristotelian conception of generation *per se*, merely about some (not central) aspects of it, especially as it compares to the pangenesis theory. (b) The author(s) of these chapters seem(s) to be working in pretty much the same context as Aristotle in *GA* 1–2, with Aristotle's own conception of generation, and the pangenesis theory he criticises, as the two main alternative or contending accounts. (c) *Pr.* 4.15 contains a rare instance (in the *Problemata physica*) of a concern for final causality, and that—all things being equal—suggests a date closer to the time Aristotle was working.[68]

---

67 In this way, I think my view is in accord with Meeusen's (2020: 85) conclusion about the discussion of pneumatic processes in the chapters of *Pr.* 4: "Their inquisitive approach clearly indicates that they were primarily intended to attach further particulars to the universals of Aristotelian (natural) science and to add, as it were, some question marks to Aristotle's words. These questions are answered with new questions, always leaving room for further inquiry."

68 Point (c) is by no means decisive, however: Note the reference to final causation in the late (2nd c. AD?) Ps.-Alex./Arist., *Suppl. Pr.* 2.158 (230.12–234.1 Kapetanaki—Sharples), which begins: "Why do boars have tusks?" After providing one answer in terms of material causation, the author continues: "Or is it that as nature has given horns for the sake of defense and assistance (ἀλκῆς χάριν καὶ βοηθείς), so it has given tusks to boars?" (transl. Kapetanaki—Sharples [2006: 230–233]). More on this work in the next paragraph and in Oikonomopoulou's chapter in this volume. The topic of horns being for the sake of defense is also found (among a wide range of similar teleological questions) in the Preface to the first Book of Ps.-Alexander's *Medical Puzzles and Natural Problems* (3.8–11 Ideler) (most likely 2nd c. AD and later; see Meeusen's chapter in this volume).

To give a more satisfactory answer to the question When were these chapters written?—to the extent that that's possible—would require comparing them not only to Aristotle's *Generation of Animals* and the Hippocratic *On Seed*, but also, on the one hand, to the sparse 'fragments' or source-texts on the generation of animals in Theophrastus and Strato,[69] and on the other, to later relevant texts—for instance, the few chapters on the nature of seed and generation in the so-called *Supplementary Problems*, most recently edited by Kapetanaki and Sharples, which date to around the time of Alexander of Aphrodisias (late second and early third century AD).[70] One could devote a whole paper to this topic (which I have not written); so I'll simply assert, for what it's worth, that I think that the three *Pr.* 4 chapters that I have examined likely fall roughly somewhere between the period when Aristotle himself was active to the time when Strato was scholarch (ca. 286–268).[71]

Appendix: *Pr.* 4.2

(a) Why do both the eyes and the haunches of those who engage in sex a great deal sink in very noticeably, though the latter are near (the sexual organs) and the former are far from them? **(b)** Is it because even during intercourse itself these parts very noticeably cooperate in the act by contracting around the time of the emission of seed? Therefore, it is especially from here that any easily melted nourishment that is present is pressed out through pressure. **(c)** Or is it because things that are overheated melt most of all, and having sex produces heat, and those parts which are moved in the act are most heated? **(d)** Now the eyes and the buttocks noticeably cooperate in sex. For it is not possible to emit (seed) without bringing the buttocks together nor when the eyes have

69 See Theophrastus frs. 376A–383 (2.178–187 Fortenbaugh—Huby—Sharples—Gutas) (the bulk of which come from Albertus Magnus, however) and Strato frs. 70–74 (156–165 Sharples). On the former, see Sharples (1995: 107–123).

70 For instance, *Suppl. Pr.* 2.10 (124.4–6 Kapetanaki—Sharples) seems to be operating according to a radically different conception of the female's role in generation: "Why do menses occur? Because females live a life with less exercise and have much more residual matter, and much blood everywhere. So the excess is excreted for the sake of relief." (Διὰ τί ἔμμηνα γίνεται; Ὅτι ταῖς θηλείαις ἀργότερον βίον ζώσαις τὸ περίττωμα πολὺ πλέον, πολὺ δὲ τὸ αἷμα πανταχοῦ. τὸ περισσὸν οὖν ἐκκρίνεται κουφισμοῦ χάριν.) Text and translation from Kapetanaki—Sharples (2006: 124–125). (See also 2.7, 2.28, 2.171.)

71 This agrees roughly with the conclusions of Louis, for *Pr.* 4 as a whole: "au troisième siècle avant J.-C.". He goes on to say of the author of *Pr.* 4 (with more certainty than I think is justified): "Sans doute était-ce un médecin de l'entourage de Straton de Lampsaque […]" (1991: 79).

been cast down; for the contraction of the buttocks exerts pressure, just as the moisture (can be emitted) from the bladder by (pressure from) the hand, while the closing of the eyes exerts pressure on the matter from the brain. **(e)** And it is clear, from the experiment with ointments of both childless and fruitful women, that the eyes and the region around them have a great potential with a view to generation, as potency must pass this way into the seed. **(f)** But both the rectum and the eyes always are fat in everyone; so owing to their cooperation in sex they share in the heat (it produces), and for this reason they become leaner and much (of this material) is secreted into the seed. **(g)** For unless a part is fat, the heat will not melt it to the same extent, nor will it do so if the part is fat but does not cooperate in sex, as in the case of the stomach; but the kidneys perceive much more than other parts, owing to their proximity (to the sexual organs). **(h)** And the mere passage of the seed through these regions, being very noticeable, is sufficient to make them lean; for it removes something, but although it is near does not add anything.

(a) Διὰ τί τῶν πλείοσιν ἀφροδισίοις χρωμένων ἐπιδηλότατα ἐνδίδωσι* τὰ ὄμματα καὶ τὰ ἰσχία, τὰ μὲν ἐγγὺς ὄντα, τὰ δὲ πόρρω; **(b)** πότερον ὅτι καὶ ἐν αὐτῇ τῇ συνουσίᾳ ἐπιδηλότατα συμπονεῖ ταῦτα τῇ ἐργασίᾳ συνιόντα περὶ τὴν πρόεσιν τοῦ σπέρματος; συνεκθλίβεται οὖν μάλιστα ἐντεῦθεν ὅσον εὔτηκτον τῆς τροφῆς ἔνεστι διὰ τὴν θλῖψιν. **(c)** ἢ διότι παραθερμαινόμενα τήκεται μάλιστα, ὁ δ' ἀφροδισιασμὸς θερμότητα ἐργάζεται, μάλιστα δὲ ταῦτα θερμαίνεται, ἃ κινεῖται ἐν τῇ ἐργασίᾳ; **(d)** οἱ δ' ὀφθαλμοὶ καὶ τὰ περὶ τὴν ἕδραν ἐπιδήλως συμπονεῖ. οὔτε γὰρ μὴ συναγαγόντι τὰ περὶ τὴν ἕδραν ἐνδέχεται προέσθαι, οὔτε [μὴ]* τῶν ὀφθαλμῶν καταβληθέντων· τὰ μὲν γὰρ περὶ τὴν ἕδραν συνιόντα θλίβει, οἷον ἐκ κύστεως τῇ χειρὶ τὸ ὑγρόν, ἡ δὲ τῶν ὀφθαλμῶν συναγωγὴ τὰ ἀπὸ τοῦ ἐγκεφάλου. **(e)** ὅτι δὲ μεγάλην ἔχουσι τὰ ὄμματα τὴν δύναμιν καὶ ὁ τόπος αὐτῶν πρὸς γένεσιν, δηλοῖ ἡ τῶν ἀτέκνων καὶ γονίμων* γυναικῶν τοῖς ἐναλείμμασι πεῖρα, ὡς δέον ταύτῃ διελθεῖν εἰς τὸ σπέρμα δύναμιν. **(f)** πίονα δὲ ἄμφω τυγχάνει ὄντα πάντων ἀεί, ἀρχός τε καὶ ὄμματα· διὰ μὲν οὖν τὴν συνεργίαν κοινωνεῖ τῆς θερμασίας, διὰ δὲ ταύτην λεπτύνεται καὶ συναποκρίνεται πολὺ εἰς τὸ σπέρμα. **(g)** οὔτε γάρ, ἂν μὴ πῖον ᾖ, ὁμοίως τήξει* ἡ θερμότης, οὔτε πῖον ὂν μὴ συμπονοῦν, οἷον ἐν τῇ κοιλίᾳ· ἀλλὰ οἱ νεφροὶ τῶν ἄλλων μάλιστα αἰσθάνονται διὰ τὴν γειτνίασιν. **(h)** καὶ αὐτὴ δ' ἡ τοῦ σπέρματος πάροδος παρὰ τοὺς τόπους τούτους οὖσα ἐπιδηλότατα ἱκανή ἐστι λεπτύνειν· ἀφαιρεῖ γάρ, ἀλλ' οὐ προστίθησι πλησιάζουσα.

ἐνδίδωσι Sylburg (cf. *GA* 2.7.747a16) : συνδίδωσι codd.   μὴ secl. Platt   γονίμων codd. : ἀγόνων Forster   τήξει conieci (cf. Barth. *solvet*) : τρήσει Ap : γρύσει cett. codd.

Acknowledgements

I would like to thank the conference attendants for their feedback on the paper I delivered in Leuven, and Michiel Meeusen for his comments on the penultimate version.

Bibliography

Primary Sources

Balme, D.M. 1972. *Aristotle's De Partibus Animalium I and De Generatione Animalium I (with passages from II.1–3)*. Oxford: Clarendon Press.

Beets, J. et al. 2010. *Aristoteles Problemen*. Budel, NL: Damon.

Bourbon, F. 2008. *Hippocrate 12.1. Nature de la femme*. Paris: Les Belles Lettres.

Bourbon, F. 2017. *Hippocrate 12.4. Femmes stériles. Maladies des jeunes filles. Superfétation. Excision du fœtus*. Paris: Les Belles Lettres.

Burguière, P.—Gourevitch, D.—Malinas, Y. 1988. *Soranos d'Ephèse 1.1. Maladies des femmes*. Paris: Les Belles Lettres.

Drossaart Lulofs, H.J. 1965. *Aristotelis De Generatione Animalium*. Oxford: Clarendon Press.

Ferrini, M. 2002. *Aristotele Problemi*. Milan: Bompiani.

Flashar, H. 1962. *Aristoteles: Problemata Physica*. Berlin: Akademie-Verlag.

Forster, E.S. 1927. *The Works of Aristotle Translated into English Under the Editorship of W.D. Ross*, vol. 7: *Problemata*. Oxford University Press.

Fortenbaugh, W.W.—Huby, P.M.—Sharples, R.W.—Gutas, D. 1992. *Theophrastus of Eresus: Sources for His Life, Writings, Thought and Influence*, 2 vols. Leiden—New York—Köln: Brill.

Giorgianni, F. 2006. *Hippokrates, über die Natur des Kindes (De genitura und De natura pueri)*. Wiesbaden: Ludwig Reichert Verlag.

Ideler, J.L. 1841. *Physici et medici Graeci minores*. Berlin: Reimer.

Ilberg, J. 1927. *Sorani Gynaeciorum libri IV* [CMG IV]. Leipzig—Berlin: Teubner.

Joly, R. 1970. *Hippocrate 11. De la génération. De la nature de l'enfant. Des maladies IV. Du foetus de huit mois*. Paris: Les Belles Lettres.

Jones, W.H.S. 1931. *Hippocrates 4. Nature of Man. Regimen in Health. Humours. Aphorisms. Regimen 1–3. Dreams. Heracleitus: On the Universe*. Cambridge, Mass.—London: Harvard University Press.

Jouanna, J. 1996. *Hippocrate 2.2. Airs, eaux, lieux*. Paris: Les Belles Lettres.

Jouanna, J. 2003. *Hippocrate 2.3. La Maladie sacrée*. Paris: Les Belles Lettres.

Kapetanaki, S.—Sharples, R.W. 2006. *Pseudo-Aristoteles (Pseudo-Alexander), Supplementa Problematorum*. Berlin—New York: de Gruyter.

Lennox, J. 2001. *Aristotle: On the Parts of Animals I–IV*. Oxford: Clarendon Press.
Littré, É. 1839–1861. *Oeuvres complètes d'Hippocrate*. Paris: J.-B. Baillière.
Lonie, I.M. 1981. *The Hippocratic Treatises On Generation, On the Nature of the Child, Diseases IV: A Commentary*. Berlin: de Gruyter.
Louis, P. 1991. *Aristote. Problèmes*, vol. 1. Paris: Les Belles Lettres.
Mayhew, R. 2011. *Aristotle: Problems*, 2 vols. Cambridge, Mass.: Harvard University Press.
Peck, A.L. 1942. *Aristotle: Generation of Animals*. Cambridge, Mass.: Harvard University Press.
Potter, P. 2012. *Hippocrates 10. Generation. Nature of the Child. Diseases 4. Nature of Women and Barrenness*. Cambridge, Mass.—London: Harvard University Press.
Sharples, R.W. 2011. 'Strato of Lampsacus. The Sources, Texts and Translations', in M.-L. Desclos—W.M. Fortenbaugh (eds.), *Strato of Lampsacus: text, translation, and discussion*. New Brunswick—London: Transaction Publishers, 5–229.
von Staden, H. 1989. *Herophilus: The Art of Medicine in Early Alexandria*. Cambridge University Press.

Secondary Sources

Balme, D.M. 1985. 'Aristotle, *Historia Animalium* Book Ten', in J. Wiesner (ed.), *Aristoteles: Werk und Wirkung*, vol. 1. Berlin: de Gruyter, 191–206.
Bodnár, I. 2015. 'The *Problemata physica*: An Introduction', in Mayhew (2015: 1–9).
Cadden, J. 1997. 'Sciences/Silences: The Natures and Languages of "Sodomy" in Peter of Abano's *Problemata* Commentary', in Karma Lochrie et al. (eds.), *Constructing Medieval Sexuality*. Minneapolis: University of Minnesota Press, 40–57.
Cantarella, E. 1992. *Secondo natura. La bisessualità nel mondo antico* (Rome: Reuniti, 1988). *Bisexuality in the Ancient World*, C. Ó Cuilleanáin (transl.). New Haven: Yale University Press.
Centrone, B. (ed.). 2011. *Studi sui Problemata Physica Aristotelici*. Naples: Bibliopolis.
Connell, S.M. 2016. *Aristotle on Female Animals: A Study of the Generation of Animals*. Cambridge University Press.
Couke, G. 2008. 'Philosophy between Text and Tradition. The Reception of Aristotle's *Problemata* in the Middle Ages: Peter of Abano's *Expositio Problematum* IV (*De Coitu*)', 2 vols. Diss. KU Leuven.
Craik, E.M. 2015. *The 'Hippocratic' Corpus: Content and Context*. London: Routledge.
Dean-Jones, L.A. 1994. *Women's Bodies in Classical Greek Science*. Oxford: Clarendon Press.
Dean-Jones, L.A. 2011. 'Clinical Gynecology and Aristotle's Biology: The Composition of *HA* X', *Apeiron* 45: 180–199.
De Ley, H. 1980. 'Pangenesis versus panspermia: Democritean notes on Aristotle's *Generation of Animals*', *Hermes* 108: 129–153.
Dover, K. 1989. *Greek Homosexuality*, 2nd ed. London: Duckworth.

van der Eijk, P. 1999. 'On Sterility ("Hist. an. 10"), a Medical Work by Aristotle?', *Classical Quarterly* 49: 490–502.

van der Eijk, P. 2007. 'Les mouvements de la matière dans la Génération des Animaux selon Aristote', in V. Boudon-Millot et al. (eds.), *La Science Médicale Antique: Nouveaux regards: Études réunies en l'honneur de Jacques Jouanna*. Paris: Beauchesne, 405–424.

Hellmann, O. 2006. 'Peripatetic Biology and the Epitome of Aristophanes of Byzantium', in W. Fortenbaugh—S. White (eds.), *Aristo of Ceos: Text, Translation, and Discussion*. New Brunswick, NJ: Transaction Publishers, 329–359.

Jouanna, J. 1999. *Hippocrate* (Paris: Fayard, 1992). *Hippocrates*, M.B. DeBevoise (transl.). Baltimore: Johns Hopkins University Press.

Lennox, J. 1994. 'The Disappearance of Aristotle's Biology: A Hellenistic Mystery', *Apeiron* 27: 7–24.

Lloyd, G.E.R. 1983. *Science, Folklore and Ideology: Studies in the Life Sciences in Ancient Greece*. Cambridge: Cambridge University Press.

Mayhew, R. 2004. *The Female in Aristotle's Biology: Reason or Rationalization*. Chicago: University of Chicago Press.

Mayhew, R. (ed.). 2015. *The Aristotelian Problemata Physica: Philosophical and Scientific Investigations*. Leiden: Brill.

Meeusen, M. 2020. 'Aristotle's Second Breath: Pneumatic Processes in the Natural Problems (on Sexual Intercourse)', in S. Coughlin et al. (eds.), *The Concept of Pneuma After Aristotle*. Berlin Studies of the Ancient World, 63–92.

Oikonomopoulou, K. 2015. 'The *Problemata*'s Medical Books: Structural and Methodological Aspects', in Mayhew (2015: 61–78).

Schleissner, M. 1994. 'Sexuality and Reproduction in the Late Medieval *Problemata Aristotelis*', in J. Domes et al. (eds.), *Licht der Natur: Medizin in Fachliteratur und Dichtung: Festschrift für Gundolf Keil zum 60 Geburtstag*. Göppingen: Kümmerle, 383–396.

Sharples, R.W. 1995. *Theophrastus of Eresus, Commentary* vol. 5: *Sources on Biology*. Leiden: Brill.

Stoyles, B. 2015. 'Material and Teleological Explanation in *Problemata* 10', in Mayhew (2015: 124–150).

Thomas, O. 2015. 'Creating *Problemata* with the Hippocratic Corpus', in Mayhew (2015: 79–99).

Ulacco, A. 2011. 'Malattia e alterazione del calore naturale: medicina ippocratica e fisiologia aristotelica negli *hosa iatrika* e in altri *Problemata* pseudo-aristotelici', in Centrone (2011: 59–88).

CHAPTER 3

Author(s) and Reader(s) in the *Supplementary Problems* (*Supplementa Problematorum*)

Katerina Oikonomopoulou

Abstract

This chapter examines the interaction between authors and readers within the medical-naturalist collection of the so-called *Supplementary Problems* (2nd century CE, or later), with the aim of reaching an understanding of how this compilatory work may have been read and evaluated by imperial readers. Like other medical-naturalist collections of *problemata*, the *Supplementary Problems* has been relatively neglected by scholarship, not least because it lacks clear contextual information regarding its origins and readership. Its purpose is surmised to be didactic,[1] but as yet no attempt has been made to address questions pertaining to its function and readership in a systematic fashion. Accordingly, the chapter seeks to track the full gamut of author-reader relationships within the *Supplementary Problems*, by focussing on first-person statements, apostrophes to the reader, and strategies of explanation that point to a shared background of knowledge between reader and author, or, on the contrary, suggest the author occupies a privileged position, in terms of his command of medical-naturalist knowledge, in comparison to his envisaged reader. As the discussion shows, while didacticism certainly pervades the collection as a whole, its envisaged readers cannot in all cases be securely identified as students of medicine. Instead, we need to place the *Supplementary Problems*' formation in a cultural context where medical-naturalist knowledge was exchanged and shared not only in the medical school, but also in other settings (such as the symposium and oral *epideixis*).

1 Medical *Problemata* and the Question of Authorship

Although a considerable segment of ancient Greek and Roman medical knowledge survives in texts written in the format of the *problemata*, understanding the contribution such writings made to the transmission and/or dissemination

1 Kapetanaki—Sharples (2006: 11).

 | DOI:10.1163/9789004442672_005

of Graeco-Roman medicine can prove a challenging task, for two principal reasons: in the first instance, we have next to no concrete historical evidence about the authors and readership of such writings or the broader socio-cultural, intellectual and institutional contexts in which they were composed, consulted or studied. Secondly, their genre itself poses problems of interpretation: *problemata*-texts exhibit such variety in style and content, it is often hard even to proclaim with certainty that the medical topics they include are meant to be approached as specialist knowledge, rather than with a broader readership in mind.

The imperial collection of *Supplementary Problems* (*Supplementa Problematorum*) is a case in point for the difficulties described above, not least because it is a text of uncertain authorship and chronology, and with a complicated manuscript tradition.[2] Much like its relatively better known literary and intellectual predecessor, the Aristotelian *Problemata*, the *Supplementary Problems* is a product of accretion,[3] and exhibits immense learning: some of its medical enquiries engage with the Hippocratic corpus, others may well go back to Aristotle, many seem derived from the Aristotelian *Problemata*, and others yet may be linked to Alexander of Aphrodisias, or to the medical school of Alexandria.[4] Issues of intellectual paternity aside, the collection also presents interpretative difficulties in terms of its organisation and style: the distribution of problems within its three books is very uneven (22 problems in book 1, 192 problems in book 2, 49 problems in book 3), and the enquiries themselves are of variable lengths, to the effect that some resemble elaborate essays in problem-form, while others are so brief or elliptical that they resemble notes. What is more, medicine and natural science are overlapping fields across the three books, and there are even instances where medical topics are discussed side-by-side with mythical stories, or using literary quotation in order to illustrate them. What this picture suggests is that the collection is most probably a product of multiple authorship, which may imply, in turn, the co-existence of different authorial agendas as well as different types of intended readers for its contents.

In what follows, my aim will be to discuss the construction of authorial identity within the *Supplementary Problems*, by following the dialogue between reader(s) and author(s) within the collection. I speak in most cases of authors

2 See Kapetanaki—Sharples (2006: 1–28), for a detailed discussion of these issues. As they establish (2006: 27), the earliest date for individual problems within the collection is the first two centuries CE.

3 Kapetanaki—Sharples (2006: 11).

4 Flashar (1962b) and Kapetanaki—Sharples (2006: 3–11). On the Alexandrian school of medicine during the early imperial period, see Nutton (2013^2: 189, 192, 219–224).

and readers in the plural because, as we will see, the unity and consistency of the authorial voice cannot be taken for granted across the collection, nor can its readers be presumed to have constituted a uniform group. My approach follows recent studies in the fields of Ancient Medicine and History of Science which investigate the construction of authority and expertise in ancient scientific texts through rhetorical means, or seek to reconstruct the profile of the (often elusive) readers of such texts.[5] Moreover, I take into account recent work that sheds light on genre as a communicative matrix between author and audience in ancient scientific writing,[6] and which also explores author-reader relationships in ancient scientific and technical texts towards the aim of understanding these texts' self-positioning between theoretical knowledge and professional practice.[7]

2 Authors and Readers in the Prefaces of the *Supplementary Problems*

Like their predecessor, the Aristotelian *Problemata*, imperial collections of *problemata* are assumed to have originated in the context of medical teaching, and to represent knowledge that circulated internally and was not meant to be published as a polished and self-standing literary product.[8] There are certainly hints of such a connection in the *Supplementary Problems*' two prefaces, which seem underpinned by a paedagogical objective. Yet their very presence indicates that, by the imperial period, medical *problemata*-writing had acquired sufficiently independent status as a scientific genre so as to include methodological prefaces. Probably because of this, prefaces are also present in the two books of *Medical Puzzles and Natural Problems* by Ps.-Alexander of Aphrodisias (2nd c. CE), whose connections to the world of medical education have been

5 See van der Eijk (1997), Asper (2005) and Mattern (2008) on Galen, as well as the studies in Taub—Doody (2009); Doody—Föllinger—Taub (2012); Asper (2013); König—Woolf (2017); Bouras-Vallianatos—Xenophontos (2018). Also Manetti (2013) on authorial presence in the *Anonymus Londiniensis*.

6 See the studies in Erler—Heßler (2013), on the connection between argument and literary form in ancient philosophical texts; Taub (2013) and (2017), on genre in ancient scientific writing.

7 See the studies in Formisano—van der Eijk (2017).

8 On the Aristotelian *Problemata*, see Flashar (1962a: 302–310); Jacob (2004); Mayhew (2011, 1: xiii–xxiv); Bodnár (2015). On Plutarch's *Quaestiones naturales*, see Meeusen (2016a: 187–233). On Ps.-Alexander's *Medical Puzzles*, see Meeusen (2018a). On the *Supplementary Problems*, see Flashar (1962b); Kapetanaki—Sharples (2006: 11, 28).

recently discussed by Michiel Meeusen.[9] In contrast, the Aristotelian *Problemata* and Plutarch's earlier imperial *Natural Questions*[10] totally lack them.

Beginning with the preface to the first book of *Supplementary Problems* (86.1–90.11 Kapetanaki—Sharples), its author appears self-consciously to place his text at the long end of a tradition of medical writing which, as he puts it, began with the older doctors discovering the parts of medicine in an unsystematic fashion (οἱ μὲν πλεῖστοι τῶν παλαιότερων ἰατρῶν σποράδην ἐξηῦρόν τινα τῆς ἰατρικῆς). Things changed when Hippocrates, as if dispatched by a provident god,[11] "gathered [medicine] together (συνάξας) when it was as one might say wandering in perplexity (πλαζομένην), and having woven it into a finished [fabric] (τελείως ὑφάνας) made it complete and fully developed by placing the head upon it (πλήρη καὶ ἀρτίαν εἰργάσατο κεφαλὴν ἐπιθείς)". The author ascribes a self-consciously systematising agenda to Hippocrates himself, by offering an extended paraphrase of *Aphorisms* 1.1 (4.458.1–4 Littré; 98.1–4 Jones):

> Perhaps he hints even at this (ἴσως γὰρ καὶ τοῦτο αἰνίττεται) in the prologue of the *Aphorisms*, when he says "Medicine can hardly be grasped by experience; for we doctors do not encounter people's afflictions at the time we wish to, for these things are subject to chance and to the infrequency of their occurrence. Moreover it involves risks, because the art of medicine is practised on a body which is on the one subject to flux, because of matter, and unstable, but which on the other hand possesses a divine power in the soul, and [is] not, like the other crafts, [practised] on [a body] which is lifeless and of small value. In addition to this afflictions are produced and intensified by many causes, and for this reason practice finds it difficult to decide the cause that produced them. Look, [for this reason] by including the whole [of medicine] in a bare account, without the underlying matter and not involving body, I will teach it in a short time, and on account of this I will make [you] possess an account based on understanding (φέρε τῷ λόγῳ ψιλῷ χωρὶς ὑποκειμένης ὕλης ἀσωμάτως πᾶσαν περιλαβὼν ἐν ὀλίγῳ χρόνῳ διδάξω καὶ διὰ τοῦτο καὶ ἐπιστημονικὸν λόγον ἔχειν ποιήσω), and I will set before you all the causes together with their diagnoses, so that you can for the rest exercise the account in practice (καὶ τὰς αἰτίας πάσας ὑποθήσομαι σὺν ταῖς διαγνώσεσι πρὸς τὸ σὲ λοιπὸν τῇ πείρᾳ γυμνάζειν τὸν λόγον), and

9 Meeusen (2018a). See also his chapter in this volume.
10 On the *Quaestiones naturales* and its relationship to the Aristotelian *Problemata*, see Meeusen (2015), (2016a) and (2016b).
11 Possibly a Stoic notion: see Flashar (1962b) and Kapetanaki—Sharples (2006: 22–23).

> whenever you encounter any affliction by chance you can fit the account to it and exercise it and find that it is true (ὅτε δ' ἂν σοι κατὰ τύχην περιπέσῃ τι πάθος ἐφαρμόζειν τὸν λόγον καὶ γυμνάζειν καὶ ἀληθῆ τοῦτον εὑρίσκειν)."
>
> transl. KAPETANAKI—SHARPLES

According to Ineke Sluiter, "by means of this paraphrase our author has put an extended version of *Aphorisms* 1.1 in the mouth of Hippocrates: a whole programme of medical teaching is hidden in its few words."[12] This teaching is construed as a dialogue between a speaker and his addressee. The speaker, Hippocrates, marked through the use of the first person, expounds the theoretical principles and limitations of the medical art to an unnamed addressee (marked through the use of the second person) in a way that specific, as well as distinct, roles are ascribed to each one of them: the teacher is someone who has mastery and overview of the subject, as well as the ability to offer a quick access route to it (πᾶσαν περιλαβὼν ἐν ὀλίγῳ χρόνῳ διδάξω). The recipient's role is to comprehend the medical art's principles in a systematic fashion (διὰ τοῦτο καὶ ἐπιστημονικὸν λόγον ἔχειν ποιήσω) in order successfully to apply them in practice, towards diagnosing diseases and understanding their causes (τῇ πείρᾳ γυμνάζειν τὸν λόγον, ἐφαρμόζειν τὸν λόγον καὶ γυμνάζειν καὶ ἀληθῆ τοῦτον εὑρίσκειν).

Through this model relationship between teacher-pupil, the process of knowledge transmission is established as key to the *Supplementary Problems*' own function: the reader of the collection can anchor his reading experience to this model relationship, by putting himself in the position of pupil-learner. The process moreover bears the stamp of Hippocrates' medical authority, and in this way grants the authorial voice that transmits this knowledge in the remainder of the collection an analogous authoritative status. The act of paraphrasing *Aphorisms* 1.1, and the use of the verb αἰνίττεσθαι in the preface, together with the rest of the Hippocrates-exegesis that we find in the preface, suggests the narrator has a privileged position in comparison to his readers: he is able to access Hippocrates' true or hidden meanings, and make them available (just like a teacher does) to those unfamiliar with them.

---

12 Sluiter (1994: 272). Cf. *Aphorisms* 1.1 (4.458.1–4 Littré; 98.1–4 Jones): "Life is short, the Art long, opportunity fleeting, experiment treacherous, judgment difficult. The physician must be ready, not only to do his duty himself, but also to secure the co-operation of the patient, of the attendants and of externals." (Ὁ βίος βραχὺς, ἡ δὲ τέχνη μακρὴ, ὁ δὲ καιρὸς ὀξὺς, ἡ δὲ πεῖρα σφαλερὴ, ἡ δὲ κρίσις χαλεπή. Δεῖ δὲ οὐ μόνον ἑωυτὸν παρέχειν τὰ δέοντα ποιεῦντα, ἀλλὰ καὶ τὸν νοσέοντα, καὶ τοὺς παρεόντας, καὶ τὰ ἔξωθεν.) Transl. Jones (1931). See also Flashar (1962b).

It is perhaps no accident that the author has chosen the Hippocratic *Aphorisms* as his reference-point: the *Aphorisms* are a collection of diverse medical knowledge, which lacks a table of contents and a clear organisational principle, much like the collection of *Supplementary Problems* itself. The author of the *Supplementary Problems*' first preface however, offers a reading programme for this text, based on which the reader gains an understanding of its contents cumulatively, through a process of consecutive reading (90.5–11 Kapetanaki—Sharples):

> They [sc. the *Aphorisms*] are both discrete and continuous (ἔχουσι δὲ καὶ τὸ διωρισμένον καὶ τὸ συνεχὲς), and this too is a token of complete excellence; for as in the case of geometry, so with them too, if it so chance, the fifth clarifies the fourth (ὁ πέμπτος τὸν τέταρτον σαφηνίζει) and the fourth the third and the third the second, and so on. And as he proceeds he makes this clear by keeping to the order of the account (τὴν τάξιν φυλάττων τοῦ λόγου) and the sequence of cause[s] in respect of periods of life or seasons and afflictions and the like.
>
> transl. KAPETANAKI—SHARPLES

It would be intriguing to consider whether this reading programme may be applying to the *Supplementary Problems*' own heterogeneous contents: how far may its author be prompting his readers to consider a similar connection between the seemingly discrete enquiries that comprise his own text? The answer, as we will see, relies on our understanding of which portion of the problems that comprise the collection the author of this preface actually has in mind.

The existence of an authorial programme may be surmised by the collection's second preface, located after the first 38 problems of book 2 (138.6–18 Kapetanaki—Sharples):

> For the rest, then, it is time to go through the common symptoms (λοιπὸν τοίνυν περὶ τῶν κοινῶν συμπτωμάτων διελθεῖν καιρός) (by common symptoms we mean those which for the most part occur at any age), for example about dizziness and sneezes and yawning, also hiccoughs and giddiness and belching and all such things, as to why they themselves come about and in what condition of body and why some of these resolve each other and some do not, and in what sort of people they cause difficulty; and after this about bald people and loss of hair, and in general why hair and nails grow and perish, and on what occasions, and why hair is black or red or white; and in addition to these about voice and the things

> that happen to voices, for example why they are high or deep and how they are fractured and why some people speak through their nostrils; and again about hearing and smell and laughter, and then about nausea and why some people suffer from it and some do not, and what sort of people [do so] most.
>
> transl. KAPETANAKI—SHARPLES

The second preface introduces the reader to a set of topics in book 2 which the narrator groups together under the label of "common symptoms" (explained as symptoms that tend to occur at any age).[13] The label itself may explain the presence of the preface at this precise point in the collection, as it helps to unify under a single rubric biological functions and pathological conditions related to them that are otherwise extremely diverse. The narrator offers an overview of the main topics the rest of the problems of book 2 will treat, in an order that, for the most part, is closely matched by the actual problems that follow (2.39–2.53: yawning, sneezing, hiccups; 2.54–2.82: hair and nails; 2.83–2.97: voice and sound; 2.98–2.104: on odour; 2.105–2.126: vomiting, excretion and purgation).[14] In this way, and as far as the aspect of textual organisation is concerned, the preface serves to underscore the author's control over his text and its contents, as well as his ability to guide his readers through the collection's heterogeneous subject-matter, by introducing scientific concepts through which diverse phenomena can be grasped, studied and perhaps also memorised (an aim hinted at in preface 1 as well).

It is clear, then, that, if taken together, the two prefaces point to a communicative framework between author and reader/addressee that grants the author a privileged standpoint in terms of his command of the text and his knowledge and understanding of the medical art itself, while placing the reader in the position of pupil or learner, who is invited to gain, for all the *Supplementary Problems*' seeming incoherence, a thorough grasp of the medical art through its contents. Yet as we will see, the didacticism that pervades both of them does not necessarily or exclusively entail a narrow association of the collection with medical teaching. Indeed, as I will argue in the next section, such a connection cannot be taken for granted for all problems, some of which may equally plausibly be associated with other contexts, such as rhetorical performance, or even with social occasions involving the display of knowledge, such as

13 On the term σύμπτωμα in ancient medical writing, see Holmes (2015).

14 This division is reflected in the subheadings added by Kapetanaki—Sharples (2006), some of which are found in the MSS.

the symposium. Indeed, we possess ample testimony on the use of *problemata*-literature in precisely such contexts during the imperial period: Plutarch's *Table Talk*, for one, embeds many naturalist and medical problems in learned conversations purported to have taken place at symposia. Moreover, both the *Table Talk* and the miscellany *Attic Nights* by Aulus Gellius depict communities of learned imperial readers engaging with collections of medical and naturalist problems attributed to Aristotle, either by teaching them to pupils of philosophy or simply by criticising and evaluating their contents and approach, in a manner that strongly suggests that medicine and natural science did not belong to the exclusive realm of specialists during their time.[15] The last point is further corroborated by the testimony of Galen, whose anatomical demonstrations and theoretical expositions of the medical art's principles often addressed the general public.[16] In light of this, it would be more productive to view the roles of teacher and pupil in the prefaces as tropes which facilitate the transmission of medical knowledge, without necessarily or always seeking to link this transmission exclusively with the medical school.

3 Discordant Authorial Agendas in the *Supplementary Problems*

Seen as a whole, the problems contained within the collection of *Supplementary Problems* exhibit a blend of medical and naturalist investigation: they explore biological functions, explain the causes of certain illnesses or pathologies, discuss anatomical features, concern themselves with the humours and with pharmaceutical or nutritional substances (milk, wine, honey) in connection to functions such as digestion, and also include enquiries into the environment or the weather (e.g., sea water, 2.22, 2.34). This approach is characteristic of book 1 and the first part of book 2 (2.1–2.38). Part of the remainder of book 2 treats the so-called "common symptoms" (2.39–2.126: see above), while 2.127–137 discuss four-footed animals in general, with 2.138–2.161 focusing on pigs, and 2.162–2.192 on horses, mules and donkeys. The topics of book 3 continue in the same style of blending medical and naturalist topics, with a special emphasis on plants and liquids (especially wine and olive oil [3.9–3.29], including prob-

15 See Oikonomopoulou (2011), (2013a), (2015); Klotz—Oikonomopoulou (2011); Meeusen (2018b). For a detailed discussion of medicine in the *Quaestiones convivales*, see Vamvouri Ruffy (2011), (2012).

16 See von Staden (1997); Asper (2005); Mattern (2008: 69–97); Gleason (2009); Nutton (2013^2: 10, 216), on the existence of such medical contests in the city of Ephesus during the imperial period.

lems pertaining to water, milk and eggs [3.30–3.42]). Its last part (3.43–3.49) includes enquiries that treat cultural practices (in relation to the use of foods or plants), ethnography, geography and meteorology.

Overall, the thematic grouping of problems is done in a manner that is reminiscent of the book-divisions found in the Aristotelian *Problemata*.[17] Moreover, one can detect a hierarchy of topics, starting from humans, continuing with animals and concluding with the plant world and inanimate substances, in a style that is akin to the hierarchy of nature that we find in encyclopaedic works such as Pliny the Elder's *Natural History*.[18] At any rate, what is clear is that neither of the two prefaces fully or accurately describes the content of the collection in its entirety: the author of the first preface, as we saw, uses Hippocrates' *Aphorisms* as a means of proclaiming his aim to teach the medical art (whose realm he appears to restrict to the investigation of afflictions and their causes). Only the first book and parts of book 2, which are devoted to the investigation of illnesses, can be plausibly argued to fulfil this aim. Similarly, the summary of contents provided by the preface to the second part of book 2 only applies to a segment of the second book's contents (up to problem 2.126; thereafter, a completely different set of topics follows, which cannot be encompassed under the label of "common symptoms"). This fact strongly cautions against hasty assumptions about the work's unity. It also means that even the paedagogical aim proclaimed in preface 1 does not necessarily apply to the work as a whole, and that we need to keep an open mind about the contexts and aims that may have underpinned the composition of its various sections.[19]

Authorial voice is a key tool which allows access to the different agendas that underpin the various problems. The evidence is unfortunately meagre, as, for the most part, the *Supplementary Problems* is composed in the impersonal, or 'objective' style that is the hallmark of antiquity's *problemata*-collections:[20] most problems are introduced as sequences of why-questions, to which the answers provide facts, without a distinctive personal self-positioning on the author's part.[21] This is especially noticeable, but not exclusively present, in the

17 See Mayhew (2011, 1: xiii–xv), for an overview.

18 Pliny's view of nature is rooted in a Stoic background, on which see esp. Beagon (1992: 26–54). Cf. the possibility of Stoic influence in the preface to book 1 of the *Supplementary Problems*, where reference is made to a provident god. See Flashar (1962b) and Kapetanaki—Sharples (2006: 22–23).

19 Cf. Flashar (1962b: 366); Kapetanaki—Sharples (2006: 3–6).

20 See Oikonomopoulou (2013b).

21 See Oikonomopoulou (2013b).

brief problems that comprise a significant portion of the collection, especially in books 2 and 3, an example of which is problem 3.8 (258.5–8 Kapetanaki—Sharples):

> Why if cold loaves (οἱ ψυχροὶ ἄρτοι) which have been wetted touch each other do they not coalesce, but hot ones do? Is it because the cold ones have emitted the sticky moisture in them along with the steam (τὸ ἐν αὐτοῖς γλίσχρον), and when this has departed they do not stick, but the hot ones have a certain stickiness?
>
> transl. KAPETANAKI—SHARPLES

In a similar fashion to several books of the Aristotelian *Problemata*, as well as Plutarch's collection of *Natural Questions*, the author of this particular enquiry poses as a natural scientist whose observations cover all activities of everyday life (such as bread-making). Moreover, given that the source of this enquiry is almost certainly Aristotelian *Problemata* 21.6.927b6–14, it is clear that the author of the enquiry is a scientist who actively engages with the Peripatetic tradition of writing scientific *problemata*, and composes his own enquiries in a style that emulates their scientific mindset and approach.

We can compare with an equally brief problem in the same book, which embeds perspective (3.2 [256.4–6 Kapetanaki—Sharples]):

> Why do they plant nut-trees especially on tombs? (Διὰ τί επὶ τῶν μνημάτων μάλιστα τὰς καρύας φυτεύουσιν;) Is it because they bear fruit that is like caskets? Or is it because it most of all trees sheds tears, which we give as a offering to the dead (ὃ τοῖς τελευτῶσιν ἀποδιδόαμεν γέρας;)?
>
> transl. KAPETANAKI—SHARPLES

The author's use of the third person plural ("they") in the first explanation that is offered effectively distances him from the community which follows the custom of planting nut-trees on tombs, while his use of the first person plural ("we") in the second explanation suggests he shares with the same community the burial custom of offering tears to the dead (notably, the shedding of tears is not referred to simply as a common human emotional response to grief: the phrasing [ἀποδιδόαμεν γέρας] is such that links tears to ritual, and therefore to practices that are culturally specific). We can explain this variant use of persons in terms of the hierarchy of roles the author assumes in this brief enquiry: even though he is clearly a member of the cultural community whose customs he observes, he foregrounds his role as a distanced observer, for whom cultural practices, insofar as they involve nature (plants) or biological functions (tears) can be subjected to scientific investigation. Yet there is a marked difference in approach, compared to the previous problem, in that the author here does not offer a rigorous scientific explanation: he does not use scientific terms (such as γλίσχρος in the problem above), and, even though he is clearly knowledgeable in plants, he does not seize the opportunity to offer (even as a side-point) a scientific explanation for the nut-tree's shedding of tears. His key priority instead is to use scientific observation as a tool for explaining cultural practice. This is a characteristic example of an enquiry which cannot be exclusively yoked to the medical school (although its provenance in the scientific interests of doctors and natural scientists cannot be denied), but resembles some of the investigations that feature in Plutarch's *Table Talk*.[22] Thus, we can surmise that especially problems such as this could be adapted to various performative contexts, one of which might well have been the learned symposium of the imperial era.

Most striking of all cases within the *Supplementary Problems* is problem 1.17 (108.11–114.8 Kapetanaki—Sharples), in which the author, in the context of a discussion that pertains to drunkenness, includes a lengthy allegorical interpretation of the myth of Dionysus:[23]

> Why does the general public (ὁ πολὺς δῆμος) say of drinking bouts that wine is dissolved by wine, [i.e.] the resultant headache? I say that this is laymen's talk, but still true (φημὶ τοῦτο ἰδιωτικὸν μέν, ἀληθὲς δὲ τυγχάνειν). The great heat of the wine produces relaxation of the [bodily] parts; more wine, entering in and expelling this [relaxation], strengthens them and equips them to chase away and beat off the vapours that have been brought together by it and weigh down the head and the body. It is the wine most mixed [with water] that removes the heat of the previous [wine] which brought about the relaxation. For a small quantity of wine when drunk produces health, a moderate amount cheerfulness, too much drunkenness and madness, as Theognis the poet said when he spoke about a moderate [amount of] wine:
>
> Much wine is bad when drunk: but if someone drinks it
> wisely, it is not bad, but good.
>
> And for this reason it is not without consideration that they say in the myths (ὅθεν οὐκ ἀσκόπως μυθεύουσι) that a Bacchant accompanies Dionysus because wine leads to dancing, the Satyrs because [it leads to] ease of movement; a Lydian female because some are relaxed (released, *eklues-*

22 See, e.g., 1.5, 1.9, 3.10, 6.6. Also Oikonomopoulou (2011: 114–117); Meeusen (2018b).

23 Kapetanaki—Sharples (2006: 22, 24).

> *thai*) by it; a leopard because of the variegated imagination of those who are drunk (for each of them takes on a different and variegated [mode of] reasoning when affected by the wine; and the skin of the animal too is variegated); a single Bacchant who went mad and committed murder, Agave the mother of Pentheus (for many when excessively drunk have turned to murder). [They speak of] Dionysus as naked because of the revelation of the thought of those who drink that is brought about by wine. [They say that] he fell in love with Aphrodite and Ariadne (for those who are drunk are characterised by very great desire for women) (τοῖς γὰρ οἰνωθεῖσι παρέπεται πλείστη γυναικῶν ἐπιθυμία). He has a certain bald person [as companion] because much wine greatly lays waste and harms and withers (*marainein*) the brain (διὰ τὸ μάλιστα τὸν ἐγκέφαλον ἐρημοῦν καὶ βλάπτειν καὶ μαραίνειν τὸν πολὺν οἶνον), for which reason they also called him Maron. He also has Pan as a companion, that is: the power of wine is universal, or again because of the differing colour and power of wine (for [Pan] too has many shapes and many colours). [They say that] Dionysus was struck by a thunderbolt and placed in a thigh because often wine which has been warmed by the sun is perfected in its blending and power while concealed in a jar (διότι πολλάκις ὁ οἶνος ἡλιαζόμενος τελειοῦται τῇ κράσει καὶ τῇ δυνάμει τοῖς κεράμοις κρυπτόμενος). [They say that] four women are his sisters because wine undergoes four changes and transformations (διὰ τὸ τέσσαρας τροπὰς ἔχειν καὶ μεταβολὰς τὸν οἶνον).
>
> Hear also concerning Pan, that they intend him to be the whole (*pan*) of the world (ἄκουε δὲ καὶ περὶ τοῦ Πανός, ὅτι βούλονται αὐτὸν εἶναι τὸ πᾶν τοῦ κόσμου). […]
>
> transl. KAPETANAKI—SHARPLES

The enquiry investigates a popular remedy for drunkenness, which involves the consumption of wine as a cure for hangover. Although the author clearly has a dismissive view of the laypeople (ὁ πολὺς δῆμος), nevertheless he finds their prescribed remedy correct (φημὶ τοῦτο ἰδιωτικὸν μέν, ἀληθὲς δὲ τυγχάνειν) and seeks to provide a scientific explanation for its efficacy. However, he does not restrict himself to scientific means of argumentation: he strengthens his point about the virtue of moderate wine consumption by quoting Theognis (*El.* 1.509–510) and then goes on to provide an allegorical reading of the myth of Dionysus, different aspects of which he interprets as allusions to wine's various effects on the human body (such as increased sexual appetite, seen to be encoded in the mythical love affairs of Dionysus with Aphrodite and Ariadne). His allegorical explanation includes etymologies of the names of Dionysus' followers (Maron's name is etymologically associated with the verb μαραίνειν, and thus thought to refer to wine's 'withering' effect on the mind, while Pan's name is derived from the adjective πᾶν, and thus thought to refer to wine's universal power, or, alternatively, to wine's many different colours). The cosmic associations of Pan's name are themselves the subject of detailed investigation (not cited here): the god's two horns stand for the dual nature of the universe (male and female, corresponding to the sun and moon, respectively); his bimorphism (half-human and half-animal) corresponds to the division of the universe into the rational (upper) and irrational (lower) part; his constant movement stands for the instability of matter; and his love for Echo stands for the heavenly sphere's love of harmony. The enquiry concludes by bringing the properties of blood into the discussion, and examining its four parts as analogous to wine's own four parts.

This remarkable use of allegory tailored to a medical explanation makes this problem unique in our collection, in that it draws a complex authorial persona in dialogue with his readers: by distancing himself from the laypeople, the author foregrounds his own self-positioning as a specialist on the one hand, and as someone who can access, thanks to his philosophical education, the hidden meanings of myths. Much like the speaker of the preface to book 1, who boasts privileged access to Hippocrates' covert meanings, our author too is able to access the medical knowledge pertaining to the effects of wine that is hidden under the surface of widely disseminated mythical stories about the god Dionysus. The author's use of allegory points to a Neoplatonist point of view (particularly evident in his discussion of the god Pan),[24] and likely also contact with Dionysian religion (particularly in the references to Semele and Dionysus' birth from Zeus' thigh, which may allude to the Orphic myth of Zagreus, itself instrumental to Neoplatonist interpreters of the Dionysus myth).[25] Further, the author's use of poetic quotation, which at first glance seems redundant in the context of his enquiry, serves to showcase his command of literary *paideia*, and thus to yield further affirmation of his authoritative credentials.

Another distinctive feature is the communicative framework that underpins the enquiry: the author underlines his personal point of view through the use of the verb φημί ("I argue"), and addresses his readers directly when he moves on to explicating the cosmic associations of Pan's name, by apostrophising them

24 Kapetanaki—Sharples (2006: 22, 24).

25 See detailed discussion of the Dionysus-myth in Neoplatonism by Hernández de la Fuente (2014), who also mentions Plut., *De Is. et Os.* 13 (where Dionysus is associated with the Egyptian god Osiris). Cf. also *Quaest. conv.* 4.6 (where Dionysus is associated with the god of the Jews).

through the use of the imperative ἄκουε ("hear"). The choice of verbs evokes a context of oral performance, perhaps connected with medical teaching, but without precluding the possibility of a wider audience.[26] The latter possibility may also be surmised from the fact that the topic—drunkenness—comes from the realm of common experience, from the elegant use of ring composition (the enquiry begins with the biological effects of wine as a remedy for drunkenness, and concludes with blood, seen as a substance that is analogous to wine, in terms of its properties), from the fact that a quotation from archaic symposiastic poetry is used in a manner that demonstrates the author's dialogue with the literary past,[27] as well as from the fact that the explanation has a clear architecture (progressing in a seamless fashion from science to philosophy) and exhibits clarity as well as precision in its scientific and philosophical language. These features render the enquiry an elegant showpiece of philosophical, as well as scientific reasoning in a style that seems well-suited to a context of epideictic display.[28]

4 Authors and Readers in Dialogue[29]

As I already mentioned, instances such as those of problems 1.17 and 3.2, where scientific enquiries are infused with perspective, are in fact a minority within the *Supplementary Problems* as a whole, in a way that they do not provide sufficient ground towards an argument for a strategic employment of the author's voice within the collection. Nevertheless, they are often revealing of the multiplicity of identities assumed by the author(s) of the collection. We can observe these by focussing on the use of persons across the collections, through which the author refers to himself, to others, or to his readers. I have collected all the relevant examples below, followed in each case by an interpretation of their rhetorical function and significance.

---

26 Flashar (1962b: 366) seems to share this view. On orality and ancient technical writing, see van der Eijk—Formisano (2017). See also Oikonomopoulou (2011), (2013a) (2013b) and (2015); and Meeusen (2018b), on the oral contexts of transmission for *problemata* in the imperial period.

27 Cf. Xen., *Smp.* 2.4.

28 On medicine and the culture of epideictic display in the imperial period, see von Staden (1997), Mattern (2008: 69–97); Gleason (2009), focusing on Galen and the Second Sophistic's culture of *epideixis* in particular.

29 All translations from the ancient Greek text of the *Supplementary Problems* in this section are cited from Kapetanaki—Sharples (2006).

TABLE 3.1 First-person singular statements

1.Preface	I say (φημί). [see above]
1.2	I say that (φημὶ ὅτι) of itself it [sc. honey] is not pungent but well-blended, but the tongue, warming it by its own heat, changes it to be more pungent […]
1.3	I say that (λέγω ὅτι) inasmuch as it has changed from blood, in this respect milk changes more easily back to this again, and is virtually blood that has been turned white.
1.12	And, if you will allow me to say it (εἴ μοι συγχωροίης εἰπεῖν), [the egg] seems to resemble the universe […]
1.15	I say that (φημὶ ὅτι) the phlegm does not rise up of itself […]
1.16	I say that (φημὶ ὅτι) as many as were allotted a short life by the movement of the stars at their birth are more swiftly tested and caught when affected by the plague […]
1.17	I say that (φημὶ ὅτι) this is laymen's talk, but still true. [see above]
1.19	For this shape [sc. the sphere] is more perfect in god's eyes than all [other] shapes, I mean (λέγω δή) square cubic pyramidal cylindrical egg-shaped lens-shaped and the like.
2.65	Or is it because the hands are hotter and moister, the feet the coldest parts of the body, and such parts are [colder] than the others, I mean (λέγω δ' οἷον) hairs and nails?
2.165	Is it because the tail gives an indication when described in this way or that, I mean for example (λέγω δ' οἷον) straight and turned up or moving or still?
Usener Appendix 46	I say that (καὶ λέγω ὅτι) it [sc. mist] is moist and cold by nature […]

The verbs λέγω and φημί, used almost formulaically, mark the author's personal viewpoint:[30] In the few examples in which they are used the author refers to himself in the first person singular either in order to clarify his scientific viewpoint or statements, introduce examples by way of illustration

30 See Manetti (2013), on similar phrasing in the *Anonymus Londiniensis* and in the *Problems* by Cassius the iatrosophist (2012). On first-person statements in ancient medical texts, see Mattern (2008: esp. 138–140); Totelin (2012); cf. Holmes (2013). On first-person statements in other *problemata*-literature, see Oikonomopoulou (2013b).

TABLE 3.2 First-person plural statements

1.7	Why, in the case of continuous fevers, do we not wash (οὐ λούομεν) [the patients] when the fever is abating?
1.17	For as we have explained (ὥσπερ γὰρ ἐξεθέμεθα) that wine has four parts, in the same way also does blood.
2.6, 2.16, 2.17, 2.27, 2.39, 2.40, 2.41, 2.84, 2.101 (in all cases, verbs are used in the first person plural to refer to biological functions common to all humans, and particularly to the function of the human senses)	E.g., 2.6: we belch (ἐρευγόμεθα); 2.16: we pass wind (ἀποπνέομεν); 2.17: we shiver slightly (ὑποφρίττομεν); 2.39: we become dizzy (ἰλιγγιῶμεν), we look up (ἄνω βλέπωμεν); 2.84: we hear (ἐξακούομεν, ἀκούομεν).
2.34	Why do we find (εὑρίσκομεν) fresh water when we dig on the sea-shore?
2.38	Why do we carry loads (τὰ φορτία φέρομεν) on our left shoulders?
2.122	Why do we not give (προσφέρομεν) food immediately to those who have engaged in gymnastics or consumed drugs?
2.123	Or is it that they [sc. physical excretions] are not up to us, and the former things [sc. the pleasures of eating and drinking] are? (Ἢ ὅτι οὐκ ἐφ' ἡμῖν, ἐκεῖνα δὲ ἐφ' ἡμῖν;)
3.31	So we say (λέγομεν οὖν) that [animals] that are white concoct the nourishment because of their heat [...]

(e.g., 1.19 and 2.165: λέγω δή, λέγω δ' οἷον, respectively), or in order rhetorically to reinforce the points that he makes. It is no accident that such statements surface in problems that are elaborate and polished compositions (hence the fact that they are located in the first two books), resembling short essays in problem-form, with ample space for expounding theoretical concepts and providing illustration through examples. In such cases, the author's voice functions as a rhetorical construct which places the reader in a context of scientific exposition delivered by an expert whose role is to argue convincingly or explain his terms. The oral context of medical teaching is a plausible context for such enquiries, although, precisely because they are rhetorically elaborate compositions, their adaptability to other contexts of oral communication

TABLE 3.3 References to opinions, viewpoints or methods of others

1.8	Why, in the case of hectic fevers, do doctors give water (ὕδωρ παρέχουσιν οἱ ἰατροὶ) shortly before food?
1.17	The general public (ὁ πολὺς δῆμος) [see above].
2.58	Why do the white marks which some people call "lovers" and others "lies" (ἃ καλοῦσιν οἱ μὲν ἐραστάς, οἱ δὲ ψεύδη) not occur in the toenails in the same way that they do in the fingernails?
2.74	As they say also (λέγουσιν) that the Illyrians who are scalped in battles and die have bushy heads within a few days [...]
2.88	[...] some say Dionysus and others Zonysus, and some Heragores and some Heragoras. (οἷον οἱ μὲν Διόνυσον οἱ δὲ Ζώνυσον, καὶ οἱ μὲν Ἡραγόρην οἱ δ' Ἡραγόραν.)
2.123	Why does everyone speak about (λέγουσι μὲν πάντες) eating or drinking with pleasure, and the rich pride themselves on it (σεμνύνονται δὲ οἱ πλούσιοι), but not also in the case of evacuations?
3.26	And for this reason some say (ἔνιοί φασιν) that the wax-ointment is the best of doctors' (τῶν ἰατρῶν) discoveries.
3.34	[...] and for this reason doctors use it [sc. goat's suet] most (οἱ ἰατροὶ [...] χρῶνται μάλιστα) as an emollient.

(such as the symposium) cannot be precluded (cf. the case of problem 2.123, partly discussed below).[31]

In this type of authorial statement, most significant are the several examples where the first-person plural is used by the author to refer to biological functions or reflexes shared by all humans: belching, breathing, digestion, shivering, hunger, vision, sneezing, hearing, sleep, smell (which partly overlap with the so-called "common symptoms" of the preface to book 2). Through its use, the author in each instance makes himself and his readers part of the human subjects whose physiological functions are under investigation, and is thus able to affirm the universal applicability of his observations and theories. In 1.7 and 2.122, next, the use of the first person plural points to the author's membership in a community of physicians who follow certain regimens in order to cure their patients or keep them healthy (namely, bathing and providing nourishment at the appropriate time). In this way, they place emphasis on his medical expertise and specialist knowledge. Problems 2.34 and 2.38 use the first-person

31 Cf. Asper (2005) on Galen and his agonistic setting. Also Mattern (2008: 69–97).

plural in order to discuss practices (namely, digging for fresh water on the shore and carrying weights on shoulders, respectively) that, albeit involving manual labour (and thus associated with the lower ranks of society), nevertheless fall within the wider realm of life experience which the author shares with his readers. In this way, they put the author's contact with and keen observation of the world of practical affairs to the fore, and suggest his theoretical observations are rooted in (and perhaps also applicable to) the practical sphere.[32] Last but not least, the use of the first-person plural in 1.17 and 3.31 is akin to the use of the first-person singular in the examples under Table 3.1, in that the author employs it in order to cross-refer to points he made earlier, or in order to introduce new points or draw emphasis to his conclusions. The variation is however significant, insofar as it invites the reader to follow the author in these textual operations and intimately involves him in the logical course of the argument.[33]

In most cases, the opinions of the general public are cited, in order to track common linguistic usage or linguistic variation (2.88), comment on cultural practice or refer to commonly held views and opinions (in a way that, as we saw in the case of problems 1.17 and 3.2, serves to differentiate them from or juxtapose them to the specialist's point of view). The opinions of other doctors (perhaps from rival schools) are never cited by way of reinforcing points or engaging in doctrinal polemics.[34] In three instances (1.8, 3.26, 3.34) mention is made of 'the doctors' in general, in a way that might suggest that the author seeks to differentiate himself from medical specialists and their discoveries or prescribed regimens (cf. 1.7 and 2.122 above): if so (and this is not simply a summary reference to his own profession), he could alternatively be posing as a natural scientist who is obviously familiar with medical practice, but perhaps not necessarily a practicing doctor himself.

Literary quotation and doxography constitute special cases of the author referring to the opinions of others (not included in table 3.3 above). Both have a very limited presence: the collection presents us with quotations from Homer (2.145, 3.34), an unidentified comic poet (2.78), Empedocles (2.102) and Hippocrates (1.Pref., 1.4), and also cites the opinions of Heraclitus (2.42) Aristotle (3.11, Usener Appendix 46) and an author named Alcimachus, who wrote on Celtic customs (2.181). In all cases, the invocation of poetic and scientific authorities invests the author's scientific views with a veneer of authority or, as in the case

32 Cf. Formisano—van der Eijk (2017).

33 Cf. Mattern (2008: 138–140), on the alternation between 'I' and 'we' statements in Galen. See also Oikonomopoulou (2013b); Lehoux (2017).

34 Cf. the frequent engagement with the opinions of adversaries in other imperial encyclopaedic and medical texts: see esp. Fögen (2013), on Pliny the Elder.

of the Theognis-quotation in problem 1.17, illustrate them in a way that makes them accessible to non-specialist readers.[35] As far as scientific authorities in particular are concerned, quoting from their works or citing their opinions joins the author and his readers in a dialogue with scientific views of the past, towards the aim of appraising them from a fresh perspective.[36]

Also not included in the tables above are the many instances in which the authors of individual problems refer to patients,[37] women, old men, children, slaves, the rich, and foreigners, as case studies distinct from themselves, on the basis of whose physiological and anatomical characteristics or illnesses they formulate their scientific theories and offer scientific explanations. Such a colourful variety of human subjects is a testament to the vast scope of the collection, transcending limits of gender, social class or culture. Discussions of foreign peoples and locations (found only in the second and third books) are especially noteworthy, as instances in which the author assumes the garb of the ethnographer. Thus, Ethiopians (2.66, 2.73) are mentioned in the context of discussing curly hair and are contrasted to Scythians, who have straight hair (2.73). The remainder of ethnographic information or references to foreign places concern animals: mention is made of the absence of asses in Scythia (2.173), the habits of wild animals in Libya (2.130), the Celts' mistaken beliefs about mules (2.181), and the Carthaginians' term for the boar's tusks (2.158). Further, they are mentioned in connection to various substances: Indian sugarcane and Lebanese, Pontic and Egyptian varieties of honey (1.2), the Phrygians' bad taste in wine (2.156), the Hyrcanian lake's cleansing properties (3.45), the Dead Sea's density (3.49). As an isolated case, the Thracians (most likely meaning Thracian slaves) are also mentioned, as people who make mistakes in speech when they grow old (3.44). Interest in ethnography is well-attested in ancient medical literature (especially the Hippocratic *Airs, Waters, Places*; the Aristotelian *Problemata* also contains ethnographic information),[38] and the authors of books 2 and 3 may well have also been influenced by paradoxographical writing, which was well-established as a genre by the imperial era.[39] But the presence of knowledge of this sort within the *Supplementary Problems* is also especially revealing

35 On poetic discourse in ancient scientific writing, see Althoff (2012); Coxhead (2012); Rosen (2013); Doxiadis—Sialaros (2013); Taub (2017: 22–49).

36 On the social and intellectual dynamics that underpin the process of becoming an authority in the ancient world, see esp. Meeusen (2016b), as well as the other studies in Boodts—Leemans—Meijns (2016).

37 Cf. Mattern (2008: 140–158), on Galen's relationship to his patients.

38 On the *Airs, Waters, Places*, see Jouanna (1996) and cf. Thomas (2000: 102–134). On ethnography in the Aristotelian *Problemata*, see Leunissen (2015).

39 On paradoxographical elements in imperial *problemata*-collections, see Meeusen (2019).

TABLE 3.4 Apostrophes to the reader

1.Pref.	Hippocrates' addressee in the paraphrase of *Aphorisms* 1.1. [see above]
1.12	You should know (γίνωσκε γὰρ) that [the egg] is made of the four elements; [...] And, if you will allow me to say it (καὶ εἴ μοι συγχωροίης εἰπεῖν), [the egg] seems to resemble the universe.
1.17	Hear (ἄκουε). [see above]

of its imperial outlook, bringing the collection's authors and their readers into contact with a wider world full of exotic marvels, rich in supply of foreign products, and cosmopolitan, in terms of its contact with foreign cultures.

The very few apostrophes to the reader occur in the first book, in lengthy problems that exhibit rhetorical elaboration. They place the reader in a position whereby he is about to be instructed on something novel or important (hence the choice of imperatives such as γίνωσκε or ἄκουε: the latter, as we already saw, also evokes an oral context of transmission). When they are used in conjunction with the first-person singular, they create a virtual dialogue between author and reader-addressee, in which the author anticipates the objections or reaction of an imagined interlocutor—as in the case of problem 1.12, where the author appeals to his reader's licence (εἴ μοι συγχωροίης εἰπεῖν), in view of the fact that he is about to assimilate the egg to the universe, and thus invest it with cosmic connotations.[40]

The sparse use of verbal adjectives (ῥητέον: 2.22, ληπτέον: 2.139), and impersonal phrases (νῦν λεχθήσεται: 2.81, ὥσπερ εἴρηται: 2.139) are also integral to the dialogue the authors conduct with their readers in the *Supplementary Problems*, in that they alert the latter to key aspects of argumentative method and procedure, cross-reference previous parts of a problem, or anticipate the topic that will follow. It is in such instances in particular that the paedagogical aim that underpins many of the problems in the collection can be observed in practice, guiding the reader through the various problems' contents.

This overview of the material has hopefully allowed us to disentangle the different identities assumed by the authors of the *Supplementary Problems*, towards penetrating into its uneven texture and richness. As expected, the normative authorial subject is in all cases male, educated, Greek, and (given the topics) a scientist. But there is significant variation in terms of the authors'

40 See Kapetanaki—Sharples (2006: 105 n. 184), on the probable Stoic or Platonic roots of this association. Cf. Plut., *Quaest. conv.* 2.3.

intellectual self-positioning and cultural outlook, which may be indicative of different contexts of composition, as well as different intended audiences. For starters, it has already become clear that the collection incorporates influences from different philosophical traditions (Peripatetic, Stoic or Platonist), which are manifest in different problems, which can, in turn, be linked to the activity and interests of different intellectual communities.[41] Secondly, it is tempting to associate problems (such as 1.17) in which the author ventures into allegorical interpretations of myths, or engages in dialogue with the literary tradition with contexts of epideictic display (such as oral performance or symposia). Further, there is a marked difference in register and outlook between problems which enrich their scientific enquiries with remarks on Greek lexical variety and difference or observations pertaining to Greek cultural practice and problems which contain ethnographic information. In the former, the author poses as a cultural insider who infuses his scientific investigations with cultural insight. In the latter, the author poses as a well-travelled physician, in the style of Hippocratic doctors, or as a collector of ethnographic curiosities, resembling Herodotus or the imperial paradoxographers. Given the popularity of cultural aetiology and ethnographic discourse in the imperial era, the presence of such themes within the *Supplementary Problems* may well seek to cater to the expectations and tastes of diverse imperial audiences or readers (not exclusively pupils of medicine). The same may well be true of the considerable proportion of problems where the author takes everyday life and its wide range of economic activities (such as animal breeding, farming, sailing, the winds and seasons) as a starting-point for his enquiries, thus posing as a scientist whose medical-naturalist point of view encompasses all aspects of life (even the most mundane), and who is, for precisely this reason, able to communicate knowledge effectively to readers of differing social or economic backgrounds.

5 Conclusions: Complexities and Problems

Most of the recent scholarship on authorial voice and authority in ancient scientific writing has so far steered clear of ancient *problemata*-collections, no doubt because of their heterogeneity and the interpretative difficulties that present themselves, when reductive readings of their contents are attempted. What I hope has become clear from the observations that have been offered in the course of this chapter is that the co-existence of multiple authorial iden-

41 Kapetanaki—Sharples (2006: 1–28) discuss the intellectual background of most enquiries.

tities (and, consequently, multiple possibilities of context and readership) in imperial *problemata*-collections like the *Supplementary Problems* need not be a prohibiting factor in our accessing their dialogue with key cultural concerns of their time. On the contrary, it would do justice to the colourful content of these writings if more systematic work could be devoted to the ways in which medicine and natural science pose within their contents both as specialist knowledge and as culturally prized discourse.

Bibliography

Primary Sources

Flashar, H. 1962a. *Aristoteles: Problemata Physica*. Berlin: Akademie-Verlag.

Garzya, A.—Masullo, R. 2004. *I Problemi di Cassio Iatrosofista* (*Quaderni dell'Accademia Pontaniana* 38). Naples: Accademia Pontaniana.

Jones, W.H.S. 1931. *Hippocrates 4. Nature of Man. Regimen in Health. Humours. Aphorisms. Regimen 1–3. Dreams. Heracleitus: On the Universe*. Cambridge, Mass.—London: Harvard University Press.

Jouanna, J. 1996. *Hippocrate 2.2. Airs, eaux, lieux*. Paris: Les Belles Lettres.

Kapetanaki, S.—Sharples, R.W. 2006. *Pseudo-Aristoteles (Pseudo-Alexander). Supplementa Problematorum*. Berlin—New York: De Gruyter.

Littré, É. 1839–1861. *Oeuvres complètes d'Hippocrate*. Paris: J.-B. Baillière.

Mayhew, R. 2011. *Aristotle: Problems*, 2 vols. Cambridge, Mass.: Harvard University Press.

Secondary Sources

Althoff, J. 2012. 'Presocratic discourse in poetry and prose: The case of Empedocles and Anaxagoras', in Doody—Föllinger—Taub (2012: 293–299).

Asper, M. 2005. '*'Un personaggio in cerca di lettore*': Galens *Großer Puls* und die ‚Erfindung' des Lesers', in Fögen (2005: 21–39).

Asper, M. (ed.). 2013. *Writing Science. Medical and Mathematical Authorship in Ancient Greece*. Berlin—New York: De Gruyter.

Beagon, M. 1992. *Roman Nature. The Thought of Pliny the Elder*. Oxford: Oxford University Press.

Bodnár, I. 2015. 'The *Problemata Physica*: an introduction', in R. Mayhew (ed.), *The Aristotelian Problemata Physica. Philosophical and Scientific Investigations*. Leiden—Boston: Brill, 1–9.

Boodts, S.—Leemans, J.—Meijns, B. (eds.). 2016. *Shaping Authority: How did a Person become an Authority in Antiquity, the Middle Ages, and the Renaissance?*. Turnhout: Brepols.

Bouras-Vallianatos, P.—Xenophontos, S. (eds.). 2018. *Greek Medical Literature and Its Readers. From Hippocrates to Islam and Byzantium*. London: Routledge.
Coxhead, M.A. 2012. 'A close examination of the pseudo-Aristotelian *Mechanical Problems*: The homology between mechanics and poetry as *techne*', in Doody—Föllinger—Taub (2012: 300–306).
Doody, A.—Föllinger, S.—Taub, L.C. (eds.). 2012. *Structures and Strategies in Ancient Greek and Roman Technical Writing. Studies in History and Philosophy of Science* 43: 233–420.
Doxiadis, A.—Sialaros, M. 2013, 'Sing, Muse, of the hypotenuse: Influences of poetry and rhetoric on the formation of Greek mathematics', in Asper (2013: 367–410).
van der Eijk, Ph.J. 1997. 'Towards a rhetoric of ancient scientific discourse: Some formal characteristics of Greek medical and philosophical texts', in E.J. Bakker (ed.), *Grammar as Interpretation: Greek Literature in Its Linguistic Contexts*. Leiden: Brill, 77–129.
van der Eijk, Ph.J.—Formisano, M. 2017. 'Introduction: From words to acts?', in Formisano—van der Eijk (2017: 1–11).
Erler, M.—Heßler, J.E. (eds.). 2013. *Argument und literarische Form in antiker Philosophie*. Berlin—New York: De Gruyter.
Flashar, H. 1962b. 'Beiträge zur spätantiken Hippokratesdeutung', *Hermes* 90.4: 402–418.
Fögen, Th. (ed.). 2005. *Antike Fachtexte/Ancient Technical Texts*. Berlin—New York: De Gruyter.
Fögen, Th. 2013. 'Scholarship and competitiveness: Pliny the Elder's attitude towards his predecessors in the *Naturalis Historia*', in Asper (2013: 83–110).
Formisano, M.—van der Eijk, Ph.J. (eds.). 2017. *Knowledge, Text and Practice in Ancient Technical Writing*. Cambridge: Cambridge University Press.
Formisano, M. 2017. 'Introduction: The poetics of knowledge', in Formisano—van der Eijk (2017: 12–26).
Gleason, M.W. 2009. 'Shock and awe: the performance dimension of Galen's anatomy demonstrations', in C. Gill—T. Whitmarsh—J. Wilkins (eds.), *Galen and the World of Knowledge*. Cambridge: Cambridge University Press, 85–114.
Hernández de la Fuente, D. 2014. 'Neoplatonic form and content in Nonnus: Towards a new reading of Nonnian poetics', in K. Spanoudakis (ed.), *Nonnus of Panopolis in Context. Poetry and Cultural Milieu in Late Antiquity*. Berlin—New York: De Gruyter, 229–250.
Holmes, B. 2013. 'In strange lands: Disembodied authority and the role of the physician in the Hippocratic Corpus and beyond', in Asper (2013: 431–472).
Holmes, B. 2015. 'Medicine and misfortune: *Symptōma* in Greek medical writing', in B. Holmes—K.-D. Fischer (eds.), *The Frontiers of Ancient Science. Essays in Honor of Heinrich von Staden*. Berlin—New York: De Gruyter, 191–209.
Jacob, C. 2004. 'Questions sur les questions: archéologie d'une pratique intellectuelle et d'une forme discursive', in A. Volgers—C. Zamagni (eds.), *Erotapokriseis. Early*

Christian Question-and-Answer Literature in Context. Proceedings of the Utrecht Colloquium, 13–14 October 2003. Leuven: Peeters, 25–54.

Klotz, F.—Oikonomopoulou, K. 2011. 'Conclusion: Reading (from) the *Table Talk* in Aulus Gellius' *Attic Nights*', in F. Klotz—K. Oikonomopoulou (eds.), *The Philosopher's Banquet: Plutarch's* Table Talk *in the Intellectual Culture of the Roman Empire*. Oxford: Oxford University Press, 233–237.

König, J.—Woolf, G. (eds.). 2017. *Authority and Expertise in Ancient Scientific Culture*. Cambridge: Cambridge University Press.

Lehoux, D. 2017. 'The authority of Galen's witnesses', in König—Woolf (2017: 260–282).

Leunissen, M. 2015. 'The ethnography of *Problemata* 14 in (its mostly Aristotelian) context', in R. Mayhew (ed.), *The Aristotelian Problemata Physica. Philosophical and Scientific Investigations*. Leiden—Boston: Brill, 190–213.

Manetti, D. 2012. 'I *Problemi* di Cassio Iatrosophista: Difficoltà di datazione e scoperte preziose'. *Medicina nei secoli: Arte e Scienza* 24.1: 423–440.

Manetti, D. 2013. 'Levels of authorial presence in *Anonymus Londiniensis* (P. Brit. Libr. Inv. 137)', *Trends in Classics* 5.1: 159–178.

Mattern, S.P. 2008. *Galen and the Rhetoric of Healing*. Baltimore: Johns Hopkins University Press.

Meeusen, M. 2015. 'Plutarch solving natural problems: for what cause? (the case of *Quaest. Nat.* 29, 919AB)', in M. Meeusen—L. Van der Stockt (eds.), *Natural Spectaculars: Aspects of Plutarch's Philosophy of Nature*. Leuven: Leuven University Press, 129–142.

Meeusen, M. 2016a. *Plutarch's Science of Natural Problems: A Study with Commentary on* Quaestiones Naturales. Leuven: Leuven University Press.

Meeusen, M. 2016b. 'Aristotle's authority in the tradition of natural problems. The case of Plutarch of Chaeronea', in Boodts—Leemans—Meijns (2016: 47–86).

Meeusen, M. 2018a. 'An interpretation of the preface to *Medical Puzzles and Natural Problems* 1 by Pseudo-Alexander of Aphrodisias in light of medical education', in Bouras-Vallianatos—Xenophontos (2018: 94–109).

Meeusen, M. 2018b. 'Aristotelian natural problems and imperial culture: Selective readings', *Schole. Ancient Philosophy and the Classical Tradition* 12.1: 28–47.

Meeusen, M. 2019. 'Unknowable Questions and Paradoxography in ps.-Alexander of Aphrodisias' *Medical Puzzles and Natural Problems*', in G. Kazantzidis (ed.), *Medicine and Paradoxography in the Ancient World*. Berlin—New York: De Gruyter, 199–214.

Nutton, V. 2013². *Ancient Medicine*. London—New York: Routledge.

Oikonomopoulou, K. 2011. 'Peripatetic knowledge in Plutarch's *Table Talk*', in F. Klotz—K. Oikonomopoulou (eds.), *The Philosopher's Banquet: Plutarch's* Table Talk *in the Intellectual Culture of the Roman Empire*. Oxford: Oxford University Press, 105–130.

Oikonomopoulou, K. 2013a. 'Plutarch's corpus of *Quaestiones* in the tradition of imperial Greek encyclopaedism', in J. König—G. Woolf (eds.), *Encyclopaedism from Antiquity to the Renaissance*. Cambridge: Cambridge University Press, 129–153.

Oikonomopoulou, K. 2013b. 'Ancient question-and-answer literature and its role in the tradition of dialogue', in S. Föllinger—G.M. Müller (eds.), *Der Dialog in der Antike. Formen und Funktionen einer literarischen Gattung zwischen Philosophie, Wissensvermittlung und dramatischer Inszenierung*. Berlin—New York: De Gruyter, 37–63.

Oikonomopoulou, K. 2015. 'Graeco-Roman imperial reading communities as agents of epistemic transfer (1st–2nd centuries CE)', in E. Cancik-Hirschbaum—A. Traninger (eds.), *Wissen in Bewegung: Institution—Iteration—Transfer*. Wiesbaden: Harrassowitz Verlag, 181–194.

Rosen, R.M. 2013. 'Galen on poetic testimony', in Asper (2013: 177–190).

Sluiter, I. 1994. 'Two problems in ancient medical commentaries', *Classical Quarterly* 44.1: 270–275.

von Staden, H. 1997. 'Galen and the "Second Sophistic"', *BICS* Supplement 68 (*Aristotle and After*): 33–54.

Taub, L.C.—Doody, A. (eds.). 2009. *Authorial Voices in Greco-Roman Technical Writing*. Trier: Wissenschaftlicher Verlag Trier.

Taub, L.C. 2013. 'On the variety of 'genres' of Greek mathematical writing: Thinking about mathematical texts and modes of mathematical discourse', in Asper (2013: 333–366).

Taub, L.C. 2017. *Science Writing in Greco-Roman Antiquity*. Cambridge: Cambridge University Press.

Thomas, R. 2000. *Herodotus in Context: Ethnography, Science and the Art of Persuasion*. Cambridge: Cambridge University Press.

Totelin, L. 2012. 'And to end on a poetic note: Galen's authorial strategies in the pharmacological books', in Doody—Föllinger—Taub (2012: 307–315).

Vamvouri Ruffy, M. 2011. 'Symposium, physical and social health in Plutarch's *Table Talk*', in F. Klotz—K. Oikonomopoulou (eds.), *The Philosopher's Banquet: Plutarch's* Table Talk *in the Intellectual Culture of the Roman Empire*. Oxford: Oxford University Press, 131–157.

Vamvouri Ruffy, M. 2012. *Les Vertus thérapeutiques du banquet: médecine et idéologie dans les* Propos de Table *de Plutarque*. Paris: Les Belles Lettres.

CHAPTER 4

Ps.-Alexander of Aphrodisias on Unsayable Properties in *Medical Puzzles and Natural Problems*

Michiel Meeusen

Abstract

The aim of this chapter is to examine one of the central explanatory—or rather anti-explanatory—concepts Ps.-Alexander of Aphrodisias expounds in the preface to the first book of his *Medical Puzzles and Natural Problems* and which he sporadically uses in addressing specific medical-naturalist problems collected in it—that is the concept of "unsayable properties" (ἰδιότητες ἄρρητοι). This concept relies on the author's conviction that for certain natural/medical phenomena the human intellect fails to provide a proper explanation due to the particular nature of the phenomenon at hand. He ascribes this failure to a lack of descriptive resources on the side of the researcher, which is symptomatic of the weakness of human intelligence and discourse more generally. Ps.-Alexander incorporates the concept in a specifically aetiological context, where it ties in closely with more meta-physical preconceptions about the world, seen as a divinely organised cosmos. By analysing and contextualising Ps.-Alexander's concept and use of ἰδιότητες ἄρρητοι, this study aims to shed a light on the ancient debate about what medical physicians were expected to know and what was knowable to them. This question is important, as it reflects on the epistemic limits of ancient medical-naturalist research as conceived by its own practitioners, thus giving a concrete idea of what kind of questions were better left unresolved.

•••

> The ingenious organisation of Nature's activities is beyond the range of words, and it is impossible to explain adequately the exact working of the instruments it employs—that is breath and warmth.[1]

∵

1 Plut., *Quaest. conv.* 7.1.699B (14.18–21 Minar—Sandbach—Helmbold; tr. Minar, adapted): ἡ γὰρ φύσις οὐκ ἐφικτὸν ἔχει τῷ λόγῳ τὸ περὶ τὰς ἐνεργείας εὐμήχανον, οὐδ' ἔστι τῶν ὀργάνων αὐτῆς τὴν ἀκρίβειαν οἷς χρῆται (λέγω δὲ τὸ πνεῦμα καὶ τὸ θερμόν) ἀξίως διελθεῖν.

 | DOI:10.1163/9789004442672_006

1 Introducing Ps.-Alexander's *Medical Puzzles and Natural Problems*

The *Medical Puzzles and Natural Problems* (ἰατρικὰ ἀπορήματα καὶ φυσικὰ προβλήματα) transmitted under the name of Alexander of Aphrodisias, the famous commentator of Aristotle (fl. 200 CE), deals with a wide gamut of particular and often quite peculiar questions pertaining to ancient medicine and natural science.[2] The work is considered spurious today and its date remains uncertain (most likely 2nd century CE, perhaps by Alexander of Damascus, Peripatetic philosopher and opponent of Galen: see the Appendix).[3] The *Natural Problems* (προβλήματα φυσικά) ascribed to Aristotle, incidentally of equally uncertain authorship and date, clearly served as Ps.-Alexander's model.[4] In both collections, questions are commonly introduced with διὰ τί; ('Why?'), by which the author inquires specifically into the material and efficient causes of the problems at hand. Notably, teleological causality is generally absent.[5]

The 228 problem chapters in Ps.-Alexander's collection are subdivided into two books, each opening with a preface. The preface to the first book propounds the types and general method of medical-naturalist problem research, indicating which topics of investigation are of interest and how they can be approached; the preface to the second book is a eulogy of the medical art, praising it as a divine gift and "a standard of knowledge" (ἐπιστήμης […] κανόνα) bearing the "tokens of philosophy" (φιλοσοφίας […] γνωρίσματα) (52.14–15; 9 Ideler).[6]

---

2 The collection was first edited by Julius Ludwig Ideler in 1841 in the first volume of his *Physici et medici Graeci minores* (3–80), but the text is in dire need of a thorough revision and re-edition that meets the standards of modern scholarship. See Silvano (2017). A new edition is currently being prepared by Carl-Gustaf Lindqvist of Gothenburg University, the forthcoming of which is still "eagerly awaited", to use the words of Kapetanaki—Sharples (2006: 1 n. 1). For an attempt to outline the collection's complex bibliographical details, see Sharples (1987: 1198–1199); see also Id. (1998), (2004), (2005), (2006). The collection should not be confused with Alexander's three books of φυσικαὶ σχολικαὶ ἀπορίαι καὶ λύσεις, which are authentic and commonly cited in modern literature as Alexander's *Quaestiones*.

3 For the date, see Bertier—Filius (2003: 582). For speculation about the authorship of the *Medical Puzzles*, see Sharples (2005: 53–56), who on the basis of epigraphical evidence attributed the work (and part of the *Supplementary Problems* and the *On Fevers*) to the Commentator's father, whose name was also Alexander and who was also a philosopher.

4 For the place of Ps.-Alexander's work in the history of the Aristotelian *Problems*, see Flashar (1962: 364–367). For recent studies on the Aristotelian *Problems*, see Centrone (2011) and Mayhew (2015); also the new Loeb edition by Mayhew (2011). For further detail on the *Problems*' Q&A style, see the contribution of Mayhew to this volume, also that of Oikonomopoulou.

5 Final causation is rare also in the Aristotelian *Problems*: see Stoyles (2015).

6 Katerina Oikonomopoulou, Luigi Silvano and I are currently collaborating on a paper about the medical and philosophical sources and traditions that Ps.-Alexander relies on in the two

The aim of this contribution is to examine one of the central explanatory—or rather anti-explanatory—concepts Ps.-Alexander expounds in the preface to the first book and which he sporadically employs in addressing specific problems: that is the concept of "unsayable properties" (ἰδιότητες ἄρρητοι: 4.37 Ideler). This concept relies on the author's conviction that for certain natural/medical phenomena the human intellect fails to provide a proper explanation due to the particular nature of the phenomenon at hand. He ascribes this failure to a lack of descriptive resources on the side of the researcher, which in turn is symptomatic of the weakness of human intelligence and discourse more generally. Although put to practice in very specific problem contexts, we will see that Ps.-Alexander's concept of ἰδιότητες ἄρρητοι ties in closely with more meta-physical preconceptions about the world, seen as a divinely organised cosmos. A proper analysis of this concept will therefore provide a better insight into the scientific method employed in the specific problem chapters as well as the worldview propagated in the collection as a whole. As such, this paper aims to contribute to the long overdue study of Ps.-Alexander's work as an important intellectual product from the Roman Empire, showing the potential of Q&A literature to provide unexpected and so far underexploited windows onto wider landscapes, including imperial period intellectual and educational culture, diffusion and repurposing of philosophical material, and the interplay of natural/medical science with theology.

I will first examine how Ps.-Alexander introduces the notion of ἰδιότητες ἄρρητοι in light of the research project set out by him in the first preface ('in theory'). Following this, I will analyse its concrete use and occurrence in the collection of medical-naturalist problems specifically ('in practice'). In conclusion, I will locate the concept in its broader intellectual context at the time ('in context'). According to Karl Deichgräber, we are dealing with "ein Begriff der Kaiserzeitlichen Medizin".[7] However, as we will see, there is reason to assume that the concept of ἰδιότητες ἄρρητοι must have been more generally in use by that time. By analysing and contextualising Ps.-Alexander's concept of ἰδιότητες

prefaces: Oikonomopoulou—Silvano—Meeusen (forthcoming). The paper will also include an English translation and critical edition of these texts. See also Silvano (2017) for a text-critical study of the *Medical Puzzles*; Silvano (2018a) for an edition and Italian translation of the first preface; Silvano (2018b) for a study of *Med. Puzz.* 1.66 with a new edition of the text (on putrefying effects of the moon on meat); Meeusen (2018) for a study of the educational purport of the first preface; and Meeusen (2019) for the collection's paradoxographical backdrop. Numerous parallels can be traced in the *Hippocratic Problems*: see Jouanna—Guardasole (2017: XXI–III).

7 Deichgräber (1957: 38).

ἄρρητοι, this study aims to shed a light on the ancient debate about what medical physicians were expected to know and what was knowable to them. This question is important, as it reflects on the epistemic limits of ancient medical-naturalist research as conceived by its own practitioners, thus giving a concrete idea of what kind of questions they found difficult to solve.

2 Unsayable Properties 'in Theory'

Scholars agree that the importance of the preface to the first book of Ps.-Alexander's *Medical Puzzles* for the history of the Aristotelian *Natural Problems* is undeniable.[8] The text is, indeed, very seminal for interpreting the scientific method and educational purpose of this genre of writing. It has a clear protreptic function as it intends to instruct the reader—who is identified as a medical student (διδασκόμενον: 5.35 Ideler) at the very end—about the proper method and procedures of 'problematic' research. By setting out the classificatory and methodological standards for this kind of inquiry, the author, thus, aims to regulate the reader's reception of the work.[9]

The argument in the preface is twofold and can be paraphrased as follows. First (and this constitutes the bulk of the text), Ps.-Alexander provides a classification of several kinds of problems based on criteria of difficulty and solubility, emphasizing the intermediate nature of the problems he is interested in. (1) He first makes a basic distinction between problems that are soluble and those that are not (3.1–5.16 Ideler; see further). (2) The type of problems that are of interest for further inquiry "have a middle position" (μέσην ἔχοντα χώραν) and are ambiguous to comprehend, meaning that they are situated between those that are "quite clear and understood by everybody" (εὔδηλα πᾶσι γινωσκόμενα) and those that are "altogether obscure and admit no solution" (πάντα κεκρυμμένα λύσιν οὐχ ὑποδεχόμενα) (5.16–24 Ideler). (3) In a final paragraph (5.24–36 Ideler), Ps.-Alexander indicates how such problems can be properly solved and provides a set of terms and principles (κανόσι) that are of general use. By following the proposed method (μεθόδῳ) the student will be able to solve any problem, so it is promised. Ps.-Alexander is aware, however, that an exposition

8 See Flashar (1962: 365) and Garzya—Masullo (2004: 13). For the text's importance in the later history of the Aristotelian *Problems* in Renaissance Europe, see Blair (1999: 174 and 176–177).

9 For the idea that the first preface promotes an 'active reading' of the problem chapters by activating the reader's/student's attentiveness to the strategies that are employed both in raising and in solving such problems, see Meeusen (2018).

of the general method does not suffice, and that the student needs concrete applications, which he gives in the individual problem chapters that follow after the preface.

The first section (1) of the preface is especially important for this study (3.1–5.16 Ideler). Ps.-Alexander opens this section with a discussion about which kind of questions are soluble (3.1–4.1 Ideler), or to be more precise which are "immediately certain and comprehensible (πιστὰ καὶ γνώριμα), and without the savour of any ambiguity or investigation (πάσης ἀμφιβολίας καὶ ζητήσεως ἄγευστα)". These are of the type of: "Why do birds have feathers?" (this is for the sake of warmth and beauty), or "Why did some animals receive horns, others stings, and still others sharp claws or the like?" (this is for the sake of defence). These problems reveal nature's providential ordering (cf. προῄδει: "nature knows beforehand"), but they do not really trigger any inquiry, since they do not really pose any difficulty, according to Ps.-Alexander. As to the insoluble questions, on the other hand, these are known only to God, who, so Ps.-Alexander notes in a Platonic vein, created the world after the manner of a craftsman (τεχνίτης), who assembles the material bits and pieces to form compound substances (οὐσίαν ὑποστήσαντι), and therefore has detailed causal knowledge of how all the machinery works:

> All those who propose such well-known and obvious problems (γνωστὰ καὶ σαφῆ) clearly have no intelligence (νοῦ), and anyone who doubts whether heat is innate to fire, lacks the sense of touch (ἁπτικῆς αἰσθήσεως). Then again, those who feel doubt, whether nature and a providential reason take care of (λόγος προνοητικὸς προμηθεύεται) the processes of generation and corruption, the order of things, their motion, position, formation, complexions and things closely related to them, should be punished (κολάσεσιν τυγχάνουσιν ἔνοχοι). In fact, these problems are completely insoluble (ἄλυτα) and comprehensible only to God (θεῷ μόνῳ γνώριμα), who also gave substance (οὐσίαν ὑποστήσαντι) to these things. After all, a craftsman (τεχνίτης), after constructing a mechanical device, knows all the causes of its actions, whereas a layman (ἰδιώτης) is completely bereft of causal insight.
>
> 4.1–11 IDELER

Ps.-Alexander's point is straightforward: he *a priori* accepts that there must be a providential ordering of the cosmos, the functioning of which should not be questioned. In fact, those who do feel doubt should be punished (κολάσεσιν τυγχάνουσιν ἔνοχοι)—presumably for reasons of godlessness (as I have shown elsewhere, Ps.-Alexander is here alluding to Aristotle's discussion of which topics of investigation are unsuitable for debate, as treated in the *Topics*).[10] The idea, moreover, that these problems are known only to God implies that their cause cannot be grasped by our human intellect. Therefore, such insoluble questions go beyond the epistemic range of the medical-naturalist research project Ps.-Alexander has in mind.

An extensive list of "insoluble questions" (ἄποροι ζητήσεις) follows to illustrate this point (4.12–35 Ideler): for instance, "Why do people laugh when one tickles their arm-pits, soles or sides?", "Why does the magnet only attract iron, and is it brought to life by the iron filings, or why does the so-called amber stone only draw up grains and straws when conjoined to them?" etc. These unexplainable, and indeed paradoxographical, phenomena are called "unsayable properties" (ἰδιότητες ἄρρητοι) by doctors, so Ps.-Alexander says.[11] They are—and this is important for later—"known only by experience" (πείρᾳ μόνον γινωσκομένων), which means that they can be apprehended empirically but cannot be explained in scientific parlance. Notably, the list of "insoluble questions" also includes the unexplainable working of a number of simple drugs (e.g., purgatives). Certain therapeutic data were, indeed, empirical and at the same time considered unknowable, because the doctors and philosophers could not entirely account for them in terms of their constitutive elements and sensible qualities. Some substances (e.g., medicines, foodstuffs, antidotes, amulets etc.) were held to work partly because of their material constituents but also partly because of their "unsayable properties" (ἰδιότητες ἄρρητοι) as Ps.-Alexander calls them, that is, (material) properties deemed beyond description.[12]

---

10 Think of the Epicureans or other atomists, such as the medical scientist Asclepiades of Bithynia (fl. 1st half of the 1st century BCE), who held that the world is the result of material and fortuitous factors only ("the processes of generation and corruption, the order of things, their motion, position, formation, complexions and things closely related to them" does sound like someone talking about the basics of atomism). Ps.-Alexander's point runs parallel to Aristotle's discussion of which topics of investigation are unsuitable for debate in *Topics* 1.11.105a3–9: see Meeusen (2018: 98–99). An example of questions which, according to Aristotle, require κόλασις is whether or not the Gods should be honoured (or parents loved). Flashar (1962: 365) interprets κόλασις in Ps.-Alexander's text in relation to the phrasing of the problems themselves, some of which would require correction ("Korrektur in ihrer Fragestellung"), but as the passage from Aristotle's *Topics* shows, it are rather the people/students who ask such 'tabooed' questions that require "Korrektur".

11 For a study of the paradoxographical backdrop of Ps.-Alexander's *Medical Puzzles*, see Meeusen (2019), where I discuss a number of parallels in the literature.

12 These are the occult properties (the *qualitates occultae*) of medieval physicians that pertained to a brand of magical thought that remained influential well until the Scientific Revolution. See Röhr (1923: 96–106) and Copenhaver (1991: esp. 380–381 on Ps.-Alexander and Galen). Also Meeusen (2019: 210 n. 30). Cf. Mareri in this volume, n. 4.

> I could present to you a catalogue of thousands of such phenomena that are known only by experience (πείρᾳ μόνον γινωσκομένων), which amongst physicians are called 'unsayable properties' (παρὰ τοῖς ἰατροῖς ἰδιότητες ἄρρητοι λέγονται): for when the peculiar character (ἴδιον) of each of these phenomena is presented it is un-sayable (ἄῤῥητον) so far as an explanation of the causes is concerned. Some people do offer a flood of solutions for those problems, albeit in a bad way, and the solutions are unsuitable and implausible (ἀσυμφόρους δὲ καὶ ἀπιθάνους).
>
> 4.35–5.3 IDELER

As I will detail later on, the ἰδιότητες ἄρρητοι are unsayable probably because they are unique to the thing they are a property of, meaning that they are singular entities. And it is precisely for that reason that these properties cannot be put into words, since language is based on generality. As such, the notion of ἰδιότητες ἄρρητοι relates to the more common philosophical idea that we can only think and speak by means of generality, and that individuality is beyond utterance (*individuum est ineffabile*).[13]

Two further points are important in this regard. First, the fact that Ps.-Alexander emphasises that these phenomena are called ἰδιότητες ἄρρητοι amongst *physicians* (plural) seems to imply that we are dealing with a concept that must have been relatively popular in medical milieus. As we will see later on, clear parallels can, indeed, be drawn with contemporary medical literature, especially the *corpus Galenicum*. However, the concept must have been popular also in other fields, since Ps.-Alexander adds, in what follows:

> There are properties (ἰδιώματα) not only among the physicians alone (παρὰ τοῖς ἰατροῖς [...] μόνοις), but also among the philosophers (φιλοσόφοις) and grammarians (γραμματικοῖς), where they are called modifications in form (πάθη λεγόμενα) and noted as exceptions by their use (σεσημειωμένα ταῖς χρήσεσι).
>
> 5.13–16 IDELER

What matters here is that the notion of ἰδιότητες ἄρρητοι must have been more generally in use in Ps.-Alexander's days to denote an aspect of unaccountable particularity, not only in medical, but also in philosophical and grammatical contexts (I will come back to this passage later).

13 See, e.g., Pieper (1973: 729–731), and more generally Franke (2007) and (2014).

Second, the fact that Ps.-Alexander notes that "some people do offer a flood of solutions for those (insoluble) problems" indicates that whether a property is strictly unsayable or not is, in fact, open to debate. Although Ps.-Alexander forcefully opposes those who advocate accountability in such cases, the implication is that consensus is not necessarily self-evident. He gives the following example to support his case:

> People claim that purgatives that are very hot draw up the humours, but this is false (ψεῦδος), because, in that case, anything hot would also necessarily have to be purgative [*quod non*]. So the pepper, although it is hot, is not fit for drawing up humours, but is digestive and strengthening. The same is true for mastics and bitter aloes. We are saying that the terms are not convertible (φαμὲν δὲ μὴ ἀντιστρέφειν τὸν λόγον), since everything purgative is, indeed, hot in its composition and depletive in its power. But everything that is hot does not also have a purgative power. They say that the ostrich concocts iron not by means of some property (ἰδιότητί τινι), but rather by heat, which is absurd. For the lion, which has a hotter temperament than that animal, does not concoct iron.
>
> 5.4–13 IDELER

In what follows, I will examine how Ps.-Alexander's theory of ἰδιότητες ἄρρητοι, as expounded in the first preface, works out 'in practice', by exploring its precise role in the individual problem chapters collected in the *Medical Puzzles*. Ps.-Alexander notes at the end of the preface that these problems serve as examples (κατὰ μέρος: 5.35 Ideler) for the aetiological programme he has just set out, so it is worthwhile to examine how his use of the concept in these individual problem chapters squares—or does not square—with the situation sketched 'in theory'. What will be of specific concern is how consistent Ps.-Alexander's application of the concept of unsayable properties really is when theory is put to practice. Three further questions are in place. These can be summarised as follows, and will be answered by means of specific case-studies in the next section:

1. How does the unsayability of properties relate to the insolubility of problems?
2. Are properties necessarily unsayable in each and every case?
3. How definite are Ps.-Alexander's claims towards properties being unsayable?

3 Unsayable Properties 'in Practice'

Strictly speaking, the kind of problems that involve ἰδιότητες ἄρρητοι fall outside the scope of Ps.-Alexander's research project. After all, by being insoluble, these problems have no "middle position" (μέσην […] χώραν, see above), which is why they are not of interest for further inquiry. This probably explains the concept's relative paucity throughout the collection. Still, there are some occasions where Ps.-Alexander, in dealing with difficult questions, puts the concept of ἰδιότητες ἄρρητοι to work as an explanatory principle. Let us take a closer look at how consistent this is with the theory set out in the preface.

3.1 *How Does the Unsayability of Properties Relate to the Insolubility of Problems?*

The fact that Ps.-Alexander does not, as he does elsewhere, offer a practical solution to some problems may suggest that he has none. Unsayability plays an important role here. This is the case most notably in *Med. Puzz.* 2.67 (74.35–76.25 Ideler), where Ps.-Alexander—in the margin of another problem which examines why oil does not mix with other liquids—deals with the mind-body problem, that is, the problem of how the physical body and the non-physical mind interconnect (75.15–76.17 Ideler). In expounding his argument, Ps.-Alexander finds much of his inspiration in Galenic pneumatology.[14] We read that the soul-body connection is realised by breath (πνεῦμα) formed from the blood. Blood is boiled in the liver and forms vaporous breath (πνεῦμα ἀτμοειδές), which is conveyed, together with the blood, through the *vena cava* towards the heart, where it is heated even more and rarefied, thus becoming airy (ἀεροειδές). This airy breath is again lifted through the carotid arteries towards the base of the brain being guided there, so we read, "in accordance with natural providence" (κατὰ πρόνοιαν φύσεως), where it throws off its immoderate boiling by the coldness of the brain "in accordance with some natural property" (κατ' ἰδιότητά τινα φυσικήν). The breath thus becomes like ether (αἰθεροειδές), which is instrumental to the soul's activity (ὅπερ ὄργανόν ἐστι ψυχῆς πρὸς ἐνέργειαν). The puzzle here—which the invocation of a natural property (ἰδιότητά τινα φυσικήν) is needed to explain—seems to be how it comes that the brain has a refrigerating property which changes airlike into etherlike breath (i.e., how contact with something cold, the brain, and consequent cooling down from 'immoderate boiling' can cause the change in state from less refined and volatile airlike

14 As pointed out by Debru (2008: 272), "one should not represent Galen's *pneuma* doctrine in the form of a tripartite pneumatology, hierarchized and dogmatic, which was a doctrine of later Galenism, and not of Galen himself".

breath to more refined and volatile etherlike breath—one might have thought that increased heat, not decreased heat, was needed to prompt the change from airlikeness to etherlikeness). The point probably is that, of all bodily organs, only the brain has this natural property and that this is part of our providential anatomical design (or, alternatively, that the breath moves and changes in the body according to some unspecifiable design and that the brain plays a particular role in the final stage of this process).

From a scientific point of view, the reference to the working of natural providence (κατὰ πρόνοιαν φύσεως) and to some undefined natural property (κατ' ἰδιότητά τινα φυσικήν)[15] in the movement and change of the breath on becoming ethereal and organic to the soul's activity results in an unsatisfactory non-explanation (at least the explanation remains rather vague). Ps.-Alexander does not—indeed, probably does not wish to—clarify this puzzle any further (i.e., the brain's natural property in effecting the mind-body connection through etherisation of airlike breath as part of some providential design). After all, so we know from the preface, no questions should be raised regarding the working of natural providence in the world of contingent natural phenomena (those who do raise such questions should be punished, see n. 10). This probably explains why the reference to the working of some natural property in the problem at issue remains rather vague. It may well suggest that Ps.-Alexander is not very certain of what is exactly happening in the physical/physiological process under examination. At any rate, the fact that he does not put it into words, implies that the natural property at issue is, indeed, of the unsayable type, as is also shown in what follows, where Ps.-Alexander goes on to draw an analogy between the change in the breath and the breaking of horses: "just as a wild horse is tamed by the bit, so the breath is guided with bit and bridle by some unsayable natural faculty (ὑπό τινος ἀρρήτου φυσικῆς δυνάμεως)". By stating that this process occurs under influence of "some unsayable natural faculty" Ps.-Alexander indicates that its efficient cause eventually remains beyond the range of words, or at least beyond the limits of his own scientific discourse and understanding. From the end of the chapter we learn that this aetiological reticence is religiously motivated. The efficient cause looked for is

15 These two phrases may imply basically the same, in that the coldness of the brain may be a result of divine providence itself. At any rate, the syntactical construction runs very parallel in both cases (κατά + acc.). The working of natural providence in the human body recurs in *Med. Puzz.* 1.12 (8.32 Ideler: ἡ προνοουμένη τοῦ σώματος δύναμις), 1.43 (15.33 Ideler: τὴν φύσιν μὲν προνοουμένην τοῦ λοιποῦ σώματος), 1.107 (36.19–20 Ideler: ἡ φύσις ἀεὶ προνοουμένη τούτου τοῦ σώματος), 2.12 (57.25 Ideler: δύναμις προνοητική), 2.47 (65.37–66.1 Ideler: τὴν γένεσιν κατὰ πρόνοιαν φύσεως).

none other than the hand of God: in dealing with the round shape of the head resembling the structure of the heavens (καθάπερ μικρὸν οὐρανόν) Ps.-Alexander emphatically speaks of "*another* work of God" (ἕτερον ἔργον θεοῦ). The idea that we are dealing here with a kind of knowledge that belongs to the cosmic creator/τεχνίτης ties in closely with the Platonic cosmological framework sketched in the first preface,[16] thus nicely illustrating that Ps.-Alexander's understanding of the mind-body problem—and his scientific enterprise more generally—is demarcated by an essentially theological framework: in a very literal sense, God knows what's going on.

3.2 *Are Properties Necessarily Unsayable in Each and Every Case?*

To ask whether some property is unsayable or not is different from asking whether each property is strictly unsayable. This does not always seem to be the case, although the situation is not always clear. An interesting case is found in *Med. Puzz.* 2.72 (78.22–79.7 Ideler), where Ps.-Alexander examines why the nerves, although sent forth from the brain and the spinal marrow to the body parts, do not all have the same activity (ἐνέργεια) but a different one. He explains that the activity of the nerves differs not only depending on their connection (συνουσίαν) with the body parts, but also on their constitution and formation (κατασκευὴ καὶ διάπλασις), which is different from nerve to nerve: for instance, the optic nerve is pierced, the acoustic nerve more stretched, the one for taste even more so, that of the mouth of the stomach is swathed, and that of the stomach is expanded spherically. He draws a comparison with the cords on a lyre and the pitch that they produce, and then generalises the phenomenon to the other organs in the body (καὶ ἐπὶ τῶν λοιπῶν δὲ ὀργάνων τὸ αὐτὸ θεωρήσεις, ἥπατος καὶ σπληνός). For instance, the porous flesh in the kidneys and the heart, which is called παρέγχυμα ("poured filling"), is "some property/peculiar kind of flesh" (σαρκός τις ἰδιότης).[17] This is not further specified, but what Ps.-Alexander probably means is that this kind of flesh is proper to the kidneys and heart and supports these organs in fulfilling their specific function in the

---

16 The idea that the round shape of the head resembles the heavenly sphere is also Platonic (cf. *Ti.* 44d). See Sharples (2005: 55).

17 LSJ, s.v. παρέγχυμα: "anything poured in beside, name given by Erasistratus to the peculiar substance of the lungs, liver, kidneys, and spleen, as if formed separately by the veins that run into them, the word σάρξ being used of the muscular flesh". The text is odd at this point, an alternative translation is: "in the case of liver and spleen, there is porous flesh, the kind which is actually called παρέγχυμα, and in the case of kidneys and heart, a distinctive kind of flesh". Based on the parallel in Galen discussed below (where παρέγχυμα is used in reference to the flesh of the liver) this may be a more plausible reading, but whatever the case may be, the main idea is the same.

body (see further). In the stomach, to give another example, the sinews that are straight pull, and those that are transverse push, whereas in other parts the oblique ones restrain, as in the womb. The veins, arteries and membranes, so Ps.-Alexander concludes, which are common (κοινὰ ὄντα) and found in all body parts, offer a measure of usefulness (χρείας λόγον ἐπέχουσι) to each of them. "But their characteristic property is also (i.e., just as the ἰδιότης of the flesh of the kidneys and heart) uncommunicable,[18] which also attributes supreme authority to their activity" (τὸ δὲ ἴδιον καὶ ἀκοινώνητόν ἐστιν, ὃ καὶ ποιεῖ κυρίως τὴν ἐνέργειαν).

The point that Ps.-Alexander is trying to make in this problem—viz. that the constitution of the nerves and by extension that of other parts in the body is subservient to their function—is very much in line with Galen's functional explanation of human anatomy (as known, e.g., from his *On the Use of the Parts*).[19] According to Galen, the parts of the body are adapted to the performance of the organism's activities (and not the other way around), which is indeed very much in line with what Ps.-Alexander is arguing in the problem at hand, where he underlines that the proper anatomical constitution of body parts (esp. of the nerves) follows their specific bodily function.

An interesting—albeit contrastive—parallel is found in Galen, *PHP* 6.8.21–25 (5.568–570 Kühn; 412.2–23 De Lacy). After noting that some physicians call the flesh of the liver παρέγχυμα (the same word as in Ps.-Alexander: see n. 17), Galen continues that each organ has its own specific substance (οὐσία) from which it acquires an activity distinct from the rest (basically the same idea as in Ps.-Alexander). However, whereas according to Galen the nerves have a *common* form (τὸ κοινόν) and thus a *common* use just like other homoiomerous parts (such as vein, artery, bone, cartilage, membrane, ligament, and fat), Ps.-Alexander emphatically rejects this for the νεῦρα, underlining the anatomical differences in the different types of nerves and the different functions based on them (he makes no further distinctions between veins, arteries and membranes though).[20] The passage in Galen runs as follows (tr. De Lacy; adapted):

---

18 I am taking ἀκοινώνητος here as synonymous with ἄρρητος. See LSJ, s.v. ἀκοινώνητος, i.2: "not to be communicated, [...] not to be shared, incommunicable [...]"—referencing this specific passage in Ps.-Alexander. However, if the opposition is not between sayability/unsayability but between individual/shared properties (cf. the parallel in Galen below), the meaning is rather: "But the individual property of each, which is what actually makes its operation what it is, is not shared with any other" (see LSJ, ibid., i.1: "not shared with, [...] not shared in common with"). Both options do not necessarily exclude one another, since arguably these properties are so individual/distinctive that they cannot be communicated (cf. *individuum est ineffabile*).

19 See Schiefsky (2007).

20 Ps.-Alexander's inconsistency with Galen in this problem does not seem to be out of tune

> For each of the organic parts of the animal, being compounded from other simpler parts, is an entirely unique thing (πάντως ἕν γέ τι), with a substance (οὐσίαν) such as no other organ possesses in the whole body of the animal. Thus the property (τὸ ἴδιον) of the body of the stomach is like none of the rest, and the same is true of the spleen, brain, kidneys, tongue, eyes, bladders, and uterus. Now arteries and nerves and veins are implanted in the organs for a common use (ἕνεκα χρείας κοινῆς), and membranes and ligaments also in some of them; but apart from these each body has its own proper (ἴδιον) character from which it acquires an activity (ἐνέργειαν) distinct from the rest. Where there is a common form (τὸ κοινόν), there must of course be a common activity (τὴν ἐνέργειαν εἶναι κοινήν); for the activity of vein or artery or nerve cannot be different in different places in the body. Whether you observe (ἐννοήσῃς) an artery in the heel or in the brain, you will immediately observe (συνεπινοήσεις) along with it also the activity common (κοινὴν […] ἐνέργειαν) to all arteries. The same is true of nerve, vein, bone, cartilage, membrane, ligament, and fat. But to the extent that each substance has its own proper form (ἴδιον εἶδος), it must also have its own proper activity (ἰδίαν […] ἐνέργειαν). The body of the lung has a substance (οὐσίαν) of a kind that you would not find in any other body, and you would find no other like the brain, just as there is also none whose substance is of exactly the same description as that of the heart or kidneys or spleen. Each of them is like no other, and therefore each has its proper activity in addition to its proper substance (ἡ ἐνέργεια καθ' ἕκαστον ἴδιος ἐπὶ τῷ τῆς οὐσίας ἰδίῳ); and so with any flesh that is markedly different in property (ἰδιότητα) from the rest.

As is well known, Galen repeatedly advocates a Demiurgic design of the human body to support his functional view of human anatomy. In so doing he assumes the work of a divine craftsman exerting providence on behalf of living things. Ps.-Alexander also subscribes to this philosophy, but whether this is why he, at-

(*mutatis mutandis*) with the critical attitude of Alexander of Damascus during Galen's dissection of the recurrent laryngeal nerves of a pig described in *On Prognosis*: see the Appendix (with a discussion of the potential identification of the two Alexanders). Ps.-Alexander is more consistent with Galen in a different context in *Med. Puzz.* 2.60: "know that for some parts the (natural) faculty is equal in degree, as is the case for nerves, veins, and bones, in which the activity is one and the same" (70.32–35 Ideler: γίνωσκε δὲ ὡς ἐπί τινων μὲν μορίων ὁμότιμον ἔχουσι τὴν δύναμιν· ὡς ἐπὶ νεύρου καὶ φλεβὸς καὶ ὀστέου, ἐν οἷς μορίοις ἡ ἐνέργεια, ἰδία μόνου ἦν).

the end of the chapter (*Med. Puzz.* 2.72), does not provide any further specification for the "uncommunicable" (ἀκοινώνητόν) character of the "characteristic property" (ἴδιον) of veins, arteries and membranes (or the "peculiar property", ἰδιότης, of the flesh of the kidneys and heart mentioned earlier) is not clear. Considering the Galenic context, this property may very well be accounted for by the working of divine providence, indeed, (which is in line with what we saw previously, sub 3.1) but this remains unspecified.

Bearing in mind the link with Galen's functional view of human anatomy, the least that can be said is that the "characteristic/peculiar property" (ἴδιον/ἰδιότης) of arteries, veins, membranes and certain types of fleshes (and by extension of the different types of nerves), indicates that their constitution is 'proper' in such a way as to fulfil a specific function in the body (or to support the organs which they constitute in doing so). This means that the 'proper' constitution of the arteries, veins, membranes, and fleshes (and nerves) has its own distinct nature by which they are adapted to their precise bodily function (or to that of the organs which they constitute). This certainly underlines the unique/exceptional property of the types of constitutions at issue, but it does not necessarily follow that these properties are, therefore, strictly 'unsayable'. In fact, Ps.-Alexander says of the flesh of the kidneys and of the heart that it is "porous" (στοιβοειδής) and that it is called "poured filling" (παρέγχυμα: see n. 17), thus demonstrating that their ἰδιότης is not strictly non-conceptual—yet to describe this ἰδιότης in its entirety would be impossible, and this is probably why it is 'uncommunicable' (ἀκοινώνητόν) for Ps.-Alexander.

A similar case is found in *Med. Puzz.* 1.88 (29.32–30.20 Ideler), where Ps.-Alexander examines why some people with a pestilential condition die when an epidemic breaks out whereas others do not. He suggests that this is "due to their peculiar bodily mixture" (ὅτι παρὰ τὴν ἰδιότητα τῆς κράσεως;). This refers to the specific physiological state, namely the particular humoural blend (κρᾶσις) present in a patient. A distinction is made between people who have "a body full and afflicted by bad humours" (τὸ σῶμα μεστὸν [καὶ] κακόχυμον) and people with a body "free from superfluity and blessed with good humours" (ἀπέριττον καὶ εὔχυμον). Ps.-Alexander explains that the former die when they inhale putrefactive air (σηπεδονώδης ἀήρ), since it corrupts whatever minute wholesome constituent there may be in their body, whereas the latter survive, since the inhaled air causes no or only little harm in them. In this case, the "property" (ἰδιότητα) is attributed to a specific bodily mixture (κρᾶσις), which can be either κακόχυμος or εὔχυμος (i.e., bad- or good-humoured), and for that precise reason is, again, not strictly 'unsayable'. However, if there is anything 'unsayable' about the property of the bodily constitution in pestilential people, it has to do with the logical follow-up question: what is it that makes this specific humoural blend causes some people to die but others to survive? Ps.-Alexander does not, however, pursue this question.[21]

In *Med. Puzz.* 2.59 (69.17–70.5 Ideler), finally, Ps.-Alexander examines why we draw up wine or other types of liquid by sucking a straw. He explains that it are not the lips that draw up the liquid, but the force of the void (ἡ βία τοῦ κενοῦ). When the air is sucked out from the straw, the liquid necessarily follows. Ps.-Alexander draws an analogy with several medical instruments, such as catheters, medicine-droppers, and cupping-glasses, which also work according to the same principle, that is, the principle of *horror vacui* (ἀπειλῇ τοῦ κενοῦ: "by the threat of the void"). In the case of the catheter, so Ps.-Alexander argues, the wool put in it draws up breath, which in turn, by the threat of the void, draws up urine. Whereas the fire put in a cupping-glass diffuses the air in it, thus rendering the air thin and leaving the cupping-glass empty. When, subsequently, the cupping-glass is applied to the body, the fire is quenched, and an empty place remains, the instrument necessarily draws up blood by the threat of the void. Ps.-Alexander concludes that all things that have an attractive power operate in this way, as in the case of these medical tools. They do not draw up by the effect of heat, nor by the sucking power of the mouth (as the catheter shows neither of these is operative). Rather, so Ps.-Alexander notes in what seems to be a general round-up, drawing up is caused by heat (as in the case of smearing on Thapsia), by the strong drawing up the weak, and by a "property" (ἰδιότητι), as in the case of iron being attracted by magnets and blood by the body parts. That we are probably dealing here with an 'unsayable property', is suggested by the fact that magnetic attraction is listed among the ἄποροι ζητήσεις in the first preface. Whether the principle of 'the threat of the void' (operative in straws and medical instruments) also belongs to this category of 'properties' remains unspecified but may very well be implied, as it would otherwise fall *hors catégorie*.

3.3 *How Definite Are Ps.-Alexander's Claims towards Properties Being Unsayable?*

As the evidence shows, there is room for debate in determining whether some problematic phenomenon involves an unsayable property or not. This is the case where Ps.-Alexander provides alternative answers to allegedly insoluble problems. It had already been suggested in the first preface that disagreement

21 Similarly, in *Med. Puzz.* 2.66 (74.11–34 Ideler), Ps.-Alexander highlights the property (ἰδιότητα) of bread and wine, amongst all foodstuffs, in relation to their nourishing and strengthening abilities when given in due proportion. This seems to indicate the particular nutritive character of these foodstuffs for the ill but is not explained further.

is, indeed, possible in such cases, but, as we will see here, Ps.-Alexander's critical position seems much more forceful 'in theory' than it is 'in practice'. Two passages can support this point.

First, in *Med. Puzz.* 1.52 (18.17–25 Ideler), Ps.-Alexander examines why many people digest foodstuffs that are actually difficult to digest and have thick humours (such as beef) more easily, whereas they cannot digest foodstuffs that are actually easy to digest and have good humours (such as rock-fish).[22] He explains that some say that this is "due to habit" (δι' ἔθος), others that it is "due to some unsayable and unexplainable natural condition" (διά τινα ἕξιν φυσικὴν ἄρρητον καὶ ἀναιτιολόγητον), and yet others that it is "due to immoderate heat in the abdomen" (δι' ἄμετρον θερμότητα κοιλίας). Only the last explanation is elaborated in further detail. Ps.-Alexander explains that easily digestible foodstuffs digest very quickly because they are easily changed and are boiled and destroyed by the heavy heat, whereas those that are difficult to digest and to alter do not undergo much change and are only concocted (compare, for instance, chaff which burns to ashes by a larger fire because it is easily affected, whereas oak-wood does not undergo this when burned). Interestingly, the contrast with Ps.-Alexander's opposite claim in the first preface that the ostrich concocts iron not by heat but rather by some property (ἰδιότητί τινι) is striking. That there is indeed room for debate in such peculiar cases is shown by the problem at hand.

Similarly, in *Med. Puzz.* 2.74 (79.29–80.7 Ideler), Ps.-Alexander examines why the season of autumn has an irregular climate with heat and cold during the same day. We read that "some say that this season has such a bad nature, in itself simply unsayable" (τινές φασι φύσιν ἔχειν τοιαύτην αὐτὸ ἄρρητον μοχθηράν). This seems to imply that they do not actually have any clue as to what causes this climatic irregularity.[23] A number of explanations follows: Ps.-Alexander writes that some natural philosophers (τινὲς δὲ τῶν φυσικῶν) say that it is due to the sun, which moves the Zodiacal belt and, thus, turns the earth. Others say that it is at that exact time (viz. in autumn) that irregular and changing winds blow. Yet others ascribe it to the fact that the earth turns cold, after being scorched by the immoderate heat of the summer sun, and releases a fresh breeze, while

22 Ideler's edition suffers from a lacuna, see Silvano (2017: 24–26), with further discussion. A parallel problem is treated in *Med. Puzz.* 2.17 (58.32–59.5 Ideler). Cf. also *Suppl. Pr.* 1.6 (98.9–100.4 Kapetanaki—Sharples), with the commentary ad loc. of Kapetanaki—Sharples (2006: 99 n. 176).

23 Conversely, ἄρρητον can also imply "horrible" here (and understandably so), but even so no further explanation is provided. See LSJ, s.v. ἄρρητος, iii.2. One wonders whether μοχθηράν is a (not completely appropriate) gloss on τοιαύτην.

the air is still hot. As to those who say that autumn is the intermediary period between summer and winter and, thus, takes part in the climate of both opposites, Ps.-Alexander is straightforward in saying that they are in error (ψεύδονται), because this counts no less for spring also. With this, however, he does not give the impression that he aims to discard the other options or to diminish their plausibility, so they remain standing.

3.4 *Intermediate Conclusion*

From the above case-studies it appears that the theory of unsayable properties is put to practice in a fairly consistent way in the individual problem chapters. The three questions raised earlier on can be answered, in summary, as follows:

1. *How does the unsayability of properties relate to the insolubility of problems?*—When the working of divine providence comes into sight, any attempt at further explanation is abandoned. It is at that point that Ps.-Alexander's scientific discourse fails him.
2. *Are properties necessarily unsayable in each and every case?*—No, properties primarily indicate particularity but they do not appear to be strictly unsayable in each and every case. At least, they are not strictly non-conceptual, since they can be named (e.g., the concept of παρέγχυμα: see n. 17).
3. *How definite are the claims towards properties being unsayable?*—These claims are not always definite, but this was already suggested by the preface, although Ps.-Alexander takes a more critical position there.

Let us now, take a closer look at the broader intellectual context of Ps.-Alexander's notion of unsayable properties. What may be the origin of this concept? In which other ancient authors and con/texts does it occur? And what does this tell us about the broader intellectual backdrop of Ps.-Alexander's *Medical Puzzles*?

4 Unsayable Properties 'in Context'

As we saw earlier on, Ps.-Alexander attributes the concept of unsayable properties to physicians in general (παρὰ τοῖς ἰατροῖς). Amongst these physicians, Galen takes first rank, who mentions ἰδιότητες ἄρρητοι throughout his oeuvre, especially in his writings on the pulse. As Reinhardt has shown, the concept relates to Galen's philosophy of perception more generally, where it is based on an awareness that the capability of our senses to perceive an object or state of affairs in full detail far outruns the ability of the mind to conceptualise it, because the impression is much too detailed.[24] Our senses are capable of clearly perceiving an object or state of affairs under normal circumstances (e.g., a patient's pulse, by means of haptic experience), but because its features are so detailed we are unable to capture them fully with our words. Notably, the same empirical aspect is highlighted by Ps.-Alexander in the first preface, when he says that unsayable properties are "known only by experience" (πείρᾳ μόνον γινωσκομένων). This implies, as we saw, that such properties can be captured by our senses (i.e., they are empirically apprehensible) but cannot be explained in scientific parlance, due to a cognitive lack of descriptive resources.

Unsayable properties are mainly properties of the objects or states of affairs that are perceived, but Galen at times implies that what is unsayable is, in fact, the experience of the perceiving subject itself. For instance, patients can feel and locate the sensation of pain in their body, but they often fail to communicate about it in clear terms. This creates problems for the doctor to make a proper diagnosis and to suggest a specific treatment for the patient, as well as to write about it in a medical textbook—a topic which Galen discusses at length in his famous critique of Archigenes of Apamea (1st–2nd century CE) in *On the Affected Parts*.[25] In Ps.-Alexander's case, however, the aspect of medical

24 Reinhardt (2011). According to Deichgräber (1957: 39), the notion of unsayability is also present in other medical authors, but the example that he gives is dubious. Cf. Ruf. Eph., *Sat. Gon.* 4.4 (65.7 Daremberg—Ruelle): ἀσῶνται πάθει τινὶ ἀρρήτῳ (the reference is most probably to "horrible" pain here: cf. n. 23). In pre-Galenic medical literature, the word is attested in the meaning of "that, which may not be expressed/divulged" only in the Hippocratic *Oath* (*Iusiur.* 7 [630.17 Littré; 5.3 Jouanna]), see Gärtner (2015: 793–794). The context is that of the doctor's discretion about what he sees or hears when on or off duty.

25 Esp. *Loc. Aff.* 2.6–9 (8.86.12–120.2 Kühn; 326.1–364.3 Gärtner). The theory, formulated by Deichgräber (1957: 37–38), that Galen became acquainted with the concept of unsayable properties via the Stoic-pneumatic 'school' of medicine—as conceived by Wellmann (1895)—, more precisely via the writings of Archigenes of Apamea, is uncertain. Essential to Deichgräber's argument is his interpretation of the phrase ἄῤῥητός ἐστιν ἡ ἰδιότης πᾶσα καὶ κατ' αὐτούς in Galen, *Loc. Aff.* 2.9 (8.117.6–7 Kühn; 360.16–17 Gärtner; the καὶ is omitted in some mss.). In this passage, Galen is criticising Archigenes for using unclear metaphors in describing specific forms of pain. The meaning of κατ' αὐτούς is seminal. According to Deichgräber (1957: 38), Galen is arguing that the *followers* ("Anhänger") of Archigenes formulate the phrase "Keine (eigentliche) Proprietät kann ausgesagt werden", but the point rather seems to be that "the *patients* cannot express each specific type of pain" (tr. Siegel; my Italics). As such, Galen's point is not of a doxographical but of a diagnostic kind. The passage runs very parallel with the previous *Loc. Aff.* 2.7, where Galen again discusses the difficulty patients have in expressing pain verbally: "it requires a considerable effort or cannot even be communicated verbally" (tr. Siegel; 8.89.2–3 Kühn; 328.8–9 Gärtner: οὐ γὰρ μικρᾶς δυνάμεως τὸ τοιοῦτον, ἢ τῷ μηδ' εἶναι ῥητὸν αὐτό). Cf. also 2.6: "a pain which cannot be expressed in words" (8.86.16 Kühn; 326.4 Gärtner: ὃ μηδὲ ἑρμηνεῦσαι λόγῳ δυνατόν ἐστι). But even so, if we may assume that Ps.-Alexander was familiar with this ambiguous passage

diagnostics is absent, leaving space only for the concept's educational relevance, as being applicable, more precisely, to medical-naturalist research.[26] Ps.-Alexander incorporates the concept in a firm aetiological framework, where unsayability relates to inexplicability.[27] For Ps.-Alexander, the category of the unsayable functions as an explanatory *carte-blanche* when dealing with, what he believes to be, insoluble problems known only to God.

Interestingly, Galen never offers a definition or typology for the concept of unsayable properties, which suggests that his audience did not really need one.[28] That the concept must have been more widely known is, indeed, confirmed by Ps.-Alexander when he says that it was present also in other fields than medicine, viz. among philosophers and grammarians (παρὰ φιλοσόφοις καὶ γραμματικοῖς). Although the notion of ἰδιότητες ἄρρητοι does not as such seem to figure in the grammarians, it does in the philosophers. As Reinhardt argues, there may be reason to assume that the concept originated with the Stoics (but he rightly points at the paucity of the available source evidence).[29] As far as the evidence shows, the Stoics did not have a pronounced theory that, via our perception, we usually receive more information than is conceptually available to us, but they did accept that properties of objects themselves are particular.[30] Hence they are called ἰδιώματα (that is, properties).[31] This is in line

in Galen, he may have misinterpreted the κατ' αὐτούς as referring to Archigenes *cum suis* (after the manner of Deichgräber). In that case, these are probably the physicians implied in his statement (in the preface) that there are unsayable properties παρὰ τοῖς ἰατροῖς, but this is uncertain. By contrast, Gärtner (2015: 798) does not reject Deichgräber's reading but argues that αὐτούς rather refers to πόνων, i.e., the pains (8.117.4 Kühn; 360.15 Gärtner). I believe it actually refers to ἐκείνων, i.e., the patients (8.116.18 Kühn; 360.12 Gärtner), which seems to be a more natural reading, considering the context.

26 See n. 9; Meeusen (2018). At the end of the preface to the second book, Ps.-Alexander emphasises the aspect of theoretical education *vis-à-vis* practical application of the problems (53.11–16 Ideler): "And so many problems have we treated (διειλήφαμεν) for the sake of thinking (διάνοιαν) but not for the usefulness (χρείαν) of inquiries, having gathered only a few sections from these. This should suffice for those who pursue this endeavour and especially for those who intend to train their theoretical insight (τοῖς τὸν λόγον ἀσκοῦσι). They provide no little benefit also for the discovery of things (τὴν τῶν πραγμάτων εὕρεσιν)."

27 Cf., e.g., *Med. Puzz.* 1.52 (18.19 Ideler): ἄρρητον καὶ ἀναιτιολόγητον (this is in the problem about digestion of foodstuffs discussed above).

28 Reinhardt (2011: 301).

29 Reinhardt (2011: 301), following Frede (1987: 161–162). Cf. n. 25. Also according to Aristotle (not to mention Plato), knowledge of particulars (as opposed to universals) is impossible, see Leszl (1972/3) and Adamson (2005).

30 See, e.g., Cic., *Acad.* 2.56 (538.10 Rackham; tr. Rackham): the Stoics hold that "particular objects possess particular properties" (*singularum rerum singulas proprietates esse*).

31 See, e.g., Sext. Emp., *Adv. Math.* 7.248 (58.16–19 Mutschmann; tr. Bett, adapted): "For since

with Ps.-Alexander's statement (also quoted above) that: "There are *properties* (ἰδιώματα) not only in the physicians alone, but also in the philosophers and grammarians [...]".

As to the grammarians, in what directly follows, Ps.-Alexander adds that "[...] they (sc. the properties) are called modifications in form (πάθη λεγόμενα) and noted as exceptions by their use (σεσημειωμένα ταῖς χρήσεσι)". I take it that this phrase strictly relates to the grammatical backdrop of the notion of unsayable properties and *not* also to its use among philosophers (although this is not impossible syntactically speaking). In any case, the concepts of πάθη ('modifications in form') and σεσημειωμένα ('notable exceptions') are relatively common in grammatical writings, where they usually denote what are claimed to be peculiar linguistic phenomena. The notion of πάθος refers to the modification in word form, especially in dialectical morphology.[32] For instance, in *Poetics* 25 Aristotle uses the phrase "modifications of language" (1460b12: πάθη τῆς λέξεως) in reference to poetic idiom. The point is that the poet uses artificial language that does not reflect normal usage, a fact that cannot be held against him, but that does reflect the peculiarity of his language.[33] On the other hand, the participle perfect σεσημειωμένον (deriving from the *nomen actionis* σημειόω, 'to mark') is commonly used in reference to grammatical phenomena that are 'noted as exceptions', for instance, apparent exceptions in accentuation (Choerob., *in Theod.* 451g.25–26 [1.405.11–12 Hilgard]).[34] Due to their alleged peculiarity, such grammatical phenomena are considered exceptional (that is, deviant from common grammatical rules and norms), which makes them a suitable parallel for Ps.-Alexander's concept of unsayable properties, indeed. But at the same time, by invoking the philosophical and grammatical backdrop Ps.-Alexander shows his wider acquaintance with the conceptual framework of intellectual fields other than medicine and natural science, thus enhancing his role as a teacher educating a student.

---

they [sc. the Stoics] trust this appearance to be capable of perfectly grasping the underlying things, and to be skilfully stamped with all the properties attaching to them, they say that it has each of these as an attribute" (ἄκρως γὰρ πιστούμενοι ἀντιληπτικὴν εἶναι τῶν ὑποκειμένων τήνδε τὴν φαντασίαν καὶ πάντα τεχνικῶς τὰ περὶ αὐτοῖς ἰδιώματα ἀναμεμαγμένην, ἕκαστον τούτων φασὶν ἔχειν συμβεβηκός).

32 LSJ, s.v. πάθος, iv.1.

33 *Poetics* 25 is the chapter on "problems and their solutions" (1460b6: περὶ δὲ προβλημάτων καὶ λύσεων). On Aristotle's lost *Homeric Problems*, see most recently Mayhew (2019).

34 LSJ, s.v. σημειόω, ii.3. The imperative σημείωσαι, used of marginal marks (equal to the Latin '*nota bene*'), is also common in the grammarians.

5 Endnote

In conclusion, it is difficult to say with any certainty how Ps.-Alexander became acquainted with the—originally Stoic?—concept of unsayable properties: most likely via Galen. But as he suggests himself, this concept must have been somehow in the air at the time, making it easy not just for himself, but for intellectuals of all plumage, to pick it up and appropriate it to their specific authorial needs.[35] In Ps.-Alexander's case, unsayable properties mark the point where science and medicine tip over to theology, where what can be said and known is differentiated from what we should remain silent about. As such, the notion shows to the medical student—the διδασκόμενος—how far the causal (Aristotelian) model of medical-naturalist problem research could be stretched and what were its conceptual limits.

Of course, in the Graeco-Roman context, the distinction between science/medicine and theology is much less strict than it is 'for us': at least for Ps.-Alexander there is no real tipping point between them. Nor should we underrate the rhetorical aspect of the concept of unsayable properties in light of Ps.-Alexander's educational ambitions in the *Medical Puzzles*. As is well known from Galen's treatise *On Examining the Physician*,[36] a proficient doctor had to be able to formulate suiting answers to the questions asked by his patients, thus demonstrating his reliability as medical expert, whilst securing an informed clientele.[37] One may wonder whether the collections of medical problems (προβλήματα) that came down to us—including, but not restricted to, the *Medical*

---

35 That imperial philosophers (esp. Platonists) were generally familiar with the concept of 'unsayability' is shown, e.g., by the opening quote to this contribution, drawn from Plutarch's *Table Talk*: for its Platonic implications there, see Meeusen (2016: 267–268). An interesting parallel is also found in Clement of Alexandria, *Strom.* 2.6.26.2 (138.22–29 Klotz; tr. Schaff, adapted): "For dry twigs, being ready to receive the power of fire, are kindled with great ease; and the far-famed stone attracts steel through affinity (διὰ συγγένειαν), as the amber tear-drop drags to itself twigs, and the amber lump sets chaff in motion. And the substances attracted obey them, drawn by an unsayable breath (ἀρρήτῳ ἑλκόμενα πνεύματι), not as a cause (αἴτια), but as a concurring cause (συναίτια)." Cf. also, e.g., Proclus, *Theologia Platonica* 1.4 (1.17.22 Saffrey—Westerink) on Plato's use of symbolic expressions to discuss the ἀρρήτους […] ἰδιότητας of divine principles, and 5.29 (5.107.28 Saffrey—Westerink) on the demiurgic cause partaking in the ἀγνώστου καὶ ἀρρήτου τῶν θεῶν ἰδιότητος, Philoponus, *Aet. Mund.* 13.17 (530.27–28 Rabe) on ἰδιότητές τινες ἄρρητοι in the heavenly body, etc. See also recently Vlad (2019).

36 Preserved in Arabic: see Iskandar (1988), with the study of Nutton (1990: esp. 244–249).

37 In addition, we have evidence that doctors were examined by official authorities in legal contexts, and they could also take an official exam for 'public doctor' (δοκιμασία): both critical situations in which their medical expertise was at stake. See Ricciardetto and Reggiani in this volume.

Puzzles—provided a virtual training for this type of debate, perhaps, indeed, with an eye towards conceptually harnessing medical students for entering the public arena? Interestingly, the medical contests held annually in Ephesus during the Great Asclepieia included a specific discipline named the πρόβλημα.[38] This speaks to the imagination: scholars have situated these competitions in the public setting of medical demonstrations (ἐπιδείξεις) and the doctors' public struggle for patients (as known from Galen's writings) arguing that oratory was probably the decisive factor in these contests, rather than medical knowledge per se.[39] In this context, it is perhaps less important to ask whether Ps.-Alexander's musings about 'insoluble problems' (ἄποροι ζητήσεις) are indicative of his scientific ignorance or of his religious devotion (or both?), than to conclude that the implied reader—the medical διδασκομένος—now has an explanatory *carte-blanche* up his sleeves when confronted with problems he finds difficult to solve, that is, the concept of ἰδιότητες ἄρρητοι.

Appendix: Alexander of Damascus as Potential Author?

As an alternative to Sharples' theory about the potential authorship of the *Medical Puzzles and Natural Problems*, identifying Alexander of Aphrodisias' father as the collection's author (see n. 3), I here examine whether Alexander of Damascus would be a suitable candidate instead. Our main source for this Alexander is Galen, who knew the man personally as a philosophy teacher of Flavius Boethus (his friend and an ex-consul). In *On Prognosis*, Galen characterises Alexander of Damascus as "an expert in the teachings of Plato but who was devoted more to those of Aristotle"[40] and also emphasises his "contentiousness" (φιλονεικίαν).[41] Interestingly, Alexander of Damascus is often confused with the commentator Alexander of Aphrodisias, probably because he also held the Peripatetic chair in Athens (as reported by Galen in *AA* 1.1 [2.218.6–8 Kühn; 5.2–4 Garofalo]; the confusion started in the Arabic tradition). Alexander of Damascus was probably the inaugural appointee to this post, which was established by Marcus Aurelius in 176 CE.[42] As Sharples points out: "There seems no reason to identify

38 *I.Eph.* 1161.5, 1162.6–7, 1166.2 (precise meaning uncertain). See Nutton (1995: 7–8) and (2013^2: 216 n. 72).

39 See Horstmanshoff (1990: 182): "I find it hard to avoid the impression that [...] bombastic, ranting speech-making won the day." Also Zimonyi (2014; esp. 369 on προβλήματα). On the 'performance' value of medical and natural scientific προβλήματα see also Oikonomopoulou in this volume.

40 Tr. Nutton, adapted; *Praen.* 5 (14.627.3–5 Kühn; 96.8–9 Nutton).

41 *Praen.* 5 (14.629.3 Kühn; 98.11 Nutton).

42 See Follet (1989) and Todd (1995).

Alexander of Aphrodisias' father with Alexander of Damascus; if we do not do so, we now have three Peripatetic Alexanders [...] in the latter half of the second century AD".[43] Sharples does not, however, pursue the possibility that Alexander of Damascus may actually be our author.

In the passage from *On Prognosis*, Galen in a lively manner describes his public dissection of a pig in Rome. It is his intention to demonstrate the function of the recurrent laryngeal nerves in the production of voice. A number of Roman notables are also attending the event, among whom Alexander of Damascus. Follet[44] mistakenly claims that Alexander was a teacher of Galen, but what the noun διδάσκαλον (in *Praen.* 5 [14.628.3 Kühn; 96.22 Nutton]) really implies is that he was appointed as Galen's philosophical "guide" (tr. Nutton) during the dissection. This did not go well. Even before the dissection could start, Galen left the scene in anger because of a sceptical intervention of Alexander of Damascus who asked him whether "we should believe in the evidence of the senses".[45] Galen had not expected to encounter such "rustic Pyrrhonists" (ἀγροικοπυῤῥωνείους).[46]

At first sight, Alexander's sceptical question does not seem to square with the point made in the preface to the first book of the *Medical puzzles* that "anyone who doubts whether heat is innate to fire, lacks the sense of touch (ἁπτικῆς αἰσθήσεως)" (4.3–4 Ideler). But whether Alexander was really the sceptic Galen tells him to be (in a fit of anger) is uncertain. As Todd[47] has convincingly argued, Galen had previously invited Alexander to "reason out the conclusions to be drawn from the *phainomena* of the vivisection", probably because his "philosophical background was 'dogmatic' enough to allow him to engage in causal analysis on the basis of observations" (he adds[48] that "If [Alexander of Damascus] was a sceptic, he would have plenty of ammunition against the forthcoming causal analysis, without needing to question the credibility of the basic observations"). This, combined with the facts (1) that Alexander of Damascus was directly involved in current medical debates and was closely engaged with Galen's medical science and public demonstrations, and (2) that he pledged allegiance to Aristotle and Plato and had some sceptical inclinations, which were not however incompatible with his Aristotelianism as Todd[49] has shown, and which, so I would add, can be expected from any (aporetic) Platonist anyway, brings us very close to the Alexander of the *Medical Puzzles*, whose Aristotelianism-*cum*-Platonism, as we saw, speaks clearly from

43 Sharples (2005: 50 n. 30).
44 Follet (1989: 140).
45 Tr. Nutton, adapted; *Praen.* 5 (14.628.14–16 Kühn; 98.5–6 Nutton): τοῖς διὰ τῶν αἰσθήσεων φαινομένοις πιστεύειν ἡμᾶς δεῖν.
46 *Praen.* 5 (14.628.18 Kühn; 98.8 Nutton).
47 Todd (1995: 125).
48 Ibid. n. 19, with further references.
49 Todd (1995: 126–128).

the preface to the first book—including his aporetic stance *vis-à-vis* certain unexplainable medical-naturalist problems[50]—, and whose engagement with Galenic thought is clearly traceable throughout the collection. Interestingly, as we have seen (sub 3.2), this engagement with Galen is at times marked by implicit criticism, as is the case in the problem about the constitution and function of the nerves (*Med. Puzz.* 2.72 [78.22–79.7 Ideler]). That this discrepancy may not be as innocent as it may seem, is suggested by the fact that Galen's fallout with Alexander of Damascus during the dissection in Rome described in *On Prognosis* specifically concerned the anatomy and function of the recurrent laryngeal nerves (see n. 20).

The distinct activities and functions which Ps.-Alexander in *Med. Puzz.* 2.72 logically infers from the differences in constitution and formation (κατασκευὴ καὶ διάπλασις) that he observes between several types of nerves is not incompatible with Galen's invitation that Alexander of Damascus help him draw the logical conclusions from the phenomena revealed by dissection (συλλογίσασθαι δὲ τὰ ἐξ αὐτῶν [sc. τὰ ἐκ τῆς ἀνατομῆς φαινόμενα] περαινόμενα: *Praen.* 5 [14.627.18–628.1 Kühn; 96.20–21 Nutton]). The aspect of observation is indeed very central in both passages: perhaps Alexander of Damascus' sceptical question to Galen (whether "we should believe in the evidence of the senses") was only meant as a leg-up for the debate, in that it was aimed at drawing attention to the observed constitution of the nerves in question (as in Ps.-Alexander's problem)? The real problem then is why the recurrent laryngeal nerves are so thin and hairlike as Galen says (νευρίων λεπτοτάτων [...] τριχοειδῆ συζυγίαν: *Praen.* 5 [14.628.8–9 Kühn; 96.27–98.1 Nutton]) and, perhaps more importantly, why they are recurrent to begin with, with the right descending further down than the left. Galen gives an account of this in *UP* 16.4 (4.281.18–289.4 Kühn; 2.389.3–394.15 Helmreich) and in *AA* 11.4 (1.108–109 Simon), where he underlines Nature's clever design. In the former passage, he emphatically says that "it is difficult to explain Nature's skill in words" (χαλεπὸν μὲν ἑρμηνεῦσαι λόγῳ τοσαύτην τέχνην: *UP* 16.4 [4.286.10–11 Kühn; 2.392.13–14 Helmreich]). This sounds all too familiar indeed and is echoed in Ps.-Alexander's concept of the ἰδιότητες ἄρρητοι, but whether this implies that there is a direct connection is difficult to say. In order to pursue the question of authorship further, it would be worthwhile to also take into account the *Supplementary Problems* and the *On Fevers*, but this requires a different study altogether.

50 See Meeusen (2019).

Acknowledgements

I would like to express my thanks to the conference attendants for their stimulating discussion of this paper. Special thanks also to Michael Trapp and Luigi Silvano for their comments on an earlier draft. Unless otherwise indicated, translations are mine.

Bibliography

Primary Sources

Bett, R. 2005. *Sextus Empiricus: Against the Logicians*. Cambridge: Cambridge University Press.

Daremberg, Ch.—Ruelle, Ch.-Ém. 1879. *Oeuvres de Rufus d'Éphèse*. Paris: Imprimerie nationale.

De Lacy, Ph. 1978–1984. *Galeni De placitis Hippocratis et Platonis* [CMG V.4.1.2]. Berlin: Akademie-Verlag.

Garofalo, I. 1986. *Galenus: Anatomicarum administrationum libri qui supersunt novem. Earundem interpretatio arabica Hunaino Isaaci filio ascripta. vol. 1, libri 1–5*. Naples: Instituto Universitario Orientale.

Gärtner, F. 2015. *Galeni De locis affectis I–II* [CMG V.6.1.1]. Berlin: De Gruyter.

Garzya, A.—Masullo, R. 2004. *I problemi di Cassio Iatrosofista* (*Quaderni dell'Accademia Pontaniana* 38). Naples: Accademia Pontaniana.

Helmreich, G. 1909. *Galeni De usu partium libri XVII*, vol. 2. Leipzig: Teubner.

Hilgard, A. 1889–1894. *Theodosii Alexandrini Canones. Georgii Choerobosci Scholia. Sophronii patriarchae Alexandrini Excerpta*, 2 vols. Leipzig: Teubner.

Ideler, J.L. 1841. *Physici et medici Graeci minores*. Berlin: Reimer.

Iskandar, A.Z. 1988. *Galeni De optimo medico cognoscendo libelli* [CMG Suppl. Or. IV]. Berlin: Akademie-Verlag.

Jouanna, J.—Guardasole, A. 2017. *Hippocrate 16. Problèmes hippocratiques*. Paris: Les Belles Lettres.

Jouanna, J. 2018. *Hippocrate 1.2. Le Serment. Les Serments chrétiens. La Loi*. Paris: Les Belles Lettres.

Kapetanaki, S.—Sharples, R.W. 2006. *Pseudo-Aristoteles* (*Pseudo-Alexander*). *Supplementa problematorum*. Berlin—New York: De Gruyter.

Klotz, R. 1831. *Titi Flaui Clementis Alexandrini opera omnia 2, continens Stromatorum libros I–IV*. Leipzig: E.B. Schwickerti.

Kühn, C.G. 1821–1833. *Claudii Galeni Opera Omnia*. Leipzig: Car. Cnoblochii.

Littré, É. 1839–1861. *Oeuvres complètes d'Hippocrate*. Paris: J.-B. Baillière.

Mayhew, R. 2011. *Aristotle 15–16. Problems*. Cambridge, Mass.—London: Harvard university press.

Minar, E.L.—Sandbach, F.H.—Helmbold, W.C. 1961. *Plutarch's Moralia 9. Table Talk 7–9*. Cambridge, Mass.—London: Harvard university press—William Heinemann Ltd.
Mutschmann, H. 1914. *Sexti Empirici opera 2. Adversus dogmaticos libros quinque* (*Adv. mathem.* VII–XI). Leipzig: Teubner.
Nutton, V. 1979. *Galeni De praecognitione* [CMG V.8.1]. Berlin: Akademie-Verlag.
Rabe, H. 1899. *Joannes Philoponus. De aeternitate mundi contra Proclum*. Leipzig: Teubner.
Rackham, H. 1933. *Cicero 19. De natura deorum; Academica*. Cambridge, Mass.—London: Harvard University Press—William Heinemann Ltd.
Saffrey, H.D.—Westerink, L.G. 1968–1997. *Proclus. Théologie platonicienne*. Paris: Les Belles Lettres.
Simon, M. 1906. *Sieben Bücher Anatomie des Galen*, vol. 1. Leipzig: J.C. Hinrichs'sche Buchhandlung.

Secondary Sources

Adamson, P. 2005. 'On Knowledge of Particulars', *Proceedings of the Aristotelian Society* 105: 257–278.
Bertier, J.—Filius, L.S. 2003. '*Problemata physica*', in R. Goulet—J.-M. Flamand—M. Aouad (eds.), *Dictionnaire des philosophes antiques, Supplément*. Paris: CNRS Editions, 575–598.
Blair, A. 1999. 'The *Problemata* as a Natural Philosophical Genre', in A. Grafton—N.G. Siraisi (eds.), *Natural Particulars. Nature and the Disciplines in Renaissance Europe*. Cambridge, Mass.: MIT Press, 171–204.
Centrone, B. (ed.). 2011. *Studi sui* Problemata Physica *aristotelici*. Naples: Bibliopolis.
Copenhaver, B.P. 1991. 'A Tale of Two Fishes: Magical Objects in Natural History from Antiquity Through the Scientific Revolution', *Journal of the History of Ideas* 52: 373–398.
Debru, A. 2008. 'Physiology', in R.J. Hankinson (ed.), *The Cambridge Companion to Galen*. Cambridge: Cambridge University Press, 263–282.
Deichgräber, K. 1957. 'Galen als Erforscher des menschlichen Pulses: Ein Beitrag zur Selbstdarstellung des Wissenschaftlers (*De dignotione pulsuum* I 1)', *Sitzungsberichte der deutschen Akademie der Wissenschaften zu Berlin, Klasse für Sprachen, Literatur, und Kunst*, 1956, 3: 1–41.
Flashar, H. 1962. *Aristoteles, Problemata physica*. Berlin: Akademie-Verlag.
Follet, S. 1989. 'Alexandros de Damas', in R. Goulet (ed.), *Dictionnaire des philosophes antiques*, vol. 1. Paris: CNRS, 140–142.
Franke, W. 2007. *On What Cannot Be Said: Apophatic Discourses in Philosophy, Religion, Literature, and the Arts*, 2 vols. Notre Dame, Indiana: University of Notre Dame Press.
Franke, W. 2014. *A Philosophy of the Unsayable*. Notre Dame, Indiana: University of Notre Dame Press.

Frede, M. 1987. 'Stoics and Skeptics on Clear and Distinct Impressions', in M. Frede (ed.), *Essays in Ancient Philosophy*. Oxford: Clarendon Press, 151–176.

Horstmanshoff, H.F.J. 1990. 'The Ancient Physician: Craftsman or Scientist?', *Journal of the History of Medicine and Allied Sciences* 45: 176–197.

Leszl, W. 1972/3. 'Knowledge of the Universal and Knowledge of the Particular in Aristotle', *Review of Metaphysics* 26: 278–313.

Mayhew, R. (ed.). 2015. *The Aristotelian* Problemata Physica*: Philosophical and Scientific Investigations*. Leiden: Brill.

Mayhew, R. 2019. *Aristotle's Lost* Homeric Problems*: Textual Studies*, Oxford: Oxford University Press.

Meeusen, M. 2016. *Plutarch's Science of Natural Problems. A Study with Commentary on* Quaestiones Naturales. Leuven: Leuven University Press.

Meeusen, M., 2018. 'An Interpretation of the Preface to *Medical Puzzles and Natural Problems* 1 by Ps.-Alexander of Aphrodisias in Light of Medical Education', in P. Bouras-Vallianatos—S. Xenophontos (eds.), *Greek Medical Literature and its Readers: From Hippocrates to Islam and Byzantium*. London: Routledge, 94–109.

Meeusen, M. 2019. 'Unknowable Questions and Paradoxography in Ps.-Alexander's *Medical Puzzles and Natural Problems*', in G. Kazantzidis (ed.), *Medicine and Paradoxography in Antiquity*. Berlin—New York: De Gruyter, 199–214.

Nutton, V. 1990. 'The Patient's Choice: a New Treatise by Galen', *Classical Quarterly* 40: 235–257.

Nutton, V. 1995. 'The Medical Meeting Place', in Ph.J. van der Eijk—H.F.J. Horstmanshoff—P.H. Schrijvers (eds.), *Ancient Medicine in Its Socio-Cultural Context*. Amsterdam—Atlanta: Rodopi, 3–26.

Nutton, V. 2013². *Ancient Medicine*. London—New York: Routledge.

Oikonomopoulou, K.—Silvano, L.—Meeusen, M. Forthcoming. 'The prefaces to pseudo-Alexander of Aphrodisias' *Medical Puzzles and Natural Problems*, books 1 and 2: relationship, and background'.

Pieper, A. 1973. '*Individuum*', in H. Krings—H.M. Baumgartner—Ch. Wild (eds.), *Handbuch philosophischer Grundbegriffe*, vol. 3. München: Kösel Verlag, 728–737.

Reinhardt, T. 2011. 'Galen on Unsayable Properties', *Oxford Studies in Ancient Philosophy* 40: 297–317.

Röhr, J. 1923. *Der okkulte Kraftbegriff im Altertum* (*Philologus Supplementband* 17.1). Leipzig: Dieterich.

Schaff, P. et al. 1885. *Ante-Nicene Fathers 2: Fathers of the Second Century*. New York: Christian Literature Publishing Co.

Schiefsky, M.J. 2007. 'Galen's Teleology and Functional Explanation', *Oxford Studies in Ancient Philosophy* 33: 369–400.

Sharples, R.W. 1987. 'Alexander of Aphrodisias: Scholasticism and Innovation', *Aufstieg und Niedergang der römischen Welt* 2.36.2: 1176–243.

Sharples, R.W. 1998. 'Alexander and pseudo-Alexanders of Aphrodisias: *Scripta minima. Questions* and *Problems, makeweights* and prospects', in W. Kullmann—J. Althoff—M. Asper (eds.), *Gattungen wissenschaftlicher Literatur in der Antike*. Tübingen: Gunter Narr Verlag, 383–403.

Sharples, R.W. 2004. 'Evidence for Theophrastus *On Hair, On Secretion, On Wine and Olive Oil?*', *Bulletin of the Institute of Classical Studies* 47: 141–151.

Sharples, R.W. 2005. 'Implications of the New Alexander of Aphrodisias Inscription', *Bulletin of the Institute of Classical Studies* 48: 47–56.

Sharples, R.W. 2006. 'Pseudo-Alexander or Pseudo-Aristotle, *Medical Puzzles and Physical Problems*', in P. De Leemans—M. Goyens (eds.), *Aristotle's* Problemata *in Different Times and Tongues*. Leuven: Leuven University Press, 21–31.

Siegel, R.E. 1976. *Galen on the Affected Parts*. Basel: Karger.

Silvano, L. 2017. 'Un'edizione da rifare: i *Problemata* dello Pseudo-Alessandro di Afrodisia', *Philologia Antiqua* 10: 19–29.

Silvano, L. 2018a. 'Studiare la natura per problemi: il proemio al primo libro dei *Dubbi medici e problemi fisici* dello Pseudo-Alessandro di Afrodisia', *Seminari Romani di Cultura Greca* 7: 89–106.

Silvano, L. 2018b. 'La luna (piena?) e la decomposizione della carne. Nota a Pseudo-Alessandro di Afrodisia, probl. i, 66 Ideler', *Revue des Études Tardo-Antiques* 7: 29–46.

Stoyles, B.J. 2015. 'Material and Teleological Explanations in *Problemata* 10', in Mayhew (2015: 124–150).

Todd, R.B. 1995. 'Peripatetic Epistemology before Alexander of Aphrodisias: the Case of Alexander of Damascus', *Eranos* 93: 122–128.

Vlad, M. 2019. *Damascius et l'ineffable: Récit de l'impossible discours*. Paris: Vrin.

Wellmann, M. 1895. *Die pneumatische Schule bis auf Archigenes*. Berlin: Weidmann.

Zimonyi, Á. 2014. 'The Context of Medical Competitions in Ephesus', *Acta Antiqua Hungarica* 54: 355–370.

CHAPTER 5

Erotetic Logic, Uncertainty and Therapy: Galen and Alexander on Logic and Medicine

Luca Gili

Abstract

Syllogistic is grounded upon dialectics. Dialectics is a version of erotetic logic, because it deals with questions and answers. This paper intends to explore the erotetic logics of Galen and of Alexander of Aphrodisias in order to establish whether the differences in their logical systems correspond to differences in their understanding of medicine. Galen and Alexander of Aphrodisias were almost contemporaries. Both of them shared the idea that doctors should know logic to practice medicine. The radical difference between Alexander and Galen consists in the fact that Alexander has a modal logic, whereas Galen does not. In other words, the premises—the answers in a dialogical exchange—include a modal operator for Alexander, but not for Galen. This absence is not without consequences. This will become clearer if one pays attention to the role of contingency syllogistic within Alexander's own account of medicine.

1 The Need for Erotetic Logic to Formalise Medical Questioning

Contemporary philosophers have paid more attention to the study of the objective features of acquired science than to the subjective process of *discovering* scientific information.[1] The underlying logic of discovery is the logic that deals with questions and answers, because the information-seeking process consists of *asking questions* to nature.[2] While Hintikka and Alqvist were developing their systems of erotetic logic, they had the impression they were

---

1 Hintikka (1981); Kleiner (1993: 87).

2 Introducing some historical antecedents for his erotetic logic, Hintikka (1981: 69) observes that "the basic idea of this approach goes back all the way to Kant and even to Francis Bacon, who proposed to consider the process of science as a series of questions put to nature. In this approach, science is considered as a process of information-gathering and problem-solving through questioning". The seminal paper on contemporary erotetic logic is Prior—Prior (1955).

 | DOI:10.1163/9789004442672_007

developing a new domain of logic.[3] Yet, the logic of questions and answers was certainly at the centre of the study of language undertaken by Plato and Aristotle. While attempting to revitalise the dialectical logic that flourished in antiquity, D. Walton gives the following explanation for the oblivion of ancient dialectic:

> With the advent of the Enlightenment model in which all reasoning was based on the scientific standards of deductive and inductive reasoning, the old idea of dialectical reasoning in Aristotle was cast aside as 'subjective.' In the twentieth century the transformation was complete—logic became a purely abstract mathematical calculus representing the kinds of propositional inferences studied by the Stoics and the syllogistic kind of logic developed by Aristotle. Dialectical arguments based on plausible reasoning no longer made sense to modern students and had no place in modern logical theory.[4]

According to Walton, a new dialectic would embrace all dialogues that display a form of reasoned argumentation.[5] Information-seeking dialogue is thus part of this dialectical enterprise.[6] It is reasonable to say that all of Plato's early dialogues present dialectical games that have the goal of gathering information about a variety of subjects.[7] Plato's dialectical practice obeyed a number of rules that Aristotle wrote down in his works on dialectics, the *Topics* and the *Sophistical Refutations*.[8] In particular, book 8 of Aristotle's *Topics* describes the rule of the information-seeking process that involves questions and answers.[9]

---

3 See Alqvist (1975); Hintikka (1981). More recent work in dialectic shows more awareness of the ancient antecedents of multi-agent arguments. Dutilh Novaes (2015) boldly, but convincingly, argues that the normativity of logic does not affect the single-agent abstract thinking, but rather the rules of multi-agent argumentative exchange.

4 Walton (1998: 16).

5 Walton—Krabbe (1995).

6 Walton (1998: 31).

7 See Robinson (1953); Giannantoni (2005).

8 Krabbe (2014).

9 See Solmsen (1929: 47–50); Moraux (1968): "mieux que toute autre source, le huitième livre des *Topiques* nous permet d'établir comment, vers le milieu du quatrième siècle, Aristote concevait la pratique de la dialectique" (277); "l'engagement se déroule par questions et réponses. Le premier partenaire soumet à l'autre une question: celui-ci peut, d'ordinaire, y répondre par oui ou par non, se disant ainsi d'accord ou non avec la proposition avancée" (281–282); Smith (1997: xiii): "what differentiates dialectical arguments from other arguments is that they take place by *question and answer*"; Slomkowski (1997: 10–15). Duncombe—Dutilh Novaes (2016) is an excellent survey on recent research on Aristotle's dialectic.

In *Top.* 8.1–3 Aristotle describes the task of the questioner; in *Top.* 8.4–10 that of the answerer.[10]

One could expect that any theoretical reflection on medical practice would make reference to the erotetic logic that Aristotle outlines in book 8 of the *Topics*, because doctors have to gather information concerning the disease they are supposed to diagnose and cure, and they often do so by asking the patient (or people around her/him) some questions. Galen himself attests to this practice in his writings.[11] Yet, we do not see any attempt of Galen at form-

10 Many scholars have written on dialectic as the argumentative method that Aristotle would extensively adopt in his theoretical works: see, e.g., Dancy (1975); Irwin (1988). On ancient dialectic see also Sichirollo (2003).

11 In a passage from the treatise *On the Affected Parts*, Galen provides us with an account of his own practice of asking questions in order to diagnose a particular condition. After having discarded the theoretical inquiry (τῶν λογικῶν προβλημάτων ἡ σκέψις) as useless for diagnosis (εἰς τὴν διάγνωσιν τῶν παθῶν), for the cure (εἰς τὴν ἴασιν) or for future prognosis (εἰς τὴν τῶν ἀποβησομένων πρόγνωσιν) (*Loc. Aff.* 1.6 [8.56.5–7 Kühn; 290.21–23 Gärtner]), Galen retorts to his habitual method of diagnosis. The passage is worth quoting in full, because it shows that the method consists of asking questions and gathering the information provided in the answers: θέασαι γοῦν, ὅπως ἐγὼ μηδ' ἁψάμενος αὐτῆς διηγήσομαι θεραπείαν ἐκ τῆς τοῦ πεπονθότος τόπου γνώσεως εὑρεθεῖσαν. ἔχων τις ἐπικείμενον φάρμακον τοῖς τρισὶ δακτύλοις τῆς χειρὸς, ἔφασκε τριάκονθ' ἡμερῶν ἤδη τὴν αἴσθησιν αὐτῶν ἀπολωλέναι, τῆς κινήσεως ἀβλαβοῦς φυλαττομένης, ὀνίνασθαί τε μηδὲν ὑπὸ τῶν ἐπιτιθεμένων φαρμάκων. ὅπερ οὖν εἴωθα ποιεῖν ἐπὶ τῶν τοιούτων, οὐδὲ τότε παρέλιπον, ἀλλ' ἠρώτησα καλέσας τὸν προνοούμενον αὐτοῦ τῶν δακτύλων ἰατρὸν, ὁποίοις τισὶ χρησάμενος εἴη φαρμάκοις· ὡς δὲ τοῖς προσήκουσιν εὗρον, ἐζήτουν τὴν αἰτίαν τοῦ μηδὲν ὠφελεῖσθαι τὸν ἄνθρωπον, ἠρώτων τε τὰ προηγησάμενα συμπτώματα. τοῦ δὲ μήτε φλεγμονήν τινα μήτε ψύξιν μήτε πληγὴν αὐτῷ προηγήσασθαι φάντος, ἀλλ' ἐκ τοῦ κατὰ βραχὺ τὴν αἴσθησιν ἀπολέσθαι, θαυμάζων πάλιν ἠρόμην, εἰ μὴ τῶν ἀνωτέρω τι μορίων ἐπλήγη. τοῦ δὲ κατὰ μὲν τὴν χεῖρα μηδὲν εἰπόντος, ἐν ἀρχῇ δὲ τοῦ μεταφρένου πληγῆναι φάσκοντος, αὖθις ἠρόμην ὅπως τε καὶ ὁπότ' ἐπλήγη. καὶ μέντοι καὶ ἀποκριναμένου, κατὰ τὴν εἰς Ῥώμην ὁδὸν ἡνίκ' ἐξέπεσε τοῦ ὀχήματος εἶναι τὸν χρόνον οὐ πολὺ πρότερον ἢ τοὺς δακτύλους ἄρξασθαι πάσχειν, ἐτεκμηράμην ἐν τῇ πρώτῃ τοῦ μετὰ τὸν ἕβδομον σπόνδυλον νεύρου διεκπτώσει μόριόν τι ἐπὶ τῇ πληγῇ φλεγμῆναν σκιῤῥώδη διάθεσιν ἐσχηκέναι. τοῦτο δ' ἐνόησα, μεμαθηκὼς διὰ τῆς ἀνατομῆς [...] (*Loc. Aff.* 1.6 [8.56.8–57.13 Kühn; 290.23–292.16 Gärtner]): "Watch now how I will explain the therapy which I found by the knowledge of the affected part, neglecting such speculations. A patient who had received some medicine for applying to three fingers of his hand told us that these fingers had already lost all feeling for thirty days, whereas the motion of the fingers had remained intact, and that the applied drug had not helped at all. The method which I customarily employ in such cases I did not neglect at that occasion either, but I summoned and asked the physician who had taken care of his fingers what kind of drugs he had used. Since I found these adequate, I searched for the reason why nothing had helped this man by inquiring about the preceding symptoms. Since he did not mention a contusion nor a chilling nor an infection but stated that he had lost the feeling gradually, I became puzzled and asked again, whether he had not received a blow in the upper parts [of his spine]. When he told me that had not at all suffered from an injury of the hand, but asserted that he had suffered a contusion of the upper midriff

alizing the information-gathering process that involves questions and answers. In his few remarks on logic, which we mostly infer from his *Institutio logica*,[12]

[the upper part of the broad of his back], I asked again how and when he was injured. And indeed he then answered that on the way to Rome he had fallen from his carriage at a point in time not long before his fingers started to suffer. I concluded that at the first issue of the nerve [from the spine] after the seventh vertebra a part had become inflamed by the injury and had become hard. I knew this from my study of dissection […]" (transl. Siegel [1976: 38], adapted by Michiel Meeusen). In the above text, Galen offers us an example of his diagnostic method without outlining the theoretical scheme of this method, but it is not difficult to infer that he aims at gathering information in a way similar to that of the dialectician. Galen guides the patient because he knows in advance what the possible cases of pathology are. He examines all options one after the other. He has a previous general knowledge of all possible pathologies that can explain the symptoms of the patient (e.g., τοῦτο δ' ἐνόησα, μεμαθηκὼς διὰ τῆς ἀνατομῆς) and this helps him to find the appropriate questions. Sometimes he is puzzled by the answers and asks again (θαυμάζων πάλιν ἠρόμην). The scheme seems to imply the presence of an implicit premise:

(Implicit premise^1) F is caused either by P or by Q or by Z
(Question^1) Is F caused by P?
(Answer^1) No
(Conclusion^1 = Implicit premise^2) F is caused either by Q or by Z
(Question^2) Is F caused by Q?
(Answer^2) No
(Conclusion^2) Hence, F is caused by Z.

The above scheme is not syllogistic, but it is not difficult to see that there is an underlying inference that guides the questioner:

(Premise 1) All Fs that are not caused by either P or by Q are caused by Z
(Premise 2) This F is one of Fs that are not caused by either P or by Q
(Conclusion) Therefore, this F is caused by Z.

Galen's passage tells us that there might be uncertainty in the attempt of subsuming the particular case under the general rule (Galen admits that he was puzzled, θαυμάζων). From a pragmatic viewpoint, the uncertainty can be overcome by simply asking more questions: the information gathered from the answer is sufficient to formulate a diagnosis. But at the theoretical level we should take into account that 'premise 2' of the above syllogism is meant to express something that is not beyond any doubt. In this paper, I will ask myself how Galen can express this uncertainty with the resources of his logic. For Galen's method involving questions and answers see also *Loc. Aff.* 1.4 (8.41.14–42.16 Kühn; 272.23–274.10 Gärtner).

12 An excellent overview of Galen's logic is Stakelum (1940) (the book is an abridged version of a PhD dissertation that I was not able to consult). Rescher (1966) discusses the hypothesis in which Galen introduced the fourth syllogistic figure. In his *Prior Analytics* (1.1–2, 4–7), Aristotle presents the logical system known as categorical syllogistic, i.e., the deductive system that includes all valid arguments in the form of syllogisms. Aristotle groups all valid syllogisms in three 'figures' (or 'schemes') depending on the position of the middle term in the premises. Medieval logicians commonly grouped syllogisms into *four* figures. It is not certain, however, whether Galen introduced the fourth figure. Rescher (1966) maintains that he did; *contra*, see Gottschalk (1987); Morison (2008). Mau (1960) offers

Galen intends to develop a logic that functions as the underlying deductive system for medicine and for other sciences. Accordingly, he criticises Stoic logic, because it is merely concerned with logical form and not with "facts" (see *Inst. Log.* 4.6.1–2 [Kalbfleisch]). Galen relies instead on Aristotle's syllogistic, but adds individual propositions (see *Inst. Log.* 2.2–6 [Kalbfleisch]),[13] presumably because medical practice is about individual patients.[14] One would expect Galen to develop a logical system that formalises the practice of information-gathering through questions and answers, especially since Aristotle appears to have already developed such a logic in book 8 of his *Topics*. Galen is certainly aware of the possibility of formalizing argumentative patterns, as is clear from *Inst. Log.* 14.1–2 (Kalbfleisch):

> What is most important and primary in regard to anything that is not apparent to perception is the question of its existence or being; in this

an excellent commentary on Galen's short logical treatise, together with a German translation of the text. For a clear English translation and an insightful commentary on Galen's *Institutio logica*, see Kieffer (1964). Pellegrin (1998) offers a readable French translation. Morison (2008) presents an overview of Galen's logic. The only critical edition available is still Kalbfleisch (1896), which is based on the only known witness of the work (Paris, Bibliothèque Nationale, *Supplementum Graecum*, 635). The manuscript is damaged and there have not been many attempts at restoring it. Another look at the manuscript and a new edition of the text is certainly a desideratum.

13 I call 'individual propositions' propositions in which the subject is a term referring to an individual, e.g., propositions like 'Socrates is a man'. In his *Prior Analytics* 2.27.70a24–38, Aristotle discusses a syllogism with an individual proposition as a premise, but in his systematic presentation of syllogistic he seems to state that only quantified propositions may be the premises of a syllogism (see *Prior Analytics* 1.2). Galen's description of propositions in the context of a treatise on deduction (*Inst. Log.* 2.2–6 [Kalbfleisch]) uses several individual propositions as examples. This choice seems to entail that individual propositions can figure *de iure* in a deductive argument, despite Aristotle's hesitation on this subject.

14 Kieffer (1964: 64) stresses that Galen detaches himself from Aristotle in adding singular propositions. Yet, Kieffer has no explanation for this and suggests that Galen might have found this addition in his sources. It should be noted that Aristotle does not use singular propositions in the section of his *Prior Analytics* devoted to the systematic presentation of categorical syllogistic (*Prior Analytics* 1.1–2, 4–7) and adds that syllogistic primarily deals with universals rather than with individuals (*Prior Analytics* 1.27.43a42–43), but we do find singular propositions as premises of syllogisms elsewhere (see *Prior Analytics* 1.33.47b22, 30; 2.27.70a16–18; the issue has been discussed by many interpreters, see Malink [2013: 48–49] for an assessment and for references to previous scholarship). Contrary to what Kieffer suggests, Galen (or his sources) might be adding singular propositions because Aristotle himself was employing them. Galen is likely to have adopted such a logic to deal with the individual features of a patient or of a disease that a medical doctor should consider, see *Sect. Int.* 3 (1.69.6–72.3 Kühn; 4.17–6.26 Helmreich); *Med. Exp.* 29.147–148 (Walzer).

> respect the following kind of problems arise: 'Does Fate exist?', 'Is there Providence?', 'Do the gods exist?', 'Is there a void?'.
>
> In these problems we use hypothetical propositions (ἐν οἷς προβλήμασι μάλιστα χρώμεθα ταῖς ὑποθετικαῖς προτάσεσιν), which the ancients divided into those by connection and those by separation; the Stoics call the connectives conditional axioms, the separatives, disjunctive, and we agree with them at least that there are two syllogisms of the conditional axiom and two of the disjunctive.[15]

Galen discusses a series of questions about the *existence* of certain objects that cannot be perceived. He argues that in dealing with such problems, we need to employ the 'hypothetical propositions' introduced by the Stoics.[16] For example, if an Epicurean were to argue for the *existence* of the void, s/he would argue as follows:

> (a) If there is motion, then there is a void in which atoms can move.
> (b) There is motion.
> Hence, (c) there is a void.

It is important to stress that these questions are referred to as 'problems' (προβλήματα). The term has a technical meaning in the context of Aristotle's *Topics* and refers to a question that needs to be posited so that both agents in a dialectical argument may agree on the premises of a syllogistic demonstration.[17] In other words, when we are facing one of Aristotle's προβλήματα, expressed in the form of a question, we have a logical tool to deal with the issue—this tool is the hypothetical proposition.

15 Kieffer (1964: 46). Ὃ δ' ἐστὶ μέγιστόν τε καὶ πρῶτον ἐφ' ἑκάστου τῶν μὴ φαινομένων αἰσθήσει, τὸ κατὰ τὴν ὕπαρξιν ἤτοι οὐσίαν † γίγνεται μὴ εἶναι ζήτημ' ἐστίν, ἐν ᾧ γε τὰ τοιαῦτα προβάλλεται· ἆρά γ' εἱμαρμένη ἔστιν; ἆρά γε πρόνοια ἔστιν; ἆρά γε θεοὶ εἰσίν; ἆρά γε κενὸν ἔστιν; ἐν οἷς προβλήμασι μάλιστα χρώμεθα ταῖς ὑποθετικαῖς προτάσεσιν, ἃς ⟨εἰς τὰς⟩ κατὰ συνέχειαν καὶ κατὰ διαίρεσιν ἔτεμον οἱ παλαιοί· καλοῦσι δὲ τὰς μὲν κατὰ συνέχειαν οἱ Στωικοὶ συνημμένα ἀξιώματα, τὰς δὲ κατὰ διαίρεσιν διεζευγμένα, καὶ συμφωνεῖταί γε αὐτοῖς δύο μὲν γίγνεσθαι συλλογισμοὺς κατὰ τὸ συνημμένον ἀξίωμα, δύο δὲ κατὰ τὸ διεζευγμένον.

16 Slomkowski (1997: 107) maintains that Galen's remarks implicitly confirm that Aristotle's dialectic also includes hypothetical syllogisms. I am not entirely persuaded by Slomkowski's remark, but his observation attests to the possibility of looking at Galen as an author who put into practice the dialectical deductive system developed by classical authors and most notably by Aristotle in his *Topics*.

17 See Slomkowski (1997: 15 ff.).

The idea that questions (and their answers) can be 'rephrased' in the formal language of logic explains why we do not have an erotetic logic in Galen.[18] We have something that is equivalent to it, which does not display the syntactic markers of a dialectical exchange.

2 Why We Do Not Find Any Erotetic Logic After Aristotle's *Topics* 8

Galen was probably not the first to implicitly renounce the idea of an erotetic logic.[19] A similar tendency can be found in Alexander of Aphrodisias' writings too. Even though he set himself the task of commenting on Aristotle's *Topics*, Alexander clearly expels questions and answers from the domain of dialectic. Alexander does so because he is faced with a problem. Aristotle states that all valid arguments are syllogisms or can be reduced to syllogistic form.[20] A syllogism, in turn, does not seem to display any structure that resembles the dialogical exchange involving questions and answers. According to Aristotle's definition,

> A syllogism is a discourse (λόγος) in which, certain things being stated, something other than what is stated follows of necessity from their being

---

18 An erotetic argument would run as follows:
Q: Is S a P?
A: Yes.
Q: What sort of P?
A: A K.
Q: Is then S a K?
A: Yes.
This argument can be rephrased as a *Barbara* syllogism:
(i) All P are K.
(ii) All S are P.
(iii) All S are K.

19 By stating that Galen gave up erotetic logic I mean that he did not include erotetic logic in his system of logic oulined in the *Institutio logica*. He clearly employed it in the context of his medical practice (cf. the passage quoted in footnote 11).

20 See *Prior Analytics* 1.23.40b17–22: Ὅτι μὲν οὖν οἱ ἐν τούτοις τοῖς σχήμασι συλλογισμοὶ τελειοῦνταί τε διὰ τῶν ἐν τῷ πρώτῳ σχήματι καθόλου συλλογισμῶν καὶ εἰς τούτους ἀνάγονται, δῆλον ἐκ τῶν εἰρημένων· ὅτι δ' ἁπλῶς πᾶς συλλογισμὸς οὕτως ἕξει, νῦν ἔσται φανερόν, ὅταν δειχθῇ πᾶς γινόμενος διὰ τούτων τινὸς τῶν σχημάτων. "It is clear from what has been said that the syllogisms in these figures are made perfect by means of the universal syllogisms in the first figure and are reduced to them. That every syllogism without qualification can be so treated, will be clear presently, when it has been proved that every syllogism is formed through one or other of these figures" (translation from Barnes [1984], slightly modified).

> so. I mean by the last phrase that it follows because of them, and by this, that no further term is required from without in order to make the consequence necessary.[21]

Aristotle's definition does not rule out questions and answers as the setting in which a syllogistic deduction can take place. Take for instance the following argument:

> A: Are all Greeks human beings?
> B: Yes.
> A: Are all human beings animals?
> B: I don't know.
> A: Is there any human being you can name who is not an animal?
> B: There isn't.
> A: Therefore, all Greeks are animals.
> B: Indeed.

The above argument is a discourse (λόγος) in which certain premises are being posited and something other than the premises is inferred by necessity. There is no reason to think that the above argument, which may display the same structure of many a reasoning in medical practice, should not be taken to be a syllogism.[22] Alexander, however, seems to assume that the premises of syllogisms do not display question marks, because there is not a single syllogistic inference in his commentary on Aristotle's *Prior Analytics* with premises in an interrogative form. He might have been led to think this was so because Aristotle's canonical moods in *Prior Analytics* 1.1–2, 4–7 do not include questions and answers. Since Alexander developed a narrower notion of syllogism, he had the problem of presenting dialectical arguments as reducible to syllogistic, because Aristotle explicitly states that arguments involving dialectical premises are syllogisms too.[23] For this reason, the thesis expounded in *Prior Analytics* 1.23.40b17–22,

---

21 *Prior Analytics* 1.1.24b18–22: συλλογισμὸς δέ ἐστι λόγος ἐν ᾧ τεθέντων τινῶν ἕτερόν τι τῶν κειμένων ἐξ ἀνάγκης συμβαίνει τῷ ταῦτα εἶναι. λέγω δὲ τῷ ταῦτα εἶναι τὸ διὰ ταῦτα συμβαίνειν, τὸ δὲ διὰ ταῦτα συμβαίνειν τὸ μηδενὸς ἔξωθεν ὅρου προσδεῖν πρὸς τὸ γενέσθαι τὸ ἀναγκαῖον. The translation is taken from Barnes (1984) and has been slightly modified.

22 Marion—Rückert (2015) maintain that universal quantification is grounded on the dialectical search for a counterexample. Their conclusion suggests that dialectic actually grounds syllogistic. For another book claiming that Aristotle's syllogistic originated out of the (dialectical) theory of predication, see Malink (2013).

23 See *Prior Analytics* 1.1.24a25–b12: οὐδὲν δὲ διοίσει πρὸς τὸ γενέσθαι τὸν ἑκατέρου συλλογισμόν· καὶ γὰρ ὁ ἀποδεικνύων καὶ ὁ ἐρωτῶν συλλογίζεται λαβών τι κατά τινος ὑπάρχειν ἢ μὴ ὑπάρ-

namely that all valid inferences can be reduced to the syllogisms expounded in *Prior Analytics* 1.1–22, plays a crucial role within Alexander's system.[24] In Alexander's view, there should be a way of translating dialectical exchanges involving questions and answers in standard syllogisms, because all arguments can be reduced to the standard moods in the three figures.[25] The solution adopted by Alexander consists of stating that the question falls out of the syllogistic machinery. A syllogism does not display any question among its premises, but rather the *answer* to a question. In fact, Alexander maintains that the preliminary step for establishing the premises of a dialectical syllogism is to ask questions,[26] because the dialectical premise can be defined as "a question concerning two contradictory statements" (ἐρώτησις ἀντιφάσεως).[27] In Alexan-

---

χειν. ὥστε ἔσται συλλογιστικὴ μὲν πρότασις ἁπλῶς κατάφασις ἢ ἀπόφασίς τινος κατά τινος τὸν εἰρημένον τρόπον, ἀποδεικτικὴ δέ, ἐὰν ἀληθὴς ᾖ καὶ διὰ τῶν ἐξ ἀρχῆς ὑποθέσεων εἰλημμένη, διαλεκτικὴ δὲ πυνθανομένῳ μὲν ἐρώτησις ἀντιφάσεως, συλλογιζομένῳ δὲ λῆψις τοῦ φαινομένου καὶ ἐνδόξου, καθάπερ ἐν τοῖς Τοπικοῖς εἴρηται. "But this will make no difference to the production of a syllogism in either case; for both the demonstrator and the dialectician argue deductively after assuming that something does or does not belong to something. Therefore a syllogistic proposition without qualification will be an affirmation or denial of something concerning something in the way we have described; it will be demonstrative, if it is true and assumed on the basis of the first principles of its science; it will be dialectical if it asks for a choice between two contradictories (if one is enquiring) or if it assumes what is apparent and reputable, as we said in the *Topics* (if one is deducing)" (translation from Barnes [1984], slightly modified).

24 On the importance of this passage of Aristotle for the structure of Alexander's commentary on Aristotle's *Prior Analytics* see Gili (2011: 37).

25 See *in An. Pr.* 340.5–20 (Wallies). The standard syllogistic moods are the valid syllogistic inferences listed by Aristotle in the first seven chapters of the first book of the *Prior Analytics*. They are grouped into three 'figures' according to the position of the middle term. In the first figure, the middle term is the grammatical subject of the major premise and the predicate of the minor premise (valid moods: *Barbara*, *Celarent*, *Darii*, *Ferio*). In the second figure the middle term is the grammatical predicate in both the major and the minor premises (valid moods: *Cesare*, *Camestres*, *Festino*, *Baroco*). In the third figure, the middle term is the grammatical subject in both premises (valid moods: *Disamis*, *Darapti*, *Felapton*, *Ferison*, *Bocardo*). For the meaning of the medieval mnemonic names for the valid moods see, among others, Lagerlund (2008).

26 See *in Top.* 518.6–9 (Wallies): παράκειται δὲ τῷ μὲν περὶ ἐρωτήσεως τά τε πρὸς κρύψιν λαμβανόμενα καὶ ὅλως δι' ὧν ἂν ὁ ἐρωτῶν ἐπάγοιτο τὸν ἀποκρινόμενον τὴν καθόλου πρότασιν αὐτῷ τιθέναι, ἐπειδὴ ἄνευ ταύτης ἀδύνατόν ἐστι συλλογίσασθαι: "as far as questioning is concerned, there is a presentation of the assumptions against obscurity and, in general, of the means by which the questioner leads the answerer to state to him a universal premise, because without that it is impossible to make a syllogism" (my translation).

27 See *in Top.* 519.14–16 (Wallies): αἴτιον δὲ τούτου, ὅτι τῷ διαλεκτικῷ πρὸς ἄλλον ὁ λόγος, καὶ ἐξ ἐρωτήσεως λαμβάνει τὰς προτάσεις δι' ὧν τὸ προκείμενον συλλογίζεται. διὰ τοῦτο γὰρ καὶ ἡ διαλεκτικὴ πρότασις ὡρίσθη ἐρώτησις ἀντιφάσεως εἶναι: "the reason is that an argument for

der's reconstruction of Aristotle's dialectic, the questioner asks the answerer to choose between contradictory alternatives.[28] Hence, we obtain premises for a deduction by answering to προβλήματα.[29] Thus, rather than identifying the premise with the answer to a dialectical question, we should suggest that Alexander's premises are propositions expressing the information that the answerer provides in his reply. In fact, all προβλήματα have the structure 'Is S a P or not?' and the answer to such question may simply be a 'Yes' or a 'No'. By choosing to only have a proposition with the syntactic structure 'S is P' as possible premise of an argument, Alexander is departing from natural linguistic practice and embarking on the journey that will eventually lead, as Walton suggested (quoted above), to the repeal of all "subjective" elements in the mathematical logic of the past century.[30]

The absence of an erotetic logic may seem to smooth the endeavour of creating a formal language which may serve science. Indeed, if the only formal language is syllogistic (Alexander) or a revised version of syllogistic with propositional additions (Galen), our logical system is less complex than the collection of systems included in Aristotle's *Organon*. Yet, this absence makes it more difficult to have a logic that captures the very action of a dialectician or of a doc-

a dialectician is against someone and he assumes from questioning the premises from which the object of dispute is inferred. For this reason, the dialectical premise is defined as 'the question concerning two contradictory statements'" (my translation).

28 It should be noted that in principle, all questions that have as an answer a quantified proposition may be construed as questions that offer an alternative between two contradictory statements. In their description of dialectic, Aristotle and Alexander present ideal rules for the most effective dialogue. This notwithstanding, these rules are embedded in every questioning that is aimed at the collection of information, because questions that are not in the form of an alternative between contradictory statements can also be rephrased as such. This idea presupposes the philosophical claim that we gather relevant information only if we are brought to assent to quantified propositions.

29 See *in Top.* 40.20ff. (Wallies).

30 Alexander is regimenting an "ideal dialogue". I do not claim that a dialogue like "Q: What is in the pond? A: A redfish" is meaningless. Rather, I maintain that in the ideal language of dialectic, such a dialogue would have to be rephrased in order to yield information that can be "relevant", i.e., that which can be the starting point of new inferences. Alexander is not devaluing ordinary language, but is rather pointing to the logical rules embedded in ordinary language that enable us to make dialectical inferences. The 20th century idea that logic had to ban every element that could not be represented in a formal language is certainly a consequence of the attention that philosophers of ordinary language like Aristotle and Alexander paid to the rules embedded in ordinary language. This consequence, however, was not intended and it is historically inaccurate to consider Aristotle or Alexander as (grand-)fathers of 20th century insistence on banning "subjective elements" from the realm of logic.

tor who asks questions in order to gather information. One particular aspect is at risk of being lost: the uncertainty of the gathered information. Whenever we are in a dialectical context in which there are questions and answers, we easily realise that all inferences are agreed upon by the two opponents of the dialogues, but this does not rule out that these inferences may actually state a falsity. The human element is shown to be present and this reminds us that we can deceive ourselves. A formal deduction with no reference to any concrete dialogical context inevitably hides the subjective and uncertain character of the deduction. Yet, it is vital to stress the uncertainty of an inference occurring in the context of medicine. In what follows, I would like to focus on the different strategies adopted by Galen and Alexander to make up for the absence of an erotetic logic in their system, in order to explain uncertainty.

3 Expressing Uncertainty. Alexander on Modal Logic as the Underlying Deductive System for Medicine

Galen and Alexander of Aphrodisias were almost contemporaries. Galen died around the year 200 CE, whereas Alexander, whose dates of birth and death are unknown, must have been active towards the end of the 2nd or the beginning of the 3rd century CE. Some Arabic biographers talk about a clash that allegedly took place between Alexander and Galen.[31] Both of them shared the idea that doctors should know logic to practice medicine. Alexander, however, does not provide a lengthy discussion of the topic, having devoted only few pages to the subject. One might be tempted to state that Alexander and Galen had a similar approach to medicine, even though the latter developed the idea that logic is necessary for medicine in more details. Despite this similar approach, however, I maintain that Galen and Alexander understood the relationship between logic and medicine in a different way. Consequently, their understanding of medicine can be said to be different too.

31 See Fazzo (2002) on this issue, also the appendix in Meeusen's chapter. Fazzo convincingly argues that the clash between Galen and Alexander, attested by some Arabic sources, is a mere legend. I share her conclusion and I would like to stress that my comparison between the two authors is a mere theoretical endeavour that aims at assessing the philosophical strength of their respective conceptions of medicine. I do not assume that Galen was in contact with Alexander, nor that he read Alexander. Similarly, there is no strong evidence that Alexander read Galen, although he does refer to Galen as an example of a philosopher in *in Top.* 549.24 (Wallies), and reactions to Galen, without naming him, have been suspected in several of Alexander's works, see Donini (1971) and (1974: 157–173). Thanks to Michiel Meeusen for pointing this out to me.

The radical difference between Alexander and Galen lies, in my opinion, in the fact that Alexander has a modal logic, whereas Galen does not.[32] As is well known, Galen's treatise *De demonstratione* is lost,[33] but we can reconstruct Galen's logical theory from his *Institutio logica*, edited by K. Kalbfleisch in 1896.[34] The *Institutio logica* has been preserved by one single manuscript, which is often corrupted, but it is sufficient for us to have a fair picture of Galen's understanding of the domains of logic. Many scholars have underlined the fusion of Peripatetic and Stoic elements in Galen's logic. Besides categorical syllogisms,[35] Galen talks about propositional inferences too—a topic that might have been inspired by Stoic logic.[36] Furthermore, Galen has an interesting section on relational logic.[37] There is, however, no section on modal logic. This absence is not without consequences. This will become clearer if one pays attention to the role of contingency syllogistic within Alexander's own account of medicine.[38] In his commentary on Aristotle's *Prior Analytics*, Alexander writes:

> For some natural events are indeed proved on such a basis, and there are some arts concerned with what is in this way contingent—for instance, the conjectural arts. A doctor assumes that someone who is ill in such-and-such a way is for the most part unwell from surfeit, and that someone who is unwell from surfeit is for the most part cured by venesection; and

32 Logic is the discipline that deals with valid inferences. Inferences may be presented as arguments with two or more premises and a conclusion. We speak of modal logic when the language in which these sentences are expressed includes modal operators, such as 'it is necessary that …' or 'it is possible that …'. In the Middle Ages, philosophers noted that, if the non-modal syntax of a proposition included a quantifier, a subject-term, a copula and a predicate-term, the copula could be *modified* by an adverb. In the sentence 'Socrates is sharply replying to Plato', the adverb 'sharply' *modifies* the copula of the sentence. Not all modifiers are *modes* considered by logicians, but only modifiers such as 'necessarily', 'contingently', 'possibly' and 'impossibly' (see, e.g., Thomas Aquinas, *De propositionibus modalibus*, ed. Gauthier).

33 On this lost work see Chiaradonna (2009).

34 For an essential bibliography on Galen's logic see footnote 12.

35 Categorical syllogisms are syllogisms without any modal qualifier. Aristotle expounds categorical syllogisms in *Prior Analytics* 1.1–2, 4–7.

36 By 'propositional inference' I refer to inferences, the validity of which does not rely on the connection of terms (as in the case of syllogisms), but rather on the connection of propositions, as in the case of the *modus ponendo ponens* (e.g., i. if it rains, I will not go to the train station; ii. it rains; hence, iii. I will not go to the train station).

37 See *Inst. Log.* 16 (Kalbfleisch).

38 Contingency syllogistic is the section of modal syllogistic that deals with syllogisms with contingency premises.

> he deduces that it is contingent that someone who is ill in this way will be cured by venesection. Taking this to be so, he performs a venesection. For this reason, there is a syllogistic utility in these things.[39]
>
> transl. BARNES et al. (1991: 98)

Medicine, Alexander states, is among the "conjectural arts" (τέχναι στοχαστικαί).[40] Alexander understands the task of the doctor as collecting certain evidence that can be employed to deduce whether a certain surgical operation or a certain cure is applicable to a particular case. In the above passage, Alexander seems to be distinguishing the task of the physician into two steps: diagnosis and therapy. Both steps lead to formulation of contingency statements, which will be the premises of a contingency syllogism. This contingency syllogism will conclude that a certain treatment is likely to cure a certain disease that manifests itself with certain symptoms. This syllogism has the following structure.

(1) A symptomatic phenomenon A is contingently caused by cause B.
(2) Cause B is contingently cured by the operation C.
(3) Therefore, a symptomatic phenomenon A is contingently cured by the operation C.[41]

On the basis of the conclusion of this syllogism, the doctor can infer the *practical* conclusion that the patient has to undergo operation C.

Modal logic is thus essential to medicine for Alexander of Aphrodisias. For medicine is defined as a conjectural art, i.e., as an art that obtains its effect in some cases, but not in all. Consequently, the underlying logic that has to be adopted by the doctors is contingency syllogistic. There are at least two philosophical reasons for this conclusion.

(1) According to Alexander, there are only two truth-values: the truth and the falsity. Consequently, there is no way to express the epistemic uncertainty of certain knowers by means of additional truth-values, like an hypothetical 'probable' (τὸ πιθανόν).[42] If a doctor does not know with certainty if 'symptom A is always caused by disease B', he or she will state that 'symptom A is caused by disease B in some cases, but not in all'.

---

39 *In An. Pr.* 39.30–40.5 (Wallies): καὶ εἰσί τινες τέχναι περὶ τὸ οὕτως ἐνδεχόμενον, ὡς αἱ στοχαστικαί· λαβὼν γὰρ ὁ ἰατρὸς τὸ τὸν οὕτως νοσοῦντα ὡς ἐπὶ τὸ πλεῖστον ὑπὸ πλήθους ἐνοχλεῖσθαι καὶ τὸ τὸν ὑπὸ τοῦ πλήθους ἐνοχλούμενον ὡς ἐπὶ τὸ πλεῖστον διὰ φλεβοτομίας θεραπεύεσθαι συνάγει τὸ τὸν οὕτως νοσοῦντα ἐνδέχεσθαι ὑπὸ φλεβοτομίας θεραπευθῆναι, ὃ λαβὼν χρῆται τῇ φλεβοτομίᾳ. διὸ καὶ ἔστιν ἐν συλλογιστικῇ χρείᾳ.

40 See *in An. Pr.* 165.8–10 (Wallies): πολλαὶ τέχναι στοχαστικαὶ [...] ὡς ἰατρική.

41 What happens 'for the most part' (ὡς ἐπὶ τὸ πλεῖστον) happens 'contingently', according to Alexander (see Gili [2012: 57–59] for this doctrine).

42 I thank Michiel Meeusen for bringing this to my attention.

(2) Within Alexander's semantic framework for modal propositions, a necessity proposition is true if the predicate *always* holds of the subject; analogously, a contingency proposition is true if the predicate holds of the subject *at least on certain occasions*. The adverb 'always' and the adverbial expression 'at least on certain occasions' refer to either instants of time or situations.

Consequently, Alexander will adopt contingency syllogistic as the logic that suits medicine, because medicine is a conjectural art. The fact that it is 'conjectural' seems to refer to the epistemic hindrances that doctors have in formulating judgements with certainty, because Alexander considers conjectural other disciplines like the art of navigation or gymnastics. In both navigation and gymnastics there are events that escape human control, such as contrary winds or the inability of a particular diet or exercise, that are proven effective in other athletes, to bring a particular athlete to the physical condition he or she desires. Referring to Aristotle's intention to talk about contingency syllogistic, Alexander notes:

> He [sc. Aristotle] promises to speak about the other kind of contingency because there are many arts which are conjectural and deduce something under consideration on the basis of what is contingent in this way, for example, medicine, navigation, gymnastics. But also, in general, things based on deliberation are proved by means of this kind of contingency. For example, if someone were to inquire whether he ought to sail now and he argued as follows: when the winds have been judged favourable, those who sail get through safely for the most part; now the winds have been judged favourable; therefore those who sail now will get through safely for the most part.[43]
>
> transl. MUELLER—GOULD (1999: 103)

In his example, Alexander does not expand the uncertainty that is related to medicine or gymnastics, but we can have a hunch on what he might have said by inspecting the example of navigation, which he develops in full.[44]

---

43 *In An. Pr.* 165.8–14 (Wallies): περὶ δὲ τοῦ ἑτέρου ἐρεῖν ἐπαγγέλλεται, ὅτι πολλαὶ τέχναι στοχαστικαὶ οὖσαι ἐκ τοῦ οὕτως ἐνδεχομένου τὸ προκείμενον συλλογίζονται, ὡς ἰατρική, κυβερνητική, γυμναστική. ἀλλὰ καὶ ὅλως τὰ ἐκ τοῦ βουλεύεσθαι λαμβανόμενα διὰ τοιούτου ἐνδεχομένου δείκνυται· οἷον εἰ ζητοίη τις, εἰ νῦν δεῖ πλεῦσαι, καὶ λάβοι, ὅτι, ὅτε κεκριμένα τὰ πνεύματά ἐστιν, οἱ πλέοντες ὡς ἐπὶ τὸ πολὺ σῴζονται· νῦν δὲ κεκριμένα τὰ πνεύματα· οἱ νῦν ἄρα πλέοντες ὡς ἐπὶ τὸ πολὺ σωθήσονται.

44 I thank Suzanne Bobzien for discussion on this point. See Ierodiakonou (1995) on Alexander's understanding of medicine as a stochastic art.

These examples are partly taken from Aristotle. In *Nichomachean Ethics* 2.2.1104a3–10 Aristotle intends to illustrate what holds ὡς ἐπὶ τὸ πολύ and points to the examples of medicine and navigation. They both involve some deliberation and do not always attain their aim—i.e., healing the patient and safely reaching the harbour. The example of gymnastics is added by Alexander, presumably because gymnastics also involves deliberation and does not always attain its aim, i.e., to build muscles or to win a sports competition. Even if the knower does not know with certainty whether any statement within medicine or navigation is *always* true, he or she knows—and with certainty—whether it is true *for the most part*. Consequently, all propositions that express the judgement of the doctor or of the helmsman or the trainer are contingency propositions.

In order to guide their actions and their decisions, doctors, as well as helmsmen or trainers, need to make inferences on the basis of what they know. The ultimate conclusion of their inferences will be a practical judgement that will guide their actions. Alexander believes that syllogistic is the system that encompasses all possible inferences.[45] Consequently, all the inferences made by a doctor are syllogisms too; more particularly, they are contingency syllogisms.

4 Galen on Uncertainty in Medicine

Galen also shares many of the points that Alexander maintains, but does not have a modal logic. We cannot reconstruct with accuracy the content of Galen's lost treatise *De demonstratione*, but R. Chiaradonna has abundantly shown that the treatise presented an 'applied epistemology'.[46] According to Chiaradonna, Galen understands logic as 'useful' to other disciplines, in the same way as Alexander does.[47] By being useful, logic plays the role of the theory of deduction in

45 See *in An. Pr.* 255.34–260.6; 340.5–341.4 (Wallies).

46 According to Chiaradonna's (2009) reconstruction, Galen's *De demonstratione* was certainly not a logic treatise, nor a general theory of science in the vein of Aristotle's *Posterior Analytics*: it was rather a treatise that aimed at showing how to do science in specific contexts.

47 See Chiaradonna (2009: 48): "Galien et Alexandre partagent la même thèse générale: dans la logique, il ne faut étudier que ce qui sert à construire des démonstrations (cf. Alex. Aphr., *in An. Pr.* 164.25–165.2 (Wallies)). Barnes souligne une différence entre les conceptions de ces deux auteurs: Alexandre est un philosophe péripatéticien qui, en tant que tel, défend le programme de son école, selon lequel la syllogistique catégorique peut satisfaire à toutes les exigences de la science. Galien, en revanche, montre une attitude éclectique, se gardant de suivre les doctrines d'une seule école."

a discipline. An art or a science is thus understood as a set of basic propositions and as a deductive system capable of inferring conclusions from this set.

Medicine can be understood in these terms, according to both Galen and Alexander. Alexander pledges allegiance to the doctrine expounded by Aristotle in his *Posterior Analytics*. Galen, on the other hand, recognises that the school of Aristotle and Theophrastus has been the best at outlining the theory of demonstration[48] and this may explain why he also adopts a deductive framework for his medical arguments. More importantly, Galen believes that the best doctor is also a philosopher, inasmuch as medicine is a 'rational' endeavour.[49]

They differ, however, in selecting the deductive system for medicine. Alexander takes it to be contingency syllogistic, i.e., a system that has as theorems a proper subset of the theorems of logic.[50] Galen, on the other hand, has an eclectic logic, that borrows Stoic and Peripatetic elements and that may be original in some points too. There are no traces of modal arguments in his extant logical writings.[51]

48 See *PHP* 2.2.4 (5.213.8–12 Kühn; 104.3–6 De Lacy).

49 Galen does so in his treatise *Quod optimus medicus sit quoque philosophus* (on which, see below). Fortuna (1987) argues that Galen states that philosophy and logic are necessary for good doctors simply because he is opposing other doctors. In other contexts, Galen criticises philosophy (especially in the *Placita Hippocratis et Platonis*). According to Fortuna, "la duplicità dello statuto della medicina in Galeno rimane, dunque, un fatto sostanzialmente aporetico: evidentemente è per Galeno nozione complessa e problematica, le cui soluzioni e formulazioni dipendono anche dagli argomenti che si trova ad affrontare e dal pubblico che vuole raggiungere" (196). In Fortuna's view, the ambiguity of Galen's notion of medicine lies in the fact that medicine is alternatively considered a productive art or a rational art. Similar remarks appear in Vegetti (1981) and Vegetti (1994). Even though I share's Fortuna's assessment of Galen's substantial ambiguity on the notion of medicine, I would like to stress that there is no conflict between a productive and a rational art, if "rational" involves making rational arguments. All doctors have to make a practical syllogism when they have to make therapeutic decisions.

50 As I stated above, Alexander understands logic to be identical with syllogistic, i.e., with the formal system(s) outlined by Aristotle in *Prior Analytics* 1.1–22. The theorems of contingency syllogistic, i.e., the valid moods with contingency premises and conclusions, are a proper subset of the theorems of logic, i.e., of the systems of categorical and of modal syllogistic.

51 I base this claim on Chiaradonna's reconstruction of the topics included in the treatise *De demonstratione* (see Chiaradonna [2009: esp. 45]) and on Galen's *Institutio logica*. It is certainly possible that Galen had a modal logic and that he expounded it in his lost logical works (for a list of his logical works see *De libris propriis* 11–12 [19.39.1–45.8 Kühn; 115.19–121.4 Müller; 164.1–169.12 Boudon-Millot]; B. Morison analyzes the list in Morison [2008: 66–70]). However, there is no evidence of the application of modal logic in his non-logical writings. This seems to suggest that Galen simply did not adopt modal logic because he did

It should be stressed that Galen maintains that logic is needed in the three essential aspects of medical practice: diagnostics, prognostics and therapy.[52] Accordingly, doctors should be trained in logic, because otherwise they cannot exercise their art.

> Most doctors, without first training in the logical methods, either attempt to demonstrate something and deceive themselves by fallacy, or else attempt to divide something into its species and differentia and then, like bad cooks, do not cut at the joints.[53]
>
> transl. BARNES (1991: 65)

Galen maintains that the starting point of an argument should be what is held to be true by all human beings, i.e., what is undisputed (see *Meth. Med.* 1.4 [10.32 Kühn], 1.5 [10.40 Kühn], 1.7 [10.50 Kühn]). Only what is commonly agreed upon by all human beings can serve as a principle of a demonstration.

In so doing, Galen clearly distances himself from the methodic and the empiricist schools of medicine. The so-called methodic school included doctors who claimed that they were not interested in the theoretical aspects of medicine, but only in the 'method' of healing the patients.[54] The empiricists, on the contrary, maintained that it is possible to diagnose diseases on the basis of their symptoms. Empiricists claim that nothing but the ability to recognise and catalogue symptoms is required from a good doctor.

Galen was the author of a treatise in which he claims that the best doctor is a philosopher too (*Quod optimus medicus sit quoque philosophus*).[55] According to Galen, a doctor has to be versed in logic, philosophy, anatomy, physiology. While expounding the method that a doctor has to follow in diagnostics and in therapeutics, Galen observes that the doctor has to yield demonstrations (this observation is similar to Alexander's claim that physicians use syllogistic in their practice). It is not surprising then to read that Galen refers to his *De demonstratione* in the treatise on the *Method of Medicine*.

---

not need it to account for the uncertainty that is embedded in the inferences that doctors do by asking questions to their patients.

52 See Barnes (1991) for this claim.

53 *Meth. Med.* 2.6 (10.123.1–6 Kühn): ὅσοι [sc. ἰατροί] πρὶν γυμνάσασθαι κατὰ τὰς λογικὰς μεθόδους ἢ ἀποδεικνύναι τι πειρώμενοι παραλογίζονται σφᾶς αὐτούς, ἢ διαιρεῖν ὁτιοῦν εἰς εἴδη τε καὶ διαφοράς, εἶτα κἀνταῦθα κακῶν μαγείρων δίκην οὐ κατ' ἄρθρα τέμνουσιν.

54 On the methodic school see Edelstein (1987), Frede (1982) and Fortuna (2001). On the empiricist 'school' and in general on the debates among ancient school of medicine see Hankinson (2008b).

55 See footnote 49.

> I shall now set out in order for you the whole argument using the methods which I established in my work *On demonstration*. It was shown in those writings that the origins of every demonstration are the things clearly apparent to sensation and reason.[56]
>
> transl. JOHNSTON—HORSLEY (2011)

As is clear from its context, the above passage deals with demonstrations that aim at diagnosing disease. Galen tackles therapeutics later on in his *Method of Medicine* 3.7 (10.204.7–211.4 Kühn). There, Galen argues against the Methodists, who were claiming that one single therapeutic method is able to heal all diseases. Contrary to the Methodists, Galen maintains that once the disease is discovered, and the condition of the patient is clear, there is a specific therapy that should be applied. Galen believes that there is an argument that has the effect of determining which specific cure should be prescribed to a particular patient.

It seems that Galen needs a logic as a frame in which these arguments are presented. He is aware of that. However, he seems not to have employed any modal logic, which would have enabled him to account for the uncertainty embedded in the premises of a medical inference. Chiaradonna observes that Galen's method includes both axiomatic and stochastic aspects.[57] As is clear from his article, Chiaradonna mistakenly maintains that a discipline is "axiomatic" if its inferences display the necessity operator in both premises and conclusions, as is the case in the paradigmatic axiomatic discipline of mathematics. Hence, Galen appears to be confused about the status of medicine because the presence of axiomatic and stochastic aspects is tantamount to confusion if one adopts Chiaradonna's interpretations. However, the references that Chiaradonna provides to substantiate his claim do not support the thesis that Galen was confused about the status of medicine.[58] In *Meth. Med.* 1.4 (10.33.7–34.5 Kühn), Galen compares medicine with logic and with geometry. The analogy is possible because all three disciplines have an underlying deductive system. This deductive system is axiomatic and, in this sense, Chiaradonna is right in claiming that Galen's understanding of medicine includes "axiomatic aspects". Galen makes the following remarks:

56 *Meth. Med.* 1.5 (10.39.5–9 Kühn): Καί σοι τὸν ἑξῆς λόγον ἤδη ἅπαντα ποιήσομαι, χρώμενος ταῖς μεθόδοις ἃς ἐν τοῖς περὶ τῆς ἀποδείξεως ὑπομνήμασι κατεστησάμην. ὅτι τε γὰρ ἀρχαὶ πάσης ἀποδείξεώς εἰσι τὰ πρὸς αἴσθησίν τε καὶ νόησιν ἐναργῶς φαινόμενα.

57 Chiaradonna (2014: 81).

58 In order to support his interpretation, Chiaradonna (2014) focuses mostly on two texts: *Meth. Med.* 1.4 (10.33.7–34.5 Kühn) and 3.9 (10.217.13–15 Kühn).

> So in the demonstrations regarding the triangle [...] the proposition itself was reached from these two premises: the first is that the area enclosed by the five feet and the twelve feet is sixty feet, and the second is the claim that the triangle is half that area, and showing that it is. However, each of these again requires certain other premises for demonstration, then those others again, until we come to those premises that are primary, which no longer have their proof from one another or from demonstration, but from themselves. The same applies too, I think, in the case of demonstrations in the medical craft. In all instances, there must be reduction to certain primary and indemonstrable premises, and from these all things must draw their proof. Indeed, if everyone attempted to say something about the therapeutic method in this way, they would be in harmony with each other in every respect, just like arithmeticians, geometers, and logicians.[59]
>
> transl. JOHNSTON—HORSLEY (2011)

In the above passage, Galen maintains that all disagreements among doctors belonging to different schools would disappear if doctors were to make inferences the way arithmeticians, geometers and logicians do. According to Galen, doctors should be able to show how a certain conclusion can be inferred from "certain primary and indemonstrable premises" (πρώτας τινὰς ἀναποδείκτους προτάσεις). The suggestion to present medicine in an axiomatic form is not an unattainable goal, otherwise Galen would not insist on this methodological proposal. Since the starting points in any process of information-gathering are the same for all human beings,[60] any disagreement among physicians would

59 *Meth. Med.* 1.4 (10.33.7–34.5 Kühn): ὡς οὖν τῆς κατὰ τὸ τρίγωνον ἀποδείξεως, [...] αὐτὸ μὲν τὸ προκείμενον ἐκ δυοῖν τούτων ἐπεραίνετο προτάσεων, μιᾶς μὲν τῆς τὸ περιεχόμενον χωρίον ὑπό τε τῆς πεντάποδος καὶ δωδεκάποδος, ἑξηκοντάπουν γίγνεσθαι, δευτέρας δὲ τῆς ἥμισυ τρίγωνον ἐκείνου τοῦ χωρίου λεγούσης καὶ δεικνυούσης ὑπάρχειν, ἑκατέρα δὲ πάλιν τούτων ἑτέρων τινῶν εἰς ἀπόδειξιν ἐδεῖτο προτάσεων, εἶτ' ἐκεῖναι πάλιν ἑτέτινῶν εἰς ἀπόδειξιν ἐδεῖτο προτάσεων, εἶτ' ἐκεῖναι πάλιν ἑτέρων, ἄχρί περ ἂν ἐπὶ τὰς πρώτας ἀνέλθωμεν, αἱ δὲ οὐκ ἐξ ἄλλων, οὐδὲ δι' ἀποδείξεως, ἀλλ' ἐξ ἑαυτῶν ἔχουσι τὴν πίστιν, οὕτως, οἶμαι, κἀπὶ τῶν τὴν ἰατρικὴν τέχνην ἀποδεικνυ μένων ἁπάντων εἰς πρώτας τινὰς ἀναποδείκτους προτάσεις καὶ ἐξ ἑαυτῶν πιστὰς ἀνάγεσθαι χρῆναι πάντα. καὶ εἴπερ οὕτως ἅπαντες ἐπεχείρησαν εἰπεῖν τι περὶ τῆς θεραπευτικῆς μεθόδου, πάντως ἄν που καὶ συνεφώνησαν ἀλλήλοις, ὥσπερ οἱ ἀριθμητικοί τε καὶ γεωμέτραι καὶ οἱ λογιστικοί.

60 Cf. *Inst. Log.* 1.1 (Kalbfleisch) for this claim. According to Galen, all knowledge is either empirical, or intuitive, or derived from experience or from intellectual intuition by means of an argument. Hence, the ultimate starting points of any demonstration that yields new information should be empirical. Empirical and intuitive data are the same for all human beings, presumably because they all have the same five senses and the same intellect.

be about the procedural ways in which a conclusion has been derived from the principles, as is the case for the disagreements among geometers, arithmeticians and logicians. They sometimes disagree as well, but there is a method to verify who is right and who is wrong, by simply examining the deductive chains that led to different conclusions. Galen's dream is to turn medicine into a discipline similar to logic or mathematics in that there is an objective procedure to solve disagreements among physicians. But the axiomatic presentation of medicine will nevertheless be compatible with a 'stochastic' conception of its results. There is no incompatibility between having an axiomatic system and inferring contingency conclusions within this system: contingency syllogistic is certainly stochastic and axiomatic in this sense. And even though Galen does not adopt contingency syllogistic as his preferred theory of deduction, he has enough logical resources to create an axiomatic system that is capable of expressing the uncertainty that is inevitably involved in the medical practice.[61] Chiaradonna seems not to be aware that axiomatic presentations and stochastic premises are compatible with each other and he confuses the necessity of the consequence (*necessitas consequentiae*), that is granted by an axiomatic system, with the necessity of the consequent (*necessitas consequentis*).[62] The other passage considered by Chiaradonna does not support any 'stochastic' reading of Galen's theory of deduction: in *Meth. Med.* 3.9 (10.217.13 Kühn) Galen simply states that some conclusions "are arrived at by guesswork (στοχασμῷ λαμβάνεται), and that someone practiced in calculations about these matters is best able to carry out the estimation" (transl. Johnston—Horsley [2011]).[63] Galen is not speaking of the formal reconstruction of the physician's argument, but is rather describing the very process of information-gathering that the doctor performs in his practice. As we stated above, this process involves uncertainty, because it relies on probable, but not necessary, foundations (e.g., among the premises of the physician's inquiry there are the answers provided by the patient, who might be mistaken about the very symptoms of her/his condition). If the doctor arrives at certain conclusions 'by guesswork', the conclu-

61 According to Chiaradonna (2014), Galen has a mere epistemic notion of contingency. This is certainly consistent with Galen's conception of causation, which does not seem to make room for any metaphysical contingency. For my present purpose it is sufficient to stress that, regardless of Galen's philosophical understanding of contingency—be it metaphysical or epistemic—, the Greek doctor has to find a way to express contingency with the linguistic resources of his logical system.

62 The *necessitas consequentiae* is a necessity that modifies the whole inference, the *necessitas consequentis* modifies the conclusion of an inference.

63 *Meth. Med.* 3.9 (10.217.13–15 Kühn): ὅτι δὲ ἅπαντα ταῦτα στοχασμῷ λαμβάνεται καὶ ὅτι κάλλιστα δυνατός ἐστι στοχάζεσθαι ὁ γεγυμνασμένος ἐν τοῖς περὶ τούτων λογισμοῖς ἄντικρυς δῆλον.

sions are uncertain. This, however, is not incompatible with the formal systematisation of the very process of information-gathering, because Galen believes that all such processes can, in principle, be expressed with the syntactic and semantic resources of his logical language.[64] Galen can thus be faithful to an axiomatic presentation of science without stating that a doctor's conclusions are necessary truths, because in the process of discovery they are "arrived at by guesswork" (στοχασμῷ λαμβάνεται). But if Galen's logic does not include contingency premises, how can he account for the epistemically weak status of certain premises and of a certain conclusion? Chiaradonna does not explicitly addresses the issue. His article, however, suggests that Galen has premises that *describe* as credible (but not necessary) the starting point of the inference. One might think that Galen would have to adopt two strategies, depending on the type of inference. In the case of a propositional inference, the uncertainty of a premise can be embedded with expressions such as 'it is probable that', 'probably' etc.[65] In the case of a syllogistic inference, the addition of an adverb like 'probably', 'contingently' etc. should be understood as a logical component of the predicate and not of the copula, because Galen's logic does not contemplate any modalised copula.[66]

---

64 Galen makes this statement in *Inst. Log.* 1.4 (Kalbfleisch): ἡ δὲ πᾶσα λέξις δι' ἧς ὁμολογηθέντων τινῶν ἐπιφέρεταί τι συμπέρασμα, συμπέρασμά τε προσαγορεύεται καὶ τοῦτ' αὐτὸ καὶ συλλογισμός.

65 An example of such an inference would be the following:
a) If it is probable that the patient suffers from illness I, the patient should probably be treated with treatment T.
b) It is probable that the patient suffers from illness I.
c) Hence, the patient should probably be treated with treatment T.
The above argument is a non-modal *modus ponendo ponens* and Galen does not need any modal operator to express the uncertainty of both premises and conclusion.

66 Consider the following example:
a) All patients who display symptom S are probably affected by illness I.
b) All patients in the waiting room are patients who display symptom S.
c) Hence, all patients in the waiting room are probably affected by illness I.
In Galen's formalisation, the predicate of the major premise and of the conclusion is 'probably affected by illness I' and the syllogism is a non-modal *Barbara*. In Alexander of Aphrodisias' formalisation, the predicate of the major premise and of the conclusion is 'affected by illness I' and the syllogism is a *Barbara* QXQ, i.e., a *Barbara* with contingency major premise, categorical minor premise and contingency conclusion. It is worth stressing that the two philosophers differ in their formal reconstruction of the physician's argument because their logical languages have different syntactic resources, but they are analyzing an identical process of information-gathering that includes a series of questions by means of which a physician tries to figure out which are the symptoms displayed by a group of patients.

5 Conclusion

The whole medical inference is a dialogue in which the doctor (or his helpers) ask questions in order to gather information from the patient. But all processes of information-gathering can be rephrased in a formal way according to both Galen and Alexander. When a doctor trained in logic rephrases in the ideal language of logic a real dialogue that took place with a concrete patient, the doctor can eliminate the question-and-answer structure from the inference, but cannot eliminate the uncertainty of the information collected from the answers of the patient. Unlike Alexander, Galen cannot formally represent with syntactic operators the epistemic discrepancy between sets of premises of different epistemic value. This, however, does not mean that Galen's medicine is a system that only includes arguments with necessary premises and necessary conclusions. Contrary to Alexander, the epistemically weak status of certain premises has to be embedded in the premises themselves. Both philosophers maintain that doctors are often *uncertain* about the truth of the premises of their inferences. The Peripatetic doctors will resort to contingency syllogisms to account for this uncertainty. The Galenic doctors will use non-modal inferences where premises are understood to be uncertain.

Even if Galen and Alexander agree in maintaining that medicine can be formally represented as an axiomatic deductive system, the logical languages of their deductive systems are different. Alexander has modal logic at his disposal, Galen does not. And this cannot but lead to radically different understandings of medicine as a deductive system.

Acknowledgements

I thank Jan Opsomer and Gerd Van Riel for their comments on my paper at the Leuven conference and Michiel Meeusen for his invaluable comments on an earlier draft of this paper. On April 15, 2019, I presented this paper a second time at the University of Verona at the kind invitation of Linda Napolitano within the framework of the Asklepios conferences. I thank Linda Napolitano and Alessandro Stavru for their comments on that occasion. Any remaining mistakes are only mine.

Bibliography

Primary Sources

Boudon-Millot, V. 2007. *Galien 1. Introduction générale. Sur l'ordre de ses propres livres. Sur ses propres livres. Que l'excellent médecin est aussi philosophe*. Paris: Les Belles Lettres.

De Lacy, P. 1978. *Galen, On the doctrines of Hippocrates and Plato* [CMG 5.4.1.2]. Berlin: Akademie-Verlag.

Gärtner, F. 2015. *Galeni De locis affectis I–II* [CMG v.6.1.1]. Berlin: De Gruyter.

Helmreich, G. 1893. *Claudii Galeni Pergameni Scripta Minora, vol. 3*. Leipzig: Teubner.

Kalbfleisch, K. 1896. *Galenus, Institutio logica*. Leipzig: Teubner.

Kühn, C.G. 1821–1833. *Claudii Galeni Opera Omnia*. Leipzig: Car. Cnoblochii.

Müller, I. 1891. *Claudii Galeni Pergameni Scripta Minora, vol. 2*. Leipzig: Teubner.

Wallies, M. 1883. *Alexandri Aphrodisiensis in Aristotelis Analyticorum Priorum librum primum commentarium*. Berlin: Reimer.

Wallies, M. 1891. *Alexandri Aphrodisiensis in Aristotelis Topicorum libros octo commentaria*. Berlin: Reimer.

Walzer, R. 1944. *Galen on Medical Experience*. Oxford: Oxford University Press.

Translations and Secondary Sources

Alqvist, L. 1975. *A New Approach to the Logical Theory of Interrogatives*. Tübingen: Günter Narr Verlag.

Barnes, J. (ed.). 1984. *The Revised Oxford Translation of Aristotle*. Princeton: Princeton University Press.

Barnes, J. 1991. 'Galen on Logic and Therapy', in F. Kudlien—R.J. Durling (eds.), *Galen's Method of Healing*. Leiden—New York—Kobenhavn—Köln: Brill, 50–102.

Barnes, J.—Bobzien, S.—Flannery, K.—Ierodiakonou, K. 1991. *Alexander of Aphrodisias. On Aristotle, Prior Analytics 1.1–7*. London: Duckworth.

Chiaradonna, R. 2009. 'Le traité de Galien *Sur la démonstration* et sa postérité tardo-antique', in R. Chiaradonna—F. Trabattoni (eds.), *Physics and Philosophy of Nature in Greek Neoplatonism*. Leiden: Brill, 43–77.

Chiaradonna, R. 2014. 'Galen on What is Persuasive (*Pithanon*) and What Approximates to Truth', in P. Adamson—R. Hansberger—J. Wilberding (eds.), *Philosophical Themes in Galen*. London: Institute of Classical Studies, 58–88.

Dancy, R. 1975. *Sense and Contradiction*. Dordrecht: D. Reidel.

Donini, P.L. 1971. 'L'anima e gli elementi nel *De Anima* di Alessandro di Afrodisia', *Atti della Academia delle Scienze di Torino, classe di scienze morali, storiche e filologiche* 105: 61–107.

Donini, P.L. 1974. *Tre studi sull' aristotelismo nel II secolo d.C.* Turin: Paravia.

Duncombe, M.—Dutilh Novaes, C. 2016. 'Dialectic and Logic in Aristotle and His Tradition', *History and Philosophy of Logic* 37: 1–8.

Dutilh Novaes, C. 2015. 'A Dialogical, Multi-Agent Account of the Normativity of Logic', *Dialectica* 69/4: 587–609.
Edelstein, L. 1987. 'The Methodists', in O. Temkin—C.L. Temkin (eds.), *Ancient Medicine. Selected Papers of Ludwig Edelstein*. Baltimore—London: John Hopkins University Press, 173–191.
Fazzo, S. 2002. 'Alexandre d' Aphrodise contre Galien: la naissance d' une légende', *Philosophie Antique* 2: 109–144.
Frede, M. 1982. 'On the So-Called Methodical School of Medicine', in J. Barnes—J. Brunschwig—M. Burnyeat—M. Schofield (eds.), *Science and Speculation. Studies in Hellenistic Theory and Practice*. Cambridge: Cambridge University Press, 1–23.
Fortuna, S. 1987. 'La definizione della medicina in Galeno', *La Parola del Passato* 234: 181–196.
Fortuna, S. 2001. 'Il metodo della diagnosi in Galeno (*De locis affectis*, VIII, 1–452 K.)', *Elenchos* 22: 281–304.
Giannantoni, G. 2005. *Dialogo socratico e nascita della dialettica nella filosofia di Platone*, edited by B. Centrone, Naples: Bibliopolis (*Elenchos* 43).
Gili, L. 2011. *La sillogistica di Alessandro di Afrodisia. Sillogistica categorica e sillogistica modale nel commento agli* Analitici Primi *di Aristotele*. Hildesheim—Zürich—New York: Georg Olms.
Gili, L. 2012. 'Alexander of Aphrodisias' Solution to the Puzzle of the Two Barbaras: A Semantic Approach', *Documenti e studi sulla tradizione filosofica medievale* 23: 35–64.
Gottschalk, H. 1987. 'Aristotelian Philosophy in the Roman World', in W. Haase (ed.), *Aufstieg und Niedergang der römischen Welt* 2.36.1. Berlin: De Gruyter, 1079–174.
Hankinson, R.J. (ed.). 2008a. *The Cambridge Companion to Galen*. Cambridge: Cambridge University Press.
Hankinson, R.J. 2008b. 'Epistemology', in Hankinson (2008a: 157–183).
Hintikka, J. 1981. 'On the Logic of an Interrogative Model of Scientific Inquiry', *Synthese* 47/1: 69–83.
Ierodiakonou, K. 1995. 'Alexander of Aphrodisias on Medicine as a Stochastic Art', in P. van der Eijk—H.F.J. Horstmanshoff—P.H. Schrijvers (eds.), *Ancient Medicine in Its Socio-Cultural Context*. Amsterdam—Atlanta: Rodopi, 473–485.
Irwin, T. 1988. *Aristotle's First Principles*. Oxford: Clarendon Press.
Johnston, I.—Horsley, G.H.R. 2011. *Galen, Method of Medicine*, 3 vols. Cambridge, Mass.: Harvard University Press.
Kieffer, J.S. 1964. *Galen's Institutio Logica*. Baltimore: The John Hopkins Press.
Kleiner, S.A. 1993. *The Logic of Discovery. A Theory of the Rationality of Scientific Research*. Dordrecht—Boston—London: Kluwer Academic Publishers.
Krabbe, E.C.W. 2014. 'Classical Backgrounds', in F.A. van Eemeren et al. (eds.), *Handbook of Argumentation Theory*. Dordrecht: Springer, 51–139.

Lagerlund, E. 2008. 'The Assimilation of Aristotelian and Arabic Logic up until the Later 13th Century', in D. Gabbay—J. Woods (eds.), *Handbook of the History of Logic: Volume 2. Medieval and Renaissance Logic*. Amsterdam: North Holland, 281–346.

Malink, M. 2013. *Aristotle's Modal Syllogistic*. Cambridge, Mass.—London: Harvard University Press.

Marion, M.—Rückert, H. 2015. 'Aristotle on Universal Quantification: A Study from the Point of View of Game Semantics', *History and Philosophy of Logic* 37: 201–229.

Mau, J. 1960. *Galen. Einführung in die Logik. Kritisch-exegetischer Kommentar mit deutschen Übersetzung*. Berlin: Akademie-Verlag.

Moraux, P. 1968. 'La joute dialectique d'après le huitième livre des *Topiques*', in G.E.L. Owen (ed.), *Aristotle on Dialectic. The Topics. Proceedings of the Third Symposium Aristotelicum*. Oxford: Clarendon Press, 277–311.

Morison, B. 2008. 'Logic', in Hankinson (2008a: 66–115).

Mueller, I.—Gould, J. 1999. *Alexander of Aphrodisias. On Aristotle, Prior Analytics 1.8–13*. London: Duckworth.

Pellegrin, P. 1998. *Galien, Traités philosophiques et logiques*. Paris: Flammarion.

Prior, M.—Prior, A. 1955. 'Erotetic Logic', *The Philosophical Review* 64: 43–59.

Rescher, N. 1966. *Galen and the Syllogism. An Examination of the Thesis that Galen Originated the Fourth Figure of the Syllogism in the Light of New Data from Arabic Sources*. Pittsburgh: University of Pittsburgh Press.

Robinson, R. 1953. *Plato's Earlier Dialectic*. Oxford: Clarendon Press.

Sichirollo, L. 2003. *Dialettica*. Rome: Editori Riuniti.

Siegel, R.E. 1976. *Galen, On the Affected Parts*. Basel—New York: S. Karger.

Slomkowski, P. 1997. *Aristotle's Topics*. Leiden—Boston—Köln: Brill.

Smith, R. 1997. *Aristotle, Topics. Books I and VIII with excerpts from related texts*. Oxford: Clarendon Press.

Solmsen, F. 1929. *Die Entwicklung der aristotelischen Logik und Rhetorik*. Berlin: Weidemann.

Stakelum, J.W. 1940. *Galen and the Logic of Proposition*. Rome: Angelicum.

Vegetti, M. 1981. 'Modelli di medicina in Galeno', in V. Nutton (ed.), *Galen: Problems and Prospects*. London: The Wellcome Institute for the History of Medicine, 47–63.

Vegetti, M. 1994. 'L'immagine del medico e lo statuto epistemologico della medicina in Galeno', in W. Haase (ed.), *Aufstieg und Niedergang der römischen Welt* 2.37.2. Berlin—New York: De Gruyter, 1672–717.

Walton, D. 1998. *The New Dialectic. Conversational Contexts of Argument*. Toronto—Buffalo—London: University of Toronto Press.

Walton, D.N.—Krabbe, E.C.W. 1995. *Commitment in Dialogue. Basic Concepts of Interpersonal Reasoning*. Albany: State University of New York Press.

CHAPTER 6

La réponse du médecin : les rapports d'inspection médicale écrits en grec sur papyrus (Ier-IVe siècles)

Antonio Ricciardetto

Résumé

Découverts dans les sables d'Égypte, où ils se sont conservés par centaines de milliers, les papyrus documentaires grecs donnent une foule d'informations sur le genre de vie, l'état sanitaire, l'alimentation, l'hygiène, les accidents, maladies et épidémies des autochtones, ainsi que sur la démographie et l'organisation de la médecine. Parmi ceux-ci, trente et un papyrus d'époques romaine et byzantine (Ier-IVe s. apr. J.-C.) contiennent le rapport d'une inspection conduite par des médecins sur le corps blessé ou malade d'hommes, de femmes et d'enfants de toutes conditions sociales. Dans quel but l'expert est-il mandaté et comment se déroule l'inspection ? À quelles questions est-il chargé de répondre ? Que nous apprennent les observations cliniques consignées sur la condition des patients examinés et sur les pratiques médicales ? Après avoir analysé la structure et le contenu de ces documents, on les comparera à ceux de textes littéraires comme les fiches de malades des *Épidémies* hippocratiques.

1 Introduction

Offrant la possibilité d'établir un contact direct avec les habitants du Pays du Nil, les papyrus apportent une contribution inégalée à la connaissance de la civilisation antique, spécialement dans l'Égypte gréco-romaine et byzantine. La médecine n'échappe pas à cette règle, puisque, parmi les centaines de milliers de papyrus tirés des sables d'Égypte, où le climat chaud et sec a permis leur conservation, plus de cinq cents documents majoritairement écrits en grec ont un contenu médical.[1] Parmi ceux-ci, 31 papyrus d'époque romaine et du début de la période byzantine (Ier-IVe siècles apr. J.-C.) contiennent le rapport (προσφώνησις) d'une inspection conduite par un ou plusieurs experts, le plus souvent

1 Pour un aperçu général sur l'apport des papyrus documentaires à la médecine dans l'Égypte romaine, voir Marganne (1996 : 2725-2733).

des médecins, qui, à partir de la seconde moitié du IIe siècle, portent le titre de « médecin public » (δημόσιος ἰατρός),[2] sur le corps d'hommes, de femmes et d'enfants de toutes conditions sociales, en majorité encore en vie, victimes d'une agression, d'une bagarre, d'un accident ou d'une maladie. Ces rapports donnent une idée d'un type de questions auxquelles l'expert devait répondre dans la pratique de sa profession. Ils s'insèrent dans une procédure administrative et légale qui, telle qu'elle a pu être reconstituée, comprend quatre documents : la pétition, l'ordre, le rapport médical, et, en cas de procès, le compte rendu d'audience.[3]

On compte à ce jour 13 pétitions (βιβλίδιον ou ἔγκλημα ; puis plus tard, λίβελλον) dans lesquelles un individu s'adresse à une autorité, expose sa plainte et demande (ἀξιοῦν) l'intervention d'un expert pour examiner (ἐπιθεωρεῖν, ἐφορᾶν, σημειοῦν) sa condition ou celle d'un de ses proches. Elles sont datées entre le 11 février 167 et le milieu du VIe siècle, et la moitié d'entre elles est antérieure à 284, date à laquelle la majorité des papyrologues font commencer la période byzantine.[4] S'il donne suite à la requête, le stratège charge alors un de ses assistants (ὑπηρέτης)[5] de trouver un expert qui examinera la victime, et de l'accompagner durant l'inspection médicale : c'est l'ordre (ἐπιστολή).[6] Une

2 Les seules exceptions sont le P.Oxy. III 476, où les experts qui inspectent la victime sont deux fossoyeurs, ainsi que le P.Mert. II 89, dans lequel on apprend que l'examen a été conduit par un assistant de l'autorité. Sur le médecin public, et sur les origines de la procédure médico-légale, cf. Ricciardetto (2013 : 109-111).

3 Sur la procédure médico-légale, cf. Ricciardetto (à paraître), qui constitue la version remaniée du chapitre II de ma thèse doctorale (Ricciardetto [2015]). Parmi les études sur les rapports médicaux, il faut citer celles de Sudhoff (1909 : 234-253) ; Nanetti (1941 : 301-314) ; Boswinkel (1956 : 181-190) ; Amundsen – Ferngren (1978 : 336-353) ; Manfredi (2004 : 153-170) ; Torallas Tovar (2004 : 183-200) ; Hirt Raj (2006 : 102-119 et tableau III) ; Mitthof (2007 : 55-63) ; Id. (2008 : 301-318), ainsi que la *Réponse* de B. Legras, dans le même volume, p. 319-324 ; Ricciardetto (2013 : 101-115).

4 Ce sont, par ordre chronologique, P.Harr. II 192 (prov. inconnue, 11 février 167), P.Oxy. XXXI 2563 (Oxyrhynchus, c. 170), C.Pap.Gr. II, app. 1 (Oxyrhynchus, entre février et mai 177), PSI inv. 4153 (identifié à tort comme un rapport médical par S. Russo, l'éditrice du papyrus, dans Ead. – Bastianini [2013 : 62-64] ; Oxyrhynchus, 215/216), P.Flor. I 59 (prov. inconnue, 225, 241 ou 279), P.Oxy. LVIII 3926 (Oxyrhynchus, 9 février 246), P.Oxy. XII 1556 (nome oxyrhynchite, 2 janvier 247), P.Oxy. LXI 4122 (Oxyrhynchus, 22 juin 305), P.Oxy. LI 3620 (Oxyrhynchus, 2 février 326), P.Gron.Amst. 1 (Oxyrhynchus, 14 mars 454), P.Bon. 22 = SB XVIII 13127 (Oxyrhynchus, Ve/VIe siècles), P.Oxy. XVI 1885 (Oxyrhynchus, 29 novembre 509), P.Oxy. XX 2268 (Oxyrhynchus, milieu du VIe siècle ?).

5 Sur l'assistant et son rôle, voir Ricciardetto (2013 : 105-106 n. 14).

6 Il existe deux types d'ordres : directs, quand ils ont été notés sur un coupon contenant aussi une copie de la pétition, et indirects, lorsqu'on ne dispose que d'une allusion à celui-ci dans le rapport médical. On ne connaît à ce jour que deux exemples d'ordre direct, dans deux papyrus d'Oxyrhynchus : P.Oxy. III 475 et LVIII 3926.

fois la victime examinée, un rapport médical, écrit par l'expert, consigne les résultats de l'inspection. Les 31 rapports connus à ce jour sont datés de c. 89/94 à 393 de notre ère, et plus de la moitié d'entre eux remonte au IVe siècle (18 rapports).[7] Même si l'on n'a pas conservé de rapport postérieur à 393, il dut y en avoir bien après cette date, puisqu'on connaît des pétitions avec demande d'inspection médicale jusqu'au VIe siècle. La plupart des rapports proviennent d'Oxyrhynchus, la métropole du nome oxyrhynchite, mais quelques-uns ont été retrouvés dans deux autres métropoles, Hermopolis et Héracléopolis, ainsi que dans le nome arsinoïte. Le nombre restreint de rapports provenant de cette région pourtant riche en découvertes papyrologiques, s'explique par le fait que celles-ci n'ont pas été faites dans la métropole du nome, où étaient conservées les archives, mais dans des villages. Jusqu'ici, aucun rapport médical n'a été découvert au sud d'Hermopolis.[8] Comme le montrent deux comptes rendus d'audience, le rapport médical, qui décrit les conséquences d'une agression, d'une maladie ou d'un accident, peut être utilisé comme preuve dans le cadre d'un procès.[9]

---

7 P.Oxy. LXXX 5254 (Oxyrhynchus, c. 89/94), P.Oslo III 95 (Oxyrhynchus, avril 96), PSI inv. 3241 (Oxyrhynchus, 13 juillet 96), PSI inv. 3242 (Oxyrhynchus, dernière décennie du Ier siècle), – ces deux derniers papyrus, publiés par Bartoletti Colombo (1971: 4-7), ne sont répertoriés, ni dans le *Sammelbuch*, ni dans la base de données *HGV* (au 1er avril 2019), mais ils figurent dans *Trismegistos*, sous les no 131604-131605 –, P.Oxy. LXXX 5255 (Oxyrhynchus, c. 118/121 ou c. 166/168), BGU II 647 (Karanis, 22 août 130), P.Oxy. III 476 (Oxyrhynchus, 159/161), P.Oxy. I 51 (Oxyrhynchus, 31 août 173), PSI V 455 (Oxyrhynchus, 8 août 178), P.Oxy. LXXX 5256 (Oxyrhynchus, 25 septembre 190), P.Oslo III 96 (Oxyrhynchus, juillet/août 252), P.Oxy. XLV 3245 (Oxyrhynchus, 297), P.Mert. II 89 (nome arsinoïte, 14 janvier 300), P.Oxy. LIV 3729 (Oxyrhynchus, 4 mai 307), BGU III 928 (Héracléopolis, 307 ou 311), P.Oxy. LXXX 5257 (Oxyrhynchus, 312), P.Oxy. LXIV 4441 col. I et II (Oxyrhynchus, janvier/février 316), P.Oxy. VI 896 col. II (Oxyrhynchus, 1 avril 316), CPR XVIIA 23 (Hermopolis, 322), P.Oxy. I 52 (Oxyrhynchus, 25 juillet/23 août 325), P.Oxy. XLIV 3195 (Oxyrhynchus, 13?-14 juin 331), P.Oxy. LXVI 4528 (Oxyrhynchus, 6 mai 336), P.Athen. 34 (Héracléopolis?, 347), P.Louvre II 116 = SB XX 14638 et son double P.Cair.Preis. 7 = SB XX 14639 (Hermopolis, c. 330/340), P.Oxy. LXIII 4370 (Oxyrhynchus, 7 novembre 354), P.Oxy. LXVI 4529 (Oxyrhynchus, 22 juin 376), P.Lips. I 42 et son double P.Lips. inv. 7 (Hermopolis, 27 mars/25 avril 391), P.Rein. II 92 (Oxyrhynchus, 25 mars/23 avril 393).

8 Je laisse de côté le SPP I, p. 8 (éd. de Ricci [1901: 8]), provenant d'Antinoopolis, et daté du 13 février 455 apr. J.-C. Comme en témoigne sa structure, ce document n'est pas un rapport médical à proprement parler (comme le pense Hirt Raj [2006: tableau III]), mais un certificat. De fait le document, qui n'est d'ailleurs pas appelé προσφώνησις, mais ἐκσφράγισμα, s'il a pour expéditeur l'expert, comme pour les rapports (à ceci près que, dans le certificat, il est mentionné en premier lieu), il a pour destinataire, non pas un fonctionnaire, mais la personne qui a été examinée. Si aucun rapport médical grec n'est attesté hors d'Égypte, c'est en raison des conditions climatiques. De fait, puisqu'ils étaient écrits sur papyrus, ils n'ont pu être conservés que là où il fait à la fois chaud et sec.

9 On connaît à ce jour deux copies d'extraits de comptes rendus d'audience, provenant

Les rapports sont écrits au recto d'un coupon de papyrus, le plus souvent par une seule main (qui est généralement soignée et ne correspond pas à celle de l'expert), sauf pour les souscriptions. Ils occupent une colonne de texte d'environ 25 à 30 lignes. Ils faisaient l'objet d'au moins une copie (ἀντίγραφον), ce qui a permis, à deux reprises, d'identifier, tantôt le rapport lui-même, tantôt sa copie.[10] Ainsi, dans un rapport provenant de Karanis (au nord du nome arsinoïte), et daté du 22 août 130 de notre ère (BGU II 647), une note dans la marge supérieure signale qu'il s'agit d'une copie; quant à l'original, à ce jour, il n'a pas été retrouvé. Le patient (ou un de ses proches) devait conserver une copie du rapport, tandis que l'original destiné à l'autorité mandante était archivé, selon la manière suivante, fréquemment utilisée dans l'administration romaine: un numéro était noté dans la marge supérieure, puis les coupons de papyrus contenant les expertises (et d'autres documents datés de la même année ou concernant une même autorité) étaient collés ensemble, par ordre croissant des numéros, de manière à former un rouleau, dénommé τόμος συγκολλήσιμος. On suppose que les coupons de papyrus étaient classés par ordre chronologique, mais les quelques fragments de τόμοι conservés à ce jour ne permettent pas d'en avoir la certitude.[11]

2 Le déroulement de l'inspection médicale: à quelles questions l'expert doit-il répondre?

L'examen de la structure des rapports permet de retracer le déroulement d'une inspection médicale. Ceux-ci suivent un schéma fixe, qui s'applique à tout type de rapport, que celui-ci émane de médecins, de charpentiers, ou encore de maçons.[12] On peut le diviser en dix points principaux: (1) informations ini-

d'Oxyrhynchus, avec mention de rapport médical: P.Oxy. XVII 2111 (c. 135) et XII 1502 (après 260). La structure des comptes rendus est analysée dans l'ouvrage, désormais classique, de Coles (1966).

10 Voyez, ainsi, les P.Cair.Preis. 7 – P.Louvre II 116 et les P.Lips. I 42 – P.Lips. inv. 7. Dans les deux cas, le rapport provient d'Hermopolis; le mot « copie » (ἀντίγραφον) n'est pas précisé dans ces papyrus.

11 On sait qu'il existait des τόμοι où les documents étaient collés dans l'ordre décroissant des numéros: voir P.Oxy. LX 4060 et les commentaires de l'éditeur, R.A. Coles.

12 Pour un rapport de charpentiers, voir le P.Oxy. I 53 (Oxyrhynchus, 25 février 316), qui concerne l'inspection d'un perséa, un arbre d'Afrique orientale et de la péninsule arabique, *Mimusops laurifolia* (Forsk.) Friis, très anciennement acclimaté en Égypte (au moins dès la Ve dynastie); pour un rapport d'architectes ou de maçons, voir le P.Oxy. LXIV 4441 col. III (Oxyrhynchus, janvier 316).

tiales, (2) praescript, qui fournit des informations sur l'autorité destinataire du rapport,[13] (3) nom de l'expéditeur, (4) motif de l'expertise, (5) introduction du rapport, (6) rapport, (7) éléments secondaires du rapport, (8) conclusion, (9) datation finale, et (10) souscription du ou des médecins, c'est-à-dire leur signature. Malgré quelques changements, notamment dans les types de magistrats auxquels sont adressés ces documents, leur structure demeurera à peu près identique du Ier au IVe siècle de notre ère. Ce sont surtout les points 4 à 6 du rapport qui retiendront mon attention.[14] Dans la partie « motif de l'expertise » (point 4), l'expert déclare avoir été chargé (Ier/IIe siècles : ἐπιτρέπειν, παραγγέλλειν, ἐπιτάττειν ; époque byzantine : ἐπιστέλλειν), par l'autorité, par le biais d'un assistant de ce dernier (διά + nom + ὑπηρέτης), et suite à une pétition qui a été remise à cette autorité, de se rendre sur le lieu où se trouve la personne à examiner, de l'examiner et de faire un rapport écrit sur sa condition (διάθεσις). Quelquefois, ce point contient aussi des informations sur le patient et sur son statut social ; on trouve des personnes libres et des esclaves, des hommes, des femmes et des enfants. La partie « motif de l'expertise » peut aussi contenir l'indication de la date à laquelle l'autorité a reçu la pétition. Cette dernière précision est particulièrement importante puisque, lorsque le rapport est lui-même daté (au neuvième point, « datation finale »), elle permet d'évaluer le délai qui s'est écoulé entre le moment de la remise de la pétition au bureau de l'autorité et celui de la rédaction de la déclaration. Souvent, ce délai est très court : l'examen a lieu le jour même de la remise de la pétition.[15] Deux raisons pourraient expliquer qu'il fallait agir vite. L'examen semble être effectué avant toute intervention thérapeutique : pour les cas les plus graves, il ne fallait donc pas traîner, et pour les blessés les plus légers non plus, de peur que les blessures s'atténuent. Pour les morts, le délai entre la remise de la pétition et l'inspection devait également être très bref. En effet, sous un climat chaud tel que l'est celui

13 Le mot « praescript » a été employé pour la première fois par Collomp (1926) ; cette terminologie est également utilisée par Martin (2007 : 661-675), (2008 : 219-223) et (à paraître). Il faut le distinguer de « prescrit », un substantif qui s'applique exclusivement aux lettres, dont la diplomatique est différente de celle des pétitions et des rapports.

14 Le septième point (« éléments secondaires du rapport ») n'est attesté que dans le BGU III 928 (Héracléopolis, 307 ou 311), où l'on a peut-être une allusion à la tenue vestimentaire du patient (voir les lignes 20-22, dont le déchiffrement est cependant incertain). Le huitième point (« conclusion ») se présente presque toujours sous la forme d'une déclaration (« ce dont je fais le rapport »).

15 Le BGU II 647 fait exception, puisque l'examen a eu lieu cinq jours après la transmission de la pétition. Cette durée s'explique probablement par le fait que la pétition devait avoir été soumise dans la métropole du nome, Arsinoé, au sud du nome arsinoïte, alors que l'expert mandaté était établi à Karanis, au nord-est du nome.

de l'Égypte, il était impératif d'examiner le corps mort au plus vite, avant que la putréfaction soit manifeste, et rende toute inspection vaine.

Dans le cinquième point, qui est celui de l'introduction du rapport, on trouve, après un connecteur qui relie cette partie du rapport à la précédente (le plus souvent, c'est l'adverbe ὅθεν, mais on trouve aussi διὰ τοῦτο), l'indication que l'expert s'est rendu sur les lieux où se trouve la personne blessée, malade ou décédée, accompagné de l'assistant; le médecin peut également préciser que la personne examinée (dans tous les cas, vivante) était alitée au moment de l'inspection.[16] La présence d'une date dans cette partie du rapport est exceptionnelle.[17]

Enfin, le sixième point, le rapport proprement dit, comprend deux parties. La première est l'indication, par l'expert, qu'il a examiné une personne, dont il ne donne généralement plus le nom (il se contente de la désigner par les mots τοῦτον ou τὸν προκείμενον), tandis que la seconde contient la description des observations médicales. En règle générale, l'examen ne concerne qu'une seule personne, mais quelquefois, il y en a plusieurs, comme dans le P.Athen. 34 (nome héracléopolite, 347), où c'est un groupe de bergers qui est inspecté, ou dans le CPR XVIIA 23 (Hermopolis, 322), qui consigne les résultats de l'examen de deux chefs de chantier naval. Quatre verbes désignent l'action d'inspecter: ἐφιδεῖν, ἐπισκέπτεσθαι, ὁρᾶν et ἐπιθεωρεῖν. Le premier, toujours écrit avec une aspiration fautive,[18] est de loin le plus fréquent. Le sujet du verbe est le médecin, qui, parfois, s'associe à l'assistant de l'autorité, qui est présent. L'expert peut aussi éventuellement indiquer le lieu où se déroule l'inspection, et si le patient est alité. Malgré quelques différences, on constate que tous les verbes employés relèvent du champ lexical de la vision. En effet, l'autopsie au sens étymologique du terme était le point capital de toute inspection médicale. C'était le résultat des observations visuelles qui était consigné par écrit dans le rapport, peut-être seulement de manière abrégée, et, en tout cas, de façon accessible à un non-spécialiste, tel qu'un fonctionnaire ou un magistrat.[19] On

16 Voir, par exemple, le PSI inv. 3241. L'indication que le blessé est alité peut figurer dans le rapport proprement dit (sixième point).

17 Seul, le BGU II 647 contient une date au cinquième point du rapport.

18 Sur cette fausse aspiration très fréquente dans les papyrus, voyez Mayser (1923^2: 201); Gignac (1976: 136-138); N. Gonis, dans P.Oxy. LXVI, p. 211. Dans son édition du PSI V 417, parue en 1917, G. Vitelli écrivait, à propos du mot ἐφιδῖν, que «nelle scritture dei medici pratici, in tutti i tempi della grecità (e forse non della grecità soltanto), abbondano volgarismi ed errori grafici. Ma questa aspirazione del tema ἰδ- (dovuta probabilmente ad influenza di ὁρα- [...]) è notissima e comunissima in ogni genere di scrittura [...]».

19 Le mot «autopsie», αὐτοψία, est attesté dans une pétition avec demande d'inspection médicale, le P.Harr. II 192, l. 19-21 (prov. inc., 167 apr. J.-C.): «Nous soumettons cette péti-

peut supposer aussi que le médecin interrogeait son patient, mais les rapports n'en conservent pas la trace.

La deuxième partie du rapport contient la description des observations médicales. L'énumération des blessures relevées par le médecin est introduite le plus souvent par une forme participiale du verbe ἔχειν.[20] Elle suit l'ordre *a capite ad calcem*. La syntaxe est elliptique : l'expert emploie la préposition ἐπί, « sur », suivie du nom de la partie du corps affectée, décliné au génitif, auquel succède le nom de la blessure, à l'accusatif. Les différentes observations sont reliées entre elles par la conjonction de coordination καί. Pour une partie du corps, le médecin peut préciser si c'est le côté gauche ou droit qui est atteint ; il peut aussi indiquer le nombre de blessures observées. Une blessure ou un trauma n'est pas toujours seul, mais s'accompagne parfois d'un gonflement ou d'un autre préjudice : dans ce cas, le scripteur utilise la préposition μετά, « avec », suivie du nom du gonflement ou du préjudice supplémentaire, au génitif.

La description clinique montre que l'examen, rudimentaire, n'était qu'externe. Le médecin se contentait de décrire ce qu'il observait, sans intervention thérapeutique. Les deux exceptions sont antérieures à la première attestation du titre de « médecin public », qui, semble-t-il, ne dispensait pas de soins, ou, si c'est le cas, du moins, ceux-ci n'étaient plus consignés dans le rapport écrit. Dans la première, le P.Oslo III 95 (Oxyrhynchus, 96 apr. J.-C.), le médecin dit avoir soigné la blessure au doigt médian (ἐπὶ τῷ μέσῳ | δακτύλῳ ṭραῦμα, ὃ καὶ θα|ραπεύω, l. θεραπεύω) d'une esclave qui s'est probablement battue. Dans la seconde, le BGU II 647 (Karanis, 22 août 130 apr. J.-C.), le médecin a traité la blessure d'un nommé Mystharion : il s'agissait d'une fracture profonde (κατέαγμα ἐπὶ βάθους), à la tempe gauche, avec de petits éclats de pierres (μικρὰ κατεάγματα λίθου). Le verbe grec utilisé pour signifier « traiter des blessures », τραυματοθεραπεύω, n'est, à ce jour, pas attesté ailleurs dans la littérature grecque.[21] Si l'on excepte ces deux verbes relevant de la thérapeutique, le vocabulaire médical des rapports peut être classé en deux catégories : anatomie (33

tion, en demandant (ἀξιοῦντες) qu'un assistant vienne pour observer directement (ἐπὶ τὴν] | αὐτοψίαν), accompagné d'un médecin public… », ainsi que dans un rapport médical, le CPR XVIIA 23, l. 15-17 (Hermopolis, 322 apr. J.-C.) : « nous étant rendus là-bas, moi (*sc.* le médecin) et l'assistant susmentionné, par observation directe ([δι' α]ὐτοψεί[ας), nous rapportons ([προσφ]ωνοῦμεν)… ».

20 Le participe du verbe ἔχειν n'est toutefois pas le seul moyen attesté pour introduire l'énumération des blessures. Dans quatre des plus anciens rapports, on trouve εὑρίσκειν, à la 1e personne de l'indicatif aoriste, ou une forme participiale de γιγνώσκειν.

21 Sur les spécificités lexicologiques des papyrus médicaux grecs, voir également la contribution d'I. Bonati dans ce volume.

mots) et pathologie (22 mots). C'est pour la tête et le cou que le lexique anatomique est le plus riche. En effet, sont mentionnés, la tête (κεφαλή), le sinciput ou bregma (βρέγμα), le sommet du crâne (κορυφή), entre le bregma et l'occiput,[22] la tempe (κρόταφος), le front (μέτωπον), l'oreille (ὠτίον, diminutif de οὖς),[23] le sourcil (ὀφρύς), la paupière, et plus précisément la paupière inférieure (τὸ κάτω βλέφαρον), la pommette (μῆλον),[24] le nez (ῥίς), les narines (ῥώθωνες),[25] la dent (ὀδούς),[26] le cou (τράχηλος). Pour les membres supérieurs, on trouve l'épaule (ὦμος), l'omoplate (ὠμοπλάτη), c'est-à-dire la scapula, l'acromion (ἀκρώμιον), le coude (ἀγκών), le bras (βραχίων), le cubitus (πῆχυς), la main (χείρ), ainsi que le doigt (δάκτυλος), en particulier le médium (μέσος δάκτυλος) et le pouce (μέγιστος δάκτυλος). En ce qui concerne le thorax, le dos et l'abdomen, on trouve quatre mots: ventre (κοιλία),[27] sein (μαστός), dos (νῶτον), flanc (πλευρά). Dans les rapports médicaux, la partie inférieure du corps est nettement moins bien représentée; à mon avis, il faudrait peut-être l'expliquer par le fait que le médecin ne ressentait pas la nécessité de décrire la

22 Arist., *HA* 1.7.491a33-34; voir également Hipp., *VC* 2 (3.190 Littré; 64 Hanson).

23 Les mots grecs désignant l'oreille et le genou sont tous deux des diminutifs, qui, dans le contexte des rapports, comment souvent dans la littérature, n'ont pas leur valeur diminutive. Dans la littérature, cf. notamment, pour l'oreille, *Anth. Pal.* 11.81.3; *1Samuel* 9.15; *Ev. Matt.* 26.51; Arr., *Epict.* 1.18; etc. Pour le genou, Ph., *Vit. Cont.* 51; Ps.-Luc., *Asin.* 10; Héliodore *ap.* Orib., *Coll. Med.* 48.66 (3.290.21 Raeder); Rufus *ap.* Orib., *Coll. Med.* 49.34 (4.52.4 Raeder); etc.

24 Le mot grec μῆλον, qui désigne ici la pommette, pourrait bien être attesté dans le P.Lips. I 42 = inv. 7 (double). L. Mitteis, l'éditeur du papyrus, interprétait μῆλον comme un phonétisme pour μῆρον, « la cuisse ». Il est vrai que la confusion entre les lettres *lambda* et *rhô* n'est pas rare dans les papyrus. Cependant, la solution μῆλον = pommette semble préférable, parce qu'elle permet de supprimer une difficulté (phonétisme) et qu'elle respecte l'ordre *a capite ad calcem* qui est en usage dans les descriptions des rapports.

25 Le déchiffrement du mot grec désignant la narine, dans le P.Oxy. LIV 3729, n'est pas assuré.

26 Le mot est attesté dans le PSI inv. 3242. Il ne reste pas grand-chose des détails du motif de l'inspection, mais on comprend que l'homme à examiner a été blessé suite à une bagarre (7-8: ἀπὸ συμπλο|[κῆς). Dans le récit des aventures survenues au patient, un mot est encore entièrement lisible à la ligne 8: οδους, qu'A.M. Bartoletti Colombo, l'éditrice, comprend comme le nominatif d'ὀδούς, la « dent »; avant ce mot, on ne déchiffre plus que les quatre dernières lettres d'un autre mot (ατος), et, après οδους, le début d'un nouveau mot, peut-être un verbe (εξε). Serait-il question d'une dent, arrachée lors de la rixe? Mais alors, étant au nominatif, le mot ὀδούς doit être le sujet de la phrase; pour εξε, peut-être faut-il restituer ἐξε|[κόπη], du verbe ἐκκόπτειν, « amputer », ce qui donnerait « une dent lui ayant été arrachée » (A.M. Bartoletti Colombo ne propose rien); comparer avec le PSI XIV 1435, l. 6-8 (prov. inconnue, début du Ier siècle), ἐκτιστὴς | δέ μοι γένηιται (lire γένηται) τοῦ προστίμου | τῆς τοῦ ὀδόντος ἐκκοπῆς, « que vengeance me soit faite pour la peine de m'avoir arraché la dent »; en dehors des papyrus, voir *Ev. Matt.* 5.30; Luc., *Cat.* 24.

27 PSI inv. 3241, 16 (Oxyrhynchus, 13 juillet 96). Le mot est cependant restitué.

totalité des blessures observées, mais ne mentionnait peut-être que celles qu'il voyait en premier, ou qui étaient les plus évidentes ou encore les plus impressionnantes. Les seuls membres inférieurs mentionnés sont le devant de la jambe (ἀντικνήμιον), le genou (γονάτιον, diminutif de γόνυ), la hanche (ἰσχίον) et la cuisse (μηρός). On trouve également une occurrence des muscles suspenseurs (κρεμαστῆρες) des testicules (ὄρχεις). Enfin, le sang (αἷμα) et «une membrane fine» (ὑμήν) sont également mentionnés une fois. Le lexique pathologique est, pour sa part, exclusivement traumatologique. On rencontre des mots qui désignent l'égratignure ou la légère déchirure (ἀμυχή), l'arrachement (ἀπόσυρμα) de la peau, la coupure (διαίρεσις), la déchirure (καταξυσμή), la fracture (κατέαγμα), la marque de coups (τύπος, τύμμα ou μώλωψ), ou l'absence de marque, sur un corps mort (ἄστιγος), le gonflement (οἴδημα), l'ecchymose (πελίωμα), qui peut être légère (πελιωμάτιον), le coup reçu (πληγή ou πλῆγμα) ou l'absence de coup, sur un corps mort (ἄπληγος), la concentration (συνδρομή), en parlant de sang, sur un sein, la blessure (τραῦμα ou τρῶσις), l'écorchure (ψῆγμα), la dénudation (ψίλωσις) d'un os. Les seuls mots qui ne relèvent pas de la traumatologie sont ceux qui désignent la maladie (νόσος et νόσημα), qui peut être aiguë (ὀξύς), l'état fiévreux (πυρέτιον; πυρέσσειν), la perte d'audition (κωφός) ou encore le fait de vomir (ἐξεμεῖν).[28] Dans son ensemble, la terminologie médicale est variée, mais si on examine les rapports séparément, on constate qu'au sein d'un même rapport, c'est souvent la même terminologie qui est attestée: c'est particulièrement évident dans le P.Athen. 34, où le seul terme de pathologie utilisé est τραῦμα.

Les causes de l'inspection peuvent être de trois sortes, auxquelles correspond une réponse écrite différente: la plus fréquente est celle qui concerne les agressions.[29] Dans ce cas, les détails médicaux sont particulièrement développés; en effet, si les agresseurs sont retrouvés et que le rapport est utilisé dans un procès, celui-ci pourra s'avérer accablant pour les coupables. L'état du corps sert de preuve de la violence subie. Pour les morts, l'état du corps (σῶμα νεκρόν)

---

28 P.Oslo III 95 et PSI inv. 3241, qui rapportent les résultats d'une inspection effectuée par le même médecin. Dans les deux cas, la forme grecque utilisée est ἐξαιμοῦσα, qui correspond probablement à un étacisme pour ἐξεμοῦσα (du verbe ἐξεμεῖν, vomir).

29 C'est le cas le plus fréquent, puisqu'il concerne 11 pétitions avec demande d'inspection médicale (P.Harr. II 192, P.Oxy. XXXI 2563, P.Flor. I 59, P.Oxy. LVIII 3926, P.Oxy. XII 1556, P.Oxy. LXI 4122, P.Oxy. LI 3620, P.Gron.Amst. 1, P.Bon. 22 = SB XVIII 13127, P.Oxy. XVI 1885, P.Oxy. XX 2268), et 26 rapports (P.Oxy. LXXX 5254 [?], P.Oslo III 95, PSI inv. 3242, P.Oxy. LXXX 5255, BGU II 647, PSI V 455, P.Oxy. LXXX 5256, P.Oslo III 96, P.Oxy. XLV 3245, P.Mert. II 89, P.Oxy. LIV 3729, BGU III 928, P.Oxy. LXXX 5257, P.Oxy. LXIV 4441 col. I et II, CPR XVIIA 23, P.Oxy. I 52, P.Oxy. XLIV 3195, P.Oxy. LXVI 4528, P.Athen. 34, P.Louvre II 116 = SB XX 14638 et P.Cair.Preis. 7 = SB XX 14639 [double], P.Oxy. LXIII 4370, P.Oxy. LXVI 4529, P.Lips. I 42 et inv. 7 [double]).

n'est généralement pas décrit avec précision[30]; seul, le P.Rein. II 92 est plus détaillé, puisqu'il y est spécifié que le mort ne porte, ni blessure, ni marque (11-12: ἄπ̣λ̣ηγον, | ἄσ̣τ̣ι̣γ̣ο̣ν̣). L'objectif est surtout de déterminer officiellement la cause de la mort, afin de se prémunir d'une action légale éventuelle (ainsi, dans le P.Rein. II 92, 12, il est conclu que l'individu est mort d'une maladie aiguë, ὀξείῳ νοσήμ̣[ατι] περιπεσών); dans certains cas, l'expertise semble aussi nécessaire pour obtenir le permis d'inhumer la victime. Enfin, le troisième cas, qui concerne un rapport suite à des maladies, est peu fréquent.[31] Là aussi, la description est relativement réduite et les objectifs des rapports ne sont pas clairement établis; l'important semble être de certifier qu'une personne est bel et bien malade, et qu'elle ne feint pas d'être malade (peut-être pour échapper aux liturgies?).

3 Comparaison avec les fiches de malades des *Épidémies* hippocratiques

Si l'on met de côté les aspects proprement légaux, qui sont communs à tout type de rapport, la description médicale, ainsi que celle du contexte de l'inspection, à savoir les points 4 à 6 du schéma, trouvent-elles des parallèles dans la littérature médicale? Par leur contenu, leur présentation et leur structure, les fiches de malades des *Épidémies* hippocratiques, qui décrivent notamment des cas traumatologiques, représentent un parallèle intéressant à exploiter.

Parmi la soixantaine de traités mis sous le nom d'Hippocrate (460-370/359 av. J.-C.), les *Épidémies* comprennent sept livres dont la rédaction s'étale entre la fin du Ve et la première moitié du IVe siècle avant notre ère.[32] Cette division est bien antérieure à Galien (129-216), puisqu'Érotien, glossateur d'Hippocrate dont l'activité se situe sous le règne de Néron, connaissait déjà sept livres des

30 Une, et peut-être deux pétitions (C.Pap.Gr. II, app. 1, PSI inv. 4153 [?]), un ordre, qui contient aussi une copie de pétition (P.Oxy. III 475), et trois rapports médicaux (P.Oxy. III 476 et I 51, ainsi que P.Rein. II 92), concernent l'inspection de corps morts. En outre, les inspections médicales mentionnées dans les deux copies d'extraits de comptes rendus d'audience (voir ci-dessus, n. 9), ont été conduites sur des personnes décédées de mort violente. Sur les inspections de corps morts, voir Ricciardetto (2013).

31 Seuls, deux rapports sont relatifs à une maladie: PSI inv. 3241 et P.Oxy. VI 896.

32 Le mot grec ἐπιδημίαι, dont le sens premier, au singulier, est «séjour dans un pays», désigne les «maladies générales qui s'installent et 'séjournent' dans le territoire»; cf. Jouanna (2017[2]: 218-219).

Épidémies. Ceux-ci ont très tôt été classés en trois groupes : le premier, qui comprend les livres 1 et 3, est le plus ancien[33] ; le deuxième regroupe les livres 2, 4 et 6, et le troisième, les livres 5 et 7.[34]

Dans les *Épidémies* hippocratiques on peut distinguer trois composantes fondamentales, qui apparaissent en proportions inégales selon les groupes : (1) des constitutions saisonnières (καταστάσεις), à savoir le tableau « climato-nosologique » d'une cité, pour une année donnée, (2) des fiches individuelles de malades, et, enfin, (3) des réflexions générales sur l'art médical. Seul, le deuxième élément m'intéresse ici. Du point de vue du contenu, les fiches de malades peuvent être, soit liées à des constitutions, soit indépendantes de celles-ci, et même n'avoir aucun rapport avec elles. Elles concernent toute une série de pathologies (folie, pleuritis, tuméfactions, péripneumonie, angine, choléra, problèmes lors de la grossesse ou de l'accouchement, etc.) et peuvent aussi être relatives à la traumatologie.[35] En règle générale, chaque fiche possède une structure relativement ordonnée qui comprend trois points[36] : une brève introduction, contenant les éléments d'identification du malade, dont son nom, sa localité ou son adresse, des précisions éventuelles sur ce qui a précédé la maladie (la « cause préalable », πρόφασις),[37] et sur ce qui a marqué son début, en particulier l'apparition d'une forte fièvre (πυρετὸς ὀξύς) et l'alitement du malade (κατακλίνεσθαι, κατακεῖσθαι) ; le cœur de la fiche, constitué par la suite chronologique des jours de la maladie ; une conclusion débutant généralement par un démonstratif en asyndète désignant le malade (comparer *supra*, le démonstratif qui peut se trouver au début du point 6 du rapport) et où sont indiqués les symptômes que le médecin considère comme les plus constants au cours de la maladie ; parfois, la conclusion comporte aussi une indication sur l'âge du malade. La description des symptômes s'accompagne parfois d'une indication du traitement ; c'est le cas, notamment, d'*Épidémies* 7, tandis que la thérapeutique est absente d'*Épidémies* 1 et 3.[38]

---

33 Sur l'auteur de ce premier groupe, qui a toujours été identifié à Hippocrate, mais qui est plus probablement « un disciple confirmé de l'école d'Hippocrate au moment où Hippocrate, ayant quitté Cos, s'est installé en Thessalie », cf. Jouanna – Guardasole – Anastassiou (2016 : cxxii).

34 Le lecteur trouvera une présentation générale de chaque groupe, avec la liste des éditions des traités, dans Jouanna (2017^2 : 544-549).

35 Les fiches relatives à la traumatologie ne sont guère nombreuses. Elles sont absentes du premier groupe.

36 Sur cette structure, voir Jouanna – Guardasole – Anastassiou (2016 : xlvi-xlix).

37 Sur cette « cause déclenchante », cf. Robert (1976 : 317-342) ; Jouanna – Grmek (2000 : lxi-lxii).

38 Jouanna – Grmek (2000 : lxviii).

Examinons maintenant de plus près les parallèles qui, par-delà les cinq siècles au moins qui les séparent, peuvent être relevés entre ces fiches et les rapports sur papyrus, en commençant tout d'abord par les éléments d'identification du malade ou du blessé. La fiche hippocratique, comme le rapport, peut commencer par l'indication du lieu où réside la personne malade : dans la première, la sphère d'activité est essentiellement la Grèce du Nord (en particulier l'île de Thasos, au sud de la Thrace, ainsi que les cités de Périnthe, en Thrace, et de Larissa, en Thessalie), tandis que, pour le second, c'est l'Égypte. Dans les deux cas, l'indication du lieu est généralement sommaire : elle ne comprend que le nom du village ou de la ville, comme, par exemple, « à Élis » (ἐν Ἤλιδι ; voir *Epid.* 5.1-2 [5.204 Littré ; 2-3 Jouanna – Grmek]), « à Athènes » (Ἀθήνησιν, *Epid.* 5.9-10 [5.208-210 Littré ; 6-7 Jouanna – Grmek]), « à Oxyrhynchus » (P.Oxy. XLV 3245, 14 : dans la même ville, ἐν τῇ αὐτῇ πόλει). Toutefois, on trouve parfois des indications plus précises, comme l'adresse, en particulier dans les fiches de malades du premier groupe (*Épidémies* 1 et 3)[39] : ainsi, Cléonactidès vivait au-dessus du sanctuaire d'Héraclès, à Thasos, que les archéologues de l'École Française d'Athènes ont réussi à identifier.[40] Le lieu indiqué correspond au lieu où s'est déroulée l'inspection, qui diffère parfois du lieu où réside la personne examinée : dans *Epid.* 3.1.9 (3.58 Littré ; 74.17-18 Jouanna – Guardasole – Anastassiou), la femme malade est couchée chez Tisamène ; dans le P.Oxy. I 51, Hiérax a été retrouvé pendu dans la maison d'Épagathos, dans le quartier de la Grand-rue, à Oxyrhynchus ; dans le P.Oxy. XLIV 3195, l'examen a lieu dans le λογιστήριον public de la ville, qui était peut-être réservé aux détentions préventives. Dans tous les cas, le médecin se déplace auprès du malade ou de la personne blessée.[41]

Généralement, fiches et rapports ne concernent qu'un seul patient. Le statut social des personnes examinées ou soignées est un autre point commun entre les deux types d'enquête. En effet, dans les deux cas, les médecins soignent ou observent tout type de malades ou de blessés, sans différenciation d'âge, de condition ou de sexe[42] : on trouve des personnes libres et des esclaves,[43] des

---

39 Sur les adresses dans les *Épidémies*, voir Robert (1975 : 173-194) ; Jouanna – Grmek (2000 : lxi) ; Jouanna – Guardasole – Anastassiou (2016 : xlvii et n. 36).

40 *Epid.* 1.27.6 (2.698 Littré ; 50-51 Jouanna – Guardasole – Anastassiou). Le sanctuaire d'Héraclès est également mentionné dans deux autres fiches de malades du premier groupe (*Epid.* 1.21 et 3.17.3 [2.666 et 3.112 Littré ; 31.8 et 96.2 Jouanna – Guardasole – Anastassiou]). Sur ce site, voir Grandjean – Salviat (2000 : 142-145) ; Jouanna (2014 : 43).

41 Voyez également Jouanna – Anastassiou – Magdelaine (2013 : xxix).

42 C'est la clientèle d'un médecin généraliste, telle qu'on la retrouve aussi dans le *Pronostic* ; cf. Jouanna – Anastassiou – Magdelaine (2013 : xxix).

43 Pour les esclaves, voir, par exemple, pour les fiches, *Epid.* 5.36 (5.230 Littré ; 19.10 Jouanna –

hommes, des femmes et des enfants, de toutes conditions sociales et nationalités. Même les barbares ne sont pas exclus. Le nom de ces personnes est généralement fourni (il l'est toujours dans les rapports)[44]; exceptionnellement, on indique aussi l'âge.[45]

Les introductions des fiches font notamment mention d'indications temporelles, exprimées au moyen de références à la saison, au lever et au coucher du soleil et des astres, ainsi qu'aux vents, comme dans *Epid.* 4.11 (5.150 Littré; 92-94 Smith), «au moment du coucher des Pléïades», c'est-à-dire au début de l'hiver (comparer *Epid.* 5.89 et 92 [5.254 Littré; 40-41 Jouanna – Grmek]), ou «à l'époque où souffle le zéphyr» (*Epid.* 7.98 [5.452 Littré; 107 Jouanna – Grmek]), c'est-à-dire au début du printemps, ou «vers Arcturus» (*Epid.* 7.2.8 [5.368.10 Littré; 50 Jouanna – Grmek]), le lever de cette étoile marquant le début de l'automne. En outre, comme les fiches notent au jour le jour les symptômes jugés signifiants, depuis le début de la maladie jusqu'à l'issue généralement fatale, d'autres indications temporelles apparaissent également au sein des fiches, comme le cours de la journée et de la nuit, et même, aux livres 5 et 7 des *Épidémies*, des indications d'heure («au moment où la place est pleine», «à l'heure où la place se vide»).[46] Les rapports aussi n'échappent pas à cette

---

Grmek, «L'homme d'Eubios», ὁ Εὐβίου ἄνθρωπος; voyez les commentaires dans Jouanna – Grmek [2000: 19 n. 6]: «Le terme ἄνθρωπος doit désigner ici un esclave, vraisemblablement un esclave âgé»); cf. aussi *Epid.* 5.37 (5.230 Littré; 19 Jouanna – Grmek), le garçon de Symmaque, ὁ Συμμάχου παῖς (Jouanna – Grmek [2000: 146 n. 9]). Les esclaves peuvent également être désignés par leur appartenance à un maître et par leur métier: voir, ainsi, le vigneron de Ménandre (*Epid.* 4.25 [5.168 Littré; 110 Smith]), ou encore le palefrenier de Palamède (*Epid.* 5.16 [5.214-216 Littré; 10 Jouanna – Grmek]). Sur les esclaves dans les fiches, Jouanna – Guardasole – Anastassiou (2016: xlviii). Pour des exemples d'esclaves dans les rapports sur papyrus, voir P.Oslo III 95; P.Oxy. LXIII 4370; etc.

44 Pour l'onomastique dans les *Épidémies*, voir la bibliographie mentionnée dans Jouanna – Grmek (2000: lxi n. 72). Sur les noms de malades dans *Épidémies* 1 et 3, et la manière de désigner les patients de sexe féminin, cf. Jouanna – Guardasole – Anastassiou (2016: xliv [tableau] et xlvii-xlviii). Dans les rapports sur papyrus, les noms des blessés, malades ou morts inspectés sont tous gréco-égyptiens.

45 *Epid.* 3.1.8 (3.56 Littré; 74 Jouanna – Guardasole – Anastassiou: un jeune homme d'environ vingt ans); 3.1.12 (3.62-66 Littré; 77-79 Jouanna – Guardasole – Anastassiou: une jeune fille d'environ dix-sept ans); 5.50 (5.236 Littré; 23-24 Jouanna – Grmek: où la «belle jeune fille, l'enfant de Nérios» avait vingt ans); *Epid.* 4.15 (5.152-154 Littré; 96-98 Smith: «il n'était pas âgé, vingt ans environ»); pour les rapports, voir P.Louvre II 116, où le blessé est peut-être dit «jeune» (17: ν[έ]ου τὴν ἡλ̣ι̣κ̣ε̣[ίαν]), mais le déchiffrement du texte est loin d'être assuré. On observera que l'âge n'est spécifié que pour des patients jeunes (une vingtaine d'années environ).

46 Voir ainsi *Epid.* 5.62.2 (5.242.5-6 Littré; 28.8 Jouanna – Grmek) et 88.3 (5.252.21 Littré; 40.8 Jouanna – Grmek); 7.25.5 (5.396.5 Littré; 67.4 Jouanna – Grmek), 31.2 (5.400.21 Littré; 71.1-2 Jouanna – Grmek), 84.4 (5.442.1 Littré; 99.13 Jouanna – Grmek), 92.3 (5.448.6 Littré; 104.10 Jouanna – Grmek).

règle : en effet, si l'on excepte la datation finale, qui se présente sous la forme régnale, et à l'époque byzantine, consulaire, le point « motif de l'expertise » des rapports médicaux peut contenir une datation, qui est alors indiquée de deux manières différentes : soit, par la date précise (année, mois, jour : voir, par exemple, P.Oslo III 95), soit par l'emploi d'adverbes tels que « aujourd'hui » (voir, par exemple, P.Oxy. I 51 et III 476). Ces dates renvoient au moment où le médecin a été chargé par l'autorité d'examiner une personne.

Du point de vue du contenu, plusieurs fiches de malades sont relatives à la traumatologie, comme c'est le cas de la majorité des rapports sur papyrus. Ces dernières peuvent être classées en deux catégories, d'une part, les accidents de la vie de tous les jours (voir, par exemple, *Epid.* 4.11 [5.150 Littré ; 92-94 Smith], où un enfant a été blessé à la tête par un autre enfant avec un tesson ; *Epid.* 5.50 [5.236 Littré ; 23-24 Jouanna – Grmek], où une « belle jeune fille », ἡ παρθένος ἡ καλή, de vingt ans a été frappée du plat de la main au bregma par « un petit bout de femme », ὑπὸ γυναίου φίλης, son amie, qui jouait ; *Epid.* 5.39 [5.230 Littré ; 20 Jouanna – Grmek], enfant frappé par un mulet au ventre et au foie),[47] y compris les accidents de travail (voir, par exemple, *Epid.* 4.20 [5.160 Littré ; 104 Smith], à propos d'un homme tombé du haut d'un four à potier ; *Epid.* 5.74 [5.246-248 Littré ; 34 Jouanna – Grmek] = 7.36 [5.404 Littré ; 74 Jouanna – Grmek], où l'intendant d'un grand navire a eu l'index et l'os inférieur de la main droite écrasés par l'ancre) et, d'autre part, les crimes et les blessures de guerre (voir *Epid.* 5.60 [5.240 Littré ; 27 Jouanna – Grmek] = 7.32 [5.400-402 Littré ; 71 Jouanna – Grmek] : un homme frappé à la tête par une pierre lancée par un Macédonien[48] ; *Epid.* 5.21 [5.220 Littré ; 13 Jouanna – Grmek] : un homme blessé par une lance large tenue à la main [crime ou blessure de guerre ?]).[49] Ces deux catégories sont bien représentées dans les rapports, comme, par exemple, pour la première, avec le P.Oxy. I 52 (Oxyrhynchus,

---

47 Les rapports médicaux ne contiennent pas d'accident survenu à cause d'un animal, mais plusieurs lettres privées écrites en grec rapportent que des hommes et des femmes ont été blessés par des chevaux. Dans le BGU XIII 2350, peut-être du IIe siècle, Aphroditè écrit à sa sœur qu'un cheval lui a marché sur le pied, et qu'il lui a fallu beaucoup de temps et d'argent pour s'en rétablir ; dans le P.Oxy. XLVI 3314, du IVe siècle, l'épouse de Judas, probablement un Juif, est tombée malade, suite à une chute de cheval, et est incapable de se mouvoir ; dans la lettre P.Abinn. 37 (= P.Gen. I 56), du milieu du IVe siècle, Abinnaeus, un militaire, rapporte à un confident diverses affaires concernant des soldats qui ne peuvent rejoindre le camp, et dont l'un souffre au flanc, suite au coup de talon d'un cheval.

48 Sur le contexte dans lequel doit se situer cette blessure, probablement dans une campagne des Macédoniens sous Philippe II, voir Jouanna – Grmek (2000 : xliii).

49 Jouanna – Grmek (2000 : 133 n. 18).

25 juillet/23 août 325 apr. J.-C.), qui contient le rapport de l'inspection médicale d'une jeune fille blessée dans l'écroulement de sa maison.

Le contenu et la présentation des fiches et des rapports présentent encore des points de contact supplémentaires en ce qui concerne le praticien et la description des observations médicales. Dans les *Épidémies*, l'observateur est un médecin, comme c'est aussi le cas dans la plupart des rapports médicaux.[50] Celui-ci peut travailler seul ou, plus rarement, en équipe,[51] auquel cas le texte est rédigé à la première personne, non plus du singulier, mais bien du pluriel. Par les fiches, on sait que certains de ces médecins étaient itinérants. Les rapports datés du Ier et du IVe siècle et provenant d'Oxyrhynchus attestent des expertises conduites par deux, trois, voire quatre médecins.[52] Même si tous ne signent pas nécessairement la déclaration, les verbes utilisés dans celle-ci sont conjugués au pluriel, comme dans les fiches; le pluriel peut aussi être attesté lorsque le médecin est seul, mais qu'il inclut dans sa déclaration l'assistant de l'autorité, témoin de l'examen.[53]

La tournure elliptique qu'adoptent les descriptions cliniques constitue un autre parallèle entre les deux types d'écrits. Dans les rapports, les observations se présentent comme des énumérations de blessures au moyen de la préposition ἐπί accompagnée du génitif de la partie du corps touchée, et suivie du nom de la blessure à l'accusatif, – les différentes blessures sont reliées entre elles par la conjonction de coordination καί –, tandis que la fiche peut parfois se borner à fournir une suite de mots en asyndète, qui indiquent tous les symptômes observés.[54] Dans les deux cas, ce qui est recherché, c'est la concision

50 Cf. *supra* n. 2 pour les exceptions.

51 Sur la médecine d'équipe dans le cinquième livre des *Épidémies*, voir Robert (1989: 20-27). Comme le remarque J. Jouanna dans Jouanna – Guardasole – Anastassiou (2016: 269), le fait que l'auteur signale, dans la fiche relative à la femme de Philinos (*Epid.* 1.27.4 [2.692.15 Littré; 47.2 Jouanna – Guardasole – Anastassiou]), qu'il a vu les urines qu'elle émettait, suggère que «ses descriptions de malades ne sont pas toutes le résultat d'observations personnelles. Le médecin devait avoir des assistants et des disciples. On peut aussi penser à plusieurs médecins de l'école hippocratique travaillant en équipe».

52 La publication, en 2014, du P.Oxy. LXXX 5254, daté de 89/94 de notre ère, qui s'avère désormais le plus ancien rapport médical connu à ce jour, a permis d'observer que des équipes de plusieurs médecins (en l'occurrence, deux) ne sont pas seulement attestées au IVe siècle, comme on le pensait jusqu'alors, mais déjà au Ier siècle de notre ère.

53 Il n'est pas question, dans les rapports, d'un emploi de la première personne du pluriel comme substitut de la première personne du singulier (un «nous d'auteur», *authorial we*), sur lequel cf. notamment von Staden (1994: 108); Hine (2009: 21).

54 Sur le style des fiches de malades, cf. Jouanna – Guardasole – Anastassiou (2016: 248-249). Voyez, ainsi, *Epid.* 5.55 (5.238 Littré; 25 Jouanna – Grmek): «La jeune fille tombée du haut du précipice: perte de la parole; l'agitation la tenait; et elle vomit dans la nuit beaucoup

et la rapidité. Les deux types d'écrits se caractérisent aussi par leur sobriété; les médecins ne font pratiquement aucun commentaire sur la signification des observations qu'ils notent. Toute considération personnelle est bannie tant des fiches que des rapports, où la plus stricte objectivité est de mise.[55]

On observera encore que, seul, ce qui est à la surface du corps et perceptible par les sens (dans les rapports médicaux, exclusivement la vision), est consigné dans les fiches et les rapports. Quant au vocabulaire utilisé, qu'il relève de l'anatomie et, dans une moindre mesure, de la traumatologie, il est en outre très similaire dans les deux types d'écrits: ainsi, la quasi-totalité des substantifs anatomiques présents dans les rapports sur papyrus est déjà attestée dans les *Épidémies* hippocratiques.[56] Les instruments qui ont blessé peuvent être indiqués (surtout dans les fiches, exceptionnellement dans les rapports).[57] En dehors des termes génériques désignant la maladie (νόσος, νόσημα), les seules observations cliniques des rapports qui ne relèvent pas du champ lexical de l'anatomie et de la traumatologie, – l'état fiévreux, l'alitement, le vomissement et la perte d'audition –, correspondent à des signes ou à des symptômes du comportement du malade régulièrement consignés dans les fiches des *Épidémies*.[58] L'apparition d'une fièvre et l'alitement du malade représentent en outre les deux signes qui indiquent fréquemment le début de la maladie.[59] C'étaient donc les premiers à être observés: aussi n'est-il sans doute pas éton-

de sang; du fait qu'elle était tombée du côté gauche, le sang s'écoula plus abondamment par là. C'est avec difficulté qu'elle avalait le mélicrat; râle, respiration précipitée comme chez les mourants; vaisseaux du visage tendus; décubitus sur le dos; pieds tièdes; fièvre légère; perte de la parole (…).» (Trad. J. Jouanna.)

55 Dans les fiches, les notations subjectives, voire «affectives», sont exceptionnelles: Jouanna (2017^2: 427-428). Voyez ainsi dans *Epid.* 7.24.2 (5.394.5 Littré; 66.2 Jouanna – Grmek), le médecin avoue ne plus se souvenir laquelle des deux joues d'une malade était rouge; ailleurs (*Epid.* 5.50 [5.236 Littré; 23-24 Jouanna – Grmek]), une fiche est consacrée à une «belle jeune fille», l'enfant de Nérios; dans *Epid.* 5.27.2 (5.226.10-12 Littré; 17.1-4 Jouanna – Grmek), le médecin reconnaît son erreur de diagnostic; enfin, il lui arrive de se demander si sa patiente dit la vérité (*Epid.* 4.6 [5.146 Littré; 88 Smith]).

56 Les exceptions sont rares: c'est le cas notamment du mot κρεμαστῆρες, absent de la *Collection* hippocratique, mais qu'on retrouve plus tard chez Galien (voir notamment *Sem.* 2.5 [4.635 Kühn; 188 De Lacy]; *Musc. Diss.* 25.7 [18b.995.3 Kühn; 178.13 Debru – Garofalo] et 26.3 [18b.998.5 Kühn; 181.8 Debru – Garofalo]).

57 Voir, par exemple, *Epid.* 5.62 (5.242 Littré; 28 Jouanna – Grmek), homme blessé au foie par un javelot; P.Mert. II 89 (nome arsinoïte, 14 janvier 300), homme frappé par une massue.

58 Sur les attestations de ces quatre signes ou symptômes dans les fiches du premier groupe des *Épidémies*, cf. Jouanna – Guardasole – Anastassiou (2016: xlviii, lx-lxi, lxxiii-lxxiv, lxxxvi, 248, 262-263, 271-272).

59 Jouanna – Guardasole – Anastassiou (2016: xlviii).

nant de les retrouver dans les rapports, où les précisions non traumatologiques sont peu fréquentes. Du reste, l'indication que le blessé/malade est couché ou alité au moment où le médecin lui rend visite est signalée, dans les rapports, comme dans les fiches, avant même d'entrer dans le détail des observations médicales.[60]

À côté de ces ressemblances, on relève aussi des différences sensibles entre les fiches hippocratiques et les rapports d'Égypte : écrites par des médecins, peut-être les mêmes que ceux qui traitent les malades, les premières s'adressent à un lectorat appartenant au même monde,[61] alors que les rapports sont avant tout destinés à des fonctionnaires et à des magistrats. C'est pourquoi, généralement plus détaillées que les rapports, les fiches ne se limitent pas à l'énumération des blessures : elles suivent l'évolution du patient sur plusieurs jours ou semaines, jusqu'à l'issue de la maladie et fournissent parfois aussi des indications de traitement. Les rapports, quant à eux, ont seulement pour but de consigner le plus rapidement possible par écrit les coups et blessures, comme pour avoir la photographie de l'état d'une personne à un moment donné ; dans le cas de décès, ils servent à établir la cause de la mort. Ces documents donnent donc un instantané de ce qui est visible et qui pourra servir à la défense de la personne blessée ou de ses proches, en cas de procès. Leur intérêt est d'éclairer éventuellement la justice. Le sort de l'individu inspecté n'est jamais précisé.

Malgré ces différences, qui tiennent essentiellement aux destinataires de ces écrits (le monde médical d'une part, et les autorités administratives d'autre part), à leur nature (littéraire d'une part, documentaire d'autre part) et à leurs objectifs (scientifique d'une part, administratif et juridique d'autre part), les rapports médicaux semblent néanmoins trouver un écho dans les fiches de malades. Leurs nombreux points de contact peuvent être regroupés en trois catégories :

(1) la rédaction, en particulier la présentation de l'identité du patient (nom, localité), le style rapide et concis, mais toujours précis, du scripteur, la description des signes observés, qui, si elle « donne l'impression d'être spontanée et prise sur le vif », n'en est pas moins vraisemblablement « guidée par un savoir préalable, une connaissance précise sur la multiplicité des points à examiner et à noter »[62] ;

---

60 Voir, par exemple, P.Oxy. LXIV 4441.

61 Jouanna – Grmek (2000 : lxv) ; Jouanna – Guardasole – Anastassiou (2016 : xxviii-xxix et lvii).

62 Jouanna (2017^2 : 430-431). Sa remarque a été faite pour les fiches de malades, mais elle s'applique aussi aux rapports.

(2) le contenu, en particulier la terminologie médicale ; la nature des signes à observer ; l'objectivité du médecin et son absence de commentaires sur les symptômes examinés ;
(3) le contexte dans lequel se pratiquait l'examen : les auteurs des rapports et des fiches, le plus souvent des médecins, travaillent généralement seuls, mais parfois aussi en équipe, et s'occupent de malades ou blessés de toutes conditions sociales ; la description clinique révèle que l'examen était seulement externe et pouvait être complété par l'interrogatoire du malade.[63]

Toutes ces ressemblances permettent de conclure vraisemblablement à un lien de parenté entre les deux types d'enquête, qui doit vraisemblablement s'expliquer par la continuité des pratiques enseignées et appliquées relativement à la sémiotique, en vue d'établir un diagnostic au sein du corps médical dans le monde gréco-romain. Tout se passe comme si le médecin avait en tête une liste de questions telles que « le patient est-il alité ? », « a-t-il de la fièvre ? », suivi de l'examen des blessures, et, si le malade est en état de répondre, de son interrogatoire.

Bibliographie[64]

Éditions et traductions des œuvres d'auteurs anciens

Debru, A. – Garofalo, I. 2005. *Galien 7. Les Os pour les Débutants. L'Anatomie des Muscles*. Paris : Les Belles Lettres.

De Lacy, Ph. 1992. *Galeni De semine* [CMG V.3.1]. Berlin : Akademie-Verlag.

Hanson, M. 1999. *Hippocratis De capitis vulneribus* [CMG I.4.1]. Berlin : Akademie-Verlag.

Jouanna, J. – Grmek, M.D. 2000. *Hippocrate 4.3. Épidémies V et VII*. Paris : Les Belles Lettres.

Jouanna, J. – Guardasole, A. – Anastassiou, A. 2016. *Hippocrate 4.1. Épidémies I et III*. Paris : Les Belles Lettres.

Kühn, C.G. 1821-1833. *Claudii Galeni Opera Omnia*. Leipzig : Car. Cnoblochii.

Littré, É. 1839-1861. *Oeuvres complètes d'Hippocrate*. Paris : J.-B. Baillière.

63 Sur l'interrogatoire du malade, complément de l'examen autoptique, chez le médecin hippocratique, cf. Jouanna – Anastassiou – Magdelaine (2013 : xxxvi-xxxviii).

64 Les abréviations employées dans cette contribution pour désigner les éditions papyrologiques sont celles de la *Checklist of Greek, Latin, Demotic and Coptic Papyri, Ostraca and Tablets*, disponible en ligne (http://papyri.info/docs/checklist) et régulièrement mise à jour.

Raeder, J. 1928-1933. *Oribasii Collectionum medicarum reliquiae*, 4 vols [CMG VI.1.1-2.2]. Leipzig – Berlin : Teubner.

Smith, W.D. 1994. *Hippocrates 7. Epidemics 2, 4-7*. Cambridge, Mass. : Harvard University Press.

Études et commentaires

Amundsen, D.W. – Ferngren, G.B. 1978. 'The Forensic Role of Physicians in Ptolemaic and Roman Egypt', *Bulletin of the History of Medicine* 52 : 336-353.

Bartoletti Colombo, A.M. 1971. *Dai papiri della Società Italiana* (*Estratto dai P.S.I.*). Florence : F. Le Monnier, 7 pp.

Bastianini, G. – Russo, S. 2013. *Comunicazioni dell'Istituto Papirologico « G. Vitelli »*, 11, Florence : Istituto Papirologico « G. Vitelli ».

Boswinkel, E. 1956. 'La médecine et les médecins dans les papyrus grecs', *Eos* 48.1 : 181-190.

Coles, R.A. 1966. *Reports of Proceedings on Papyri*, Papyrologica Bruxellensia 4. Bruxelles : Fondation égyptologique Reine Élisabeth.

Collomp, P. 1926. *Recherches sur la chancellerie et la diplomatique des Lagides*. Strasbourg – Paris : Les Belles Lettres.

Gignac, F.T. 1976. *A Grammar of the Greek Papyri of the Roman and Byzantine Period*. I. *Phonology*. Milan : Istituto editoriale Cisalpino-La Goliardica.

Grandjean, Y. – Salviat, F. 2000. *Guide de Thasos*, Sites et monuments 3. Paris : De Boccard, 2e éd.

Hine, H. 2009. 'Subjectivity and Objectivity in Latin Scientific and Technical Literature', in L. Taub – A. Doody (éds.), *Authorial Voices in Greco-Roman Technical Writing*. Trèves : Wissenschaftlicher Verlag Trier, 13-30.

Hirt Raj, M. 2006. *Médecins et malades de l'Égypte romaine. Étude socio-légale de la profession médicale et de ses praticiens du Ier au IVe siècle ap. J.-C.*, SAM 32. Leyde – Boston : Brill.

Jouanna, J. 2014. 'Philologie et archéologie : la médecine hippocratique et les fouilles de Thasos', *Revue des Études Grecques* 127 : 29-54.

Jouanna, J. 2017^2. *Hippocrate*. Paris : Les Belles Lettres, 2e éd.

Jouanna, J. – Anastassiou, A. – Magdelaine, C. 2013. *Hippocrate. 3.1. Pronostic*. Paris : Les Belles Lettres.

Legras, B. 2008. 'Réponse' à Mitthof (2008), in E.M. Harris – G. Thür (éds.), *Symposion 2007. Vorträge zur griechischen und hellenistischen Rechtsgeschichte* (*Durham, 2.-6. September 2007*). *Papers on Greek and Hellenistic Legal History* (*Durham, September 2-6 2007*), Akten der Gesellschaft für Griechische und Hellenistische Rechtsgeschichte 20. Vienne : Verlag der Österreichischen Akademie der Wissenschaften, 319-324.

Manfredi, M. 2004. 'Qualche osservazione sui referti medici nei papiri', in I. Andorlini (éd.), *Testi medici su papiro. Atti del Seminario di studio (Firenze, 3-4 giugno 2002)*. Florence : Istituto Papirologico « G. Vitelli », 153-170.

Marganne, M.-H. 1996. 'La médecine dans l'Égypte romaine : les sources et les méthodes', in W. Haase – H. Temporini (éds.), *Aufstieg und Niedergang der Römischen Welt* 2.37.3. Berlin – New York : W. de Gruyter, 2709-2740.

Martin, A. 2007. 'Τῷ δεῖνι παρὰ τοῦ δεῖνος. Réflexions à propos d'un type documentaire', in *Proceedings of the 24th International Congress of Papyrology, Helsinki, 1-7 August, 2004*, II, Comm. Hum. Litt., 122.2. Helsinki : Societas Scientiarum Fennica, 661-675.

Martin, A. 2008. 'Le « praescript » de P. Yale Inv. 443', *Chronique d'Égypte* 83 : 219-223.

Martin, A. à paraître. 'Le *vacat*, un silence souvent éloquent', in N. Carlig et al. (éds.), *Signes dans les textes. Recherches sur les continuités et les ruptures des pratiques scribales en Égypte pharaonique, gréco-romaine et byzantine. Actes du colloque international. Liège, 2-4 juin 2016*, Papyrologica Leodiensia 9. Liège : Presses Universitaires de Liège.

Mayser, E. 1923². *Grammatik der griechischen Papyri aus der Ptolemäerzeit*. I. *Laut- und Wortlehre*. Berlin – Leipzig : W. de Gruyter, 2e éd.

Mitthof, F. 2007. 'Forensische Medizin im römischen Ägypten', in H. Froschauer – C. Römer (éds.), *Zwischen Magie und Wissenschaft. Ärzte und Heilkunst in den Papyri aus Ägypten*, Nilus 13. Vienne : Phoibos, 55-63.

Mitthof, F. 2008. 'Forensische Medizin in römischen und spätantiken Ägypten', in E.M. Harris – G. Thür (éds.), *Symposion 2007. Vorträge zur griechischen und hellenistischen Rechtsgeschichte (Durham, 2.-6. September 2007). Papers on Greek and Hellenistic Legal History (Durham, September 2-6 2007)*, Akten der Gesellschaft für Griechische und Hellenistische Rechtsgeschichte 20. Vienne : Verlag der Österreichischen Akademie der Wissenschaften, 301-318.

Nanetti, O. 1941. 'Ricerche sui medici e sulla medicina nei papiri', *Aegyptus* 21 : 301-314.

de Ricci, S. 1901. 'Trois papyrus du musée Guimet trouvés à Antinoé', in C. Wessely (éd.), *Studien zur Palaeographie und Papyruskunde*. Leipzig : E. Avenarius, 6-8.

Ricciardetto, A. 2013. '"Inspecter un corps mort" : contribution des rapports médicaux sur papyrus (Ier-IVe siècles de notre ère) à l'histoire de la pratique médico-légale antique', in Ph. Charlier – D. Gourevitch (éds.), *Actes du 4e Colloque international de Pathographie. Saint Jean de Cole, Mai 2011*. Paris : De Boccard, 101-115.

Ricciardetto, A. 2015a. *Recherches sur la typologie des papyrus documentaires grecs en rapport avec la profession médicale (IIIe s. av. J.-C.-VIIe siècle apr. J.-C.) : contrats, pétitions, rapports médicaux et lettres*. Diss. Université de Liège.

Ricciardetto, A. 2015b. 'Y a-t-il une filiation entre la structure des fiches de malades dans les *Épidémies* hippocratiques et celle des rapports médicaux grecs d'Égypte (Ier-IVe siècles) conservés sur papyrus ?', in Ph. Charlier – D. Gourevitch (éds.), *Actes du 5e Colloque international de Pathographie. Bergues, Mai 2013*. Paris : De Boccard, 53-68.

Ricciardetto, A. à paraître. *La médecine et le droit. La procédure médico-légale dans l'Égypte romaine et byzantine d'après la documentation papyrologique grecque*, Papyrologica Leodiensia. Liège : Presses Universitaires de Liège.

Robert, F. 1975. 'Les adresses des malades dans les *Épidémies* II, IV et VI', in L. Bourgey – J. Jouanna (éds.), *La Collection hippocratique et son rôle dans l'histoire de la médecine, Colloque de Strasbourg (23-27 octobre 1972)*. Leyde : Brill, 173-194.

Robert, F. 1976. 'Prophasis', *Revue des Études Grecques* 89 : 317-342.

Robert, F. 1989. 'Médecine d'équipe dans les *Épidémies V*', in G. Baader – R. Winau (éds.), *Die hippokratischen Epidemien. Theorie – Praxis – Tradition, Verhandlungen des Ve Colloque international hippocratique (10.-15. 9. 1984)*, Sudhoffs Archiv, Beiheft 27. Stuttgart : F. Steiner, 20-27.

von Staden, H. 1994. 'Author and Authority. Celsus on the Construction of a Scientific Self', in M.E. Vázquez Buján (éd.), *Tradición e Innovación de la Medicina Latina de la Antigüedad y de la Alta Edad Media*. Saint-Jacques-de-Compostelle : Servicio de publicacións e intercambio científico da Universidade de Santiago de Compostela, 103-117.

Sudhoff, K. 1909. *Ärztliches aus griechischen Papyrus-Urkunden. Bausteine zu einer medizinischen Kulturgeschichte des Hellenismus*, Studien zur Geschichte der Medizin, 5/6. Leipzig : J.A. Barth.

Torallas Tovar, S. 2004. 'La práctica forense en el Egipto romano', *CFC (G)* 14 : 183-200.

CHAPTER 7

Definitions and Technical Terminology in the *Erôtapokriseis* on Papyrus

Isabella Bonati

Abstract

The aim of this contribution is to analyse some specific aspects of catechisms on papyrus mainly devoted to individual diseases, by focusing more precisely on the definition of the pathology and the technical terminology employed to express it. After providing a general introduction to papyri preserving medical catechisms, the chapter will illustrate the divergences and similarities in the definition of identical medical topics by means of selected *specimina*. This will be done between both papyrus catechisms and medical literature, especially compared to the tradition of the *definitiones* and *quaestiones medicinales*, and among different catechisms on papyrus. Finally, the investigation of technical vocabulary and certain expressions used to define pathologies and medical procedures in the papyri, but unparalleled in medical authors, can provide interesting insights into the language of medical question-and-answer texts. This raises the innovative question as to whether there was a sort of lexical 'particularisation' in the catechistic genre, maybe influenced by the concrete nature of the context in which the *erôtapokriseis* on papyrus were copied and used, be it for didactic purposes in medical education or during the exercise of the doctor's profession.

1 Introduction: Medical Catechisms on Papyrus*

Medical texts in question-and-answer format are a genre, the *erôtapokrisis*, which provided an excellent method to articulate and transfer medical knowledge in Antiquity. This genre is well represented among Greek medical papyri

* The present contribution falls into the DIGMEDTEXT project (ERC-2013-AdG no. 339828) funded by the European Research Council at the University of Parma (Principal Investigator: Prof. Isabella Andorlini; see http://www.papirologia.unipr.it/ERC), but the work for this contribution has been carried out during my Post-doctoral Fellowship at the North-West University of Potchefstroom, South Africa.

 | DOI:10.1163/9789004442672_009

from Egypt.[1] Medical papyri represent a complex corpus of texts that ranges from fragments belonging to the 'official' or 'formal' medical literature (i.e., medical writers whose works have also been transmitted through the Byzantine and medieval manuscript tradition: e.g., fragments of Hippocratic and Galenic treatises), and *adespota*, to proper documentary texts (e.g., physicians' reports, petitions of private individuals and private correspondence concerning health matters).[2] This corpus mostly includes technical texts conceived to convey technical knowledge. Among them, the catechisms are a representative example together with other kinds of school manuals, technical handbooks and collections of recipes. The papyri of this group occupy a sort of 'twilight zone' in the canonical separation between literary and documentary texts. Due to their 'borderline' nature, they have been conventionally categorised as 'paraliterary' or—in a somewhat pejorative way—'subliterary',[3] in comparison to the more sophisticated and 'formal' writings which came down to us via the manuscript transmission (most notably the Hippocratic and Galenic corpora, as already mentioned).

The number of papyrus catechisms known so far is quite conspicuous. The most up-to-date list enumerates 23 items, among which only one is still unpublished.[4] These catechisms range in date from the II century BCE[5] to the early IV century CE. The majority dates back to the II and III century CE. This fact attests to the long-lived popularity and the role of catechistic texts especially in Roman Egypt.[6]

The content of these texts on papyrus is traditionally divided into a series of entries each introduced by a question (ἐρώτημα), that is either indented from

1 General studies on papyri in question-and-answer format include: Zalateo (1961: 160–235) and (1964: 52–57); Ieraci Bio (1995: 187–207); Andorlini (1999: 7–15); Hanson (2003: 199–217); Leith (2009a: 107–123). On medical definitions and some particular cases, see, e.g., Kollesch (1973); Papadoyannakis (2006: 91–106); Jouanna (2008: 86–102); Maire (2008: 103–115). Studies on specific catechistic texts on papyrus are: Nicole (1903: 1–3); Bäckström (1904: 158–162); Barns (1949: 1–8); Manetti (1973: 46–49); Marganne (1978: 313–320), as well as (1986: 65–73) and (1987: 189–200); Andorlini (1992: 375–390) and (1997: 153–168); Manfredi (1997: 73–79); Maravela—Leith (1997: 637–650); Hanson—Mattern (2001: 71–83); Magdelaine (2004: 63–77); Leith (2007: 125–134), as well as (2009b: 60–66) and (2009c: 211–218).

2 See Ricciardetto's contribution to this volume.

3 Cf. Reggiani (2017: 78).

4 See the list at the end of Reggiani's contribution to this volume, and also *MedOn* s.v. catechism. The catechism on papyrus known but unpublished is P.Oxf.Ash. inv. 28 of the II–IV cent. CE (MP3 2353.8, LDAB 4226, TM 63033).

5 The only fragment dating back to the Ptolemaic period is P.Oxf.Sackler inv. s.n. of the II cent. BCE (MP3 2370, LDAB 6884, TM 65633).

6 Cf. Hanson (2001: 72) and Leith (2009a: 108).

left, or centered at mid-column, and followed by a response (ἀπόκρισις).[7] This structure is systematically employed to describe and approach the subjects according to a fixed set of topics that, in the case of *erôtapokriseis* on individual diseases, includes:[8] a definition introduced by the question τί ἐστιν (what is …?); an aetiological question inquiring the cause with expressions such as τίς αἰτία (what is the cause of …?) and πῶς γίνεται (how does … occur?); often a question on the signs, the σημεῖα (e.g., τίνα σημεῖα, what are the signs of …?); a question asking how many different forms the disease has and what differentiates these forms (e.g., τίνες διαφοραί, what are the different forms of …?, πόσαι διαφοραί, how many different forms are there of …?); a final question or section concerning the therapy (e.g., τίς θεραπεία, what is the treatment of …?, χειρουργία, surgery). Sometimes, some of these topics may be omitted, whilst other times some of them are not dealt with separately but their relevant elements are tied up together in one entry. This reveals a certain flexibility, manageability and the possibility of keeping the material updated according to the compiler's needs and the specific purpose of the papyrus.[9]

Given their formal layout, the medical texts in question-and-answer format have traditionally been considered as a form of teaching manuals used to introduce students of medicine and aspiring practitioners "to a store of medical knowledge and professional terminology",[10] but also as reference tools employed by established doctors to retain and improve information essential to their professional practice.[11] A more recent hypothesis identifies in their format and methodology a way to systematise medical knowledge through an approach which finds close parallels in the Aristotelian scientific method and maybe ultimately derived from it.[12] According to this hypothesis, such texts are connected with a wider intellectual tradition and should be regarded as "a distinct form of scientific writing".[13] This would suggest that the primary purpose

7 On the layout of *erôtapokriseis* on papyrus and the way to edit them digitally, see Reggiani's contribution to this volume.

8 See Leith (2009a: 110–111).

9 Cf. Hanson (2010: 194): "even if the ordering of topics was fixed. The format for inclusion of definitions was flexible, allowing for addition and subtraction to keep the material up-to-date and manageable. Some *erôtapokriseis* were fuller or more complete than others, with a compiler omitting or including topic's various aspects, such as differentiation and therapy, as each compiler saw fit". On the variety of kinds of question-and-answer texts on papyrus, presenting different levels of content and details, see Andorlini (1997: 160), Leith (2007: 132–134), as well as Reggiani's contribution to this volume.

10 Hanson (2003: 199). Cf. especially Andorlini (1999: 7–9).

11 Cf. Hanson (2003: 199).

12 Leith (2009a: 108–122).

13 Leith (2009a: 122).

of the papyri in question-and-answer format was practical rather than exclusively educational, presuming that they "have been used by physicians in the actual practice of their profession, which is implied especially by the inclusion of information on diagnostic signs and therapy".[14]

The fragmentary copies of *erôtapokriseis* on papyrus cover a variety of topics pertaining to ophthalmology, anatomy, pathology, gynecology and surgery. The vast majority of them preserve sections on individual diseases, especially eye conditions; other fragments are anatomical and describe various parts of the body, with no pathological content; other texts are exclusively concerned with the description of some forms of therapy, whereas some *specimina* seem to focus on the explanation of medical technical terminology.[15]

The papyrus catechisms often exhibit textual affinities with didactic treatises, teaching manuals and collections of definitions preserved in the manuscript tradition, such as the *Definitiones medicae* and the *Introductio* ascribed to Galen[16] and the Latin Ps.-Soranian *Quaestiones medicinales*. Seeing that the copies on papyrus are always fragmentary and inevitably lacunose, these more "traditional" collections of medical definitions are sometimes very useful for restoring the content of the questionnaires on papyrus. They offer striking textual parallels and also give an idea of how extensive the catechistic texts on papyrus might originally have been. It is indeed likely that the anonymous compilers of the papyrus catechisms had access, either directly or indirectly, to treatises and definitions elaborated by the traditional medical authors of the past centuries, or at least that they relied on a variety of sources that displayed close affinities with (or were among the sources of) these formal and more sophisticated works.

Furthermore, in spite of the fragmentary condition of the papyri, comparing what has survived in these fragments with the formal medical literature just mentioned, it appears evident that the ordering of the entries in the sets of question-and-answers and the arrangement of topics are not accidental, but follow a fixed scheme. This conservative tendency in ordering materials, as well as their characteristic layout, surely contributed to the usability of the papyrus catechisms: "arrangement and ordering of topics was an important aspect of what students were to learn and the sequence in which they were to learn data, while the fixed ordering *a capite ad calcem* made the information easy to consult in extensive copies of medical material",[17] thus facilitating the process of

14 Ibid.

15 For this categorisation of papyrus catechisms, see Leith (2009a: 109 and 122).

16 For the didactic purposes of these Ps.-Galenic works, see Kollesch (1973: 13–46).

17 Hanson (2010: 192).

seeking and acquiring specific details. At the same time, such a conservative approach appears to be in relative contrast with the freedom compilers had in selecting what they wrote in their definitions.[18]

2 Illustrative Cases

The starting point of this study will be a thorough examination of a selection of medical terms—especially names of pathologies—that I carried out in the frame of the project *Medicalia Online*, a lexicographical database of technical terms attested in the Greek medical papyri.[19] It is significant to point out that the definitions of pathologies given in the questionnaires on papyrus provide useful lexical information that contributes to the study of the words analysed in *Medicalia Online*. At the same time, an accurate lexical study contributes to highlighting the interest of the question-and-answer format, as well as the nature of the definitions that it preserves. I have selected some *specimina* to illustrate relevant aspects.

The first issue that I will consider concerns the content and the kind of information provided in the medical definitions. As noted before, the compilers displayed a certain freedom in choosing and arranging both the medical concepts and the way to express them. Some illustrative cases will be presented to outline similarities and differences on the same topic: firstly (A1) between catechisms on papyrus and medical literature, especially—but not only—compared to the tradition of the *definitiones* and *quaestiones medicinales*, and secondly (A2) among catechisms on papyrus. Finally (B), I will deal with lexical and linguistic matters.

A1 *Catechisms on Papyrus and Medical Literature*

In order to illustrate the divergences and similarities in the definitions of pathologies between the *erôtapokriseis* on papyrus and the medical literature a useful case is found in GMP I 6 (MP3 2340.01, LDAB 10278, TM 69007). This papyrus

18 Cf. Hanson (2003: 201).

19 Both the lexical project *Medicalia Online* and the main project *Corpus of the Greek Medical Papyri Online* (CPGM), a textual database aimed at providing comprehensive digital editions of the Greek medical papyri, have been supported by the grant ERC-2013-AdG no. 339828 of the European Research Council. See at http://www.papirologia.unipr.it/CPGM/medicalia/vocab/index.php. On the aims, structure, methodology and outcomes of *Medicalia Online*, see also Bonati (2018), (2019a) and (2019b). On the digitisation of the *CPGM* see Andorlini (2017), Reggiani (2015: 341–352), (2017: 273–275) and (2019), and Bertonazzi (2019).

scrap (4,8×11,6 cm), dating back to the end of the II or to the very beginning of the III century CE, contains a fragment of a medical catechism on some afflictions of the head and is copied on the back of a documentary roll. Three topics are discussed in this fragment. The first one is completely lost and reaches its conclusion in l. 2. The second one deals with hydrocephalus (ὑδροκέφαλον),[20] the condition characterised by an accumulation of watery fluid in the head, which is discussed in ll. 3–18 and is explicitly mentioned in ll. 5 and 7. The last topic concerns the caries of the skull known as τερηδών (a metaphorical noun of pathology named after the worm which bores holes through wood).[21] It is introduced in l. 19, very likely in the form of a question "what is teredon?", but the papyrus breaks off just after another mention of τερηδών in l. 20, the beginning of its definition.

As has been pointed out by the *editores principes*, Hanson and Mattern,[22] the text of this *erotapokrisis* on papyrus displays close affinities with the so called 'continental version' of the Latin Ps.-Soranian *Quaestiones medicinales* as preserved in a manuscript from Chartre (MS Carnotensis 62, fol. 13r–v; X cent.).[23] Indeed, these texts have the same formal layout and only in these two copies of medical questions the discussions of hydrocephalus and τερηδών are directly juxtaposed. Furthermore, since the question-answer set (entry 233) that precedes hydrocephalus (entries 234–235) and τερηδών (entries 236–237) in MS Carnotensis (62, fol. 13r–v) concerns calcification (*oporeis* cod., *l. porosis*, i.e., Greek πώρωσις), i.e., the "process by which the extremities of fractured bones are reunited by a callus" (LSJ[9] 1561 s.v.), one might presume that this was the topic lost in the upper lacuna of the papyrus.[24] By contrast, in the 'insular' tradition of the Pseudo-Soranian *Quaestiones medicinales* (MS Cottonianus Galba E IV [early XIII cent.] and MS Lincoloniensis 220 [XII cent.]) the discussion of τερηδών sits at some distance prior to hydrocephalus.[25] On the other hand, these three topics are placed in close proximity also in Ps.-Galen's *Definitiones*

20 See *MedOn* s.v. ὑδροκέφαλον.

21 See *MedOn* s.v. τερηδών.

22 Hanson—Mattern (2001).

23 The manuscript tradition of the Ps.-Soranian *Quaestiones medicinales* has been divided into two branches: MS Carnotensis 62 represents the 'continental' tradition, whereas the 'insular' tradition includes MS Cottonianus Galba E IV, fol. 238vb–244vb (early XIII cent.) and MS Lincoloniensis 220, fol. 22r–44r (XII cent.). On these manuscripts and their interrelationships, see Fischer (1998: 1–19).

24 See Hanson—Mattern (2001: 73–74).

25 Teredon is entry 227 in the Rose edition (2.270.28–29 Rose), drawn from MS Cottonianus Galba E IV and entry 313 in MS Lincolonensis 220, fol. 38r, whereas hydrocephalus is, respectively, entries 250–251 (2.273.25–274.3 Rose) and entries 336–337 in MS Lincolonensis 220, fol. 39v.

medicae, where they constitute entries 389 (πῶρός ἐστιν οὐσία λιθώδης καὶ ἀπόκριτος: "a callus is a tissue hard like a stone and thickened"), 390 (ὑδροκέφαλόν ἐστιν ὑδατώδους ὑγροῦ ἢ αἵματος τοῦ τρυγώδους συλλογὴ κατά τι μέρος τῶν τὴν κεφαλὴν πλεκόντων σωμάτων: "hydrocephalus is the accumulation of watery fluid or thick blood in a part of the bodies surrounding the head"), and 395 (τερηδών ἐστιν ὀστοῦ κατάτρησις ἀπὸ φθορᾶς: "teredon is the cavity of the bone due to deterioration") (19.442.14, 442.15–17 and 443.11–13 Kühn respectively). The similarities between the text on papyrus and the 'continental version' of Ps.-Soranus might lead to suppose that, at least in the section on description and diagnosis of hydrocephalus and perhaps τερηδών, the source of the Ps.-Soranian Latin translation was the Greek *erôtapokrisis* of which the papyrus is a lacunose copy.[26]

Focusing on the questions and answers about hydrocephalus is particularly useful since it is the most fully preserved section in the papyrus. Accounts on hydrocephalus are well represented in Greek medical literature. The earliest scientific description of hydrocephalus is found in a long passage ascribed to Hippocrates (*Morb.* 2.15 [7.26.24–28.21 Littré; 149.1–150.7 Jouanna]). Here the compound ὑδροκέφαλον is never mentioned explicitly, but the Hippocratic author refers to this condition with the periphrasis ὕδωρ ἐπὶ τῷ ἐγκεφάλῳ (water on the brain). Among the several sources on this topic, the fullest and most elaborate accounts of hydrocephalus are gathered in late antique medical compendia that often draw on earlier physicians, whose writings have otherwise gone lost: Oribasius (*Coll. Med.* 46.28 [3.237.25–239.7 Raeder]) preserves a long account by the Greek surgeon Antyllus (II cent. CE); Aëtius of Amida preserves two versions of the account by Leonidas (middle-end of the I cent. CE: cf. 6.1 [2.123.1–125.3 Olivieri] and 15.12.1–80 [34.12–37.18 Zervos]), which are quite similar in content, even if the latter is more than 30 lines longer and much more detailed; Paul of Aegina (*Medical Epitome* 6.3 [2.46.9–47.14 Heiberg]) presents an extract from an anonymous author very similar to the accounts of the other physicians. For the purpose of outlining affinities and differences between catechisms on papyrus and medical literature, it is especially relevant to compare the papyrus with the aforementioned 'continental version' of the Latin Ps.-Soranian *Quaestiones medicinales* and some Galenic passages.

In the *erôtapokrisis* on papyrus the discussion is punctuated into three sections each introduced by a question-heading:

– the first question-answer set involves the definition (ll. 3–6): the introductory question asks for the name of the condition that involves fluid or moisture in the head; the answer is that this collection of fluid is named hydrocephalus;

26 See Hanson—Mattern (2001: 75 and 80) and (2010: 193–194).

- the second set calls for the different types of hydrocephalus according to the four loci where fluid accumulations gather, moving from outermost locus, the subcutaneous layer between the scalp and the pericranium, to innermost, that between the meninges and the brain (ll. 7–10);[27]
- the final question (l. 11) seems to inquire into the aetiology of hydrocephalus; the response follows in ll. 12–18, interspersing information on symptoms and treatment, but little can be read with confidence due to the fragmentary condition of the papyrus.[28] Therefore, we will focus our attention only on the first and second question-answer set, corresponding to ll. 3–10, i.e., definition and differentiation.

	GMP I 6.3–10 (text and translation by Hanson—Mattern [2001: 81])	Ps.-Sor., *Quaest. Med.* (MS Carnot. 62, fol. 13r–v)	Ps.-Galen
Definition	ll. 3–6 [τί ἐστι τὸ ὑγρὸν ὄν] (vac.) | (vac.) [ἔν τινι μέρει τῆς κεφ]α̣λῆς; (vac.) | [τὸ πάθος προσαγορεύεται] ὑδροκέ[φαλον] | [διὰ τὸ ὑγρὸν ἐν κεφαλῇ συ]λλεγόμενον 'What is the moisture that is in some part of the head?' The disease is called hydrocephalus because of the moisture being collected in the head.	234 *Quid est hydrocefalon? aquati humores collectio uel sanguinolentum uel fecilentum semper tamen humidum.* 234 What is hydrocephalus? Accumulation of watery fluids, it is full of blood or dregs, yet always moist.	*Def. Med.* 390 (19.442.15–17 Kühn) ὑδροκέφαλον ἐστιν ὑδατώδους ὑγροῦ ἢ αἵματος τοῦ τρυγώδους συλλογὴ κατά τι μέρος τῶν τὴν κεφαλὴν πλεκόντων σωμάτων. Hydrocephalus is the accumulation of watery fluid or thick blood in a part of the bodies surrounding the head.

27 For discussion of ll. 7–10 and their restoration, see Hanson—Mattern (2001: 82–83) comm. *ad l.*

28 The editorial restoration of the question in l. 11 [πόσαι εἰσὶν] α̣ἱ̣ [αἰτί]α̣[ι]; ("how many are the causes?") derives from ll. 13–14 [λέ]γ̣ε̣τ̣αι τὴ̣ν̣ συλλ̣ο̣|[γὴν εἶναι ἐξ ἀδήλου αἰτία]ς ἢ ἐκ πρ[ο]δ̣ήλου ("it is said that the accumulation exists from either an unclear cause or from a clear one"). The supplement for these lines has been offered by the aforementioned account by Leonidas preserved by Aëtius, cf. 6.1 (2.123.5–6 Olivieri): γίγνεται δὲ τοῦτο ἢ ἐξ ἀδήλου ἢ ἐκ προδήλου αἰτίας. See Hanson—Mattern (2001: 79 and 82).

(cont.)

	GMP I 6.3–10 (text and translation by Hanson—Mattern [2001: 81])	Ps.-Sor., *Quaest. Med.* (MS Carnot. 62, fol. 13r–v)	Ps.-Galen
Differentiation	ll. 7–10 [πόσαι αἱ διαφοραὶ τῶν ὑδρ]ọκεφάλων; (vac.) | [τέσσαρες ἢ γὰρ μεταξὺ τοῦ] δέρματος καὶ | [περι-κρανίου ἢ καὶ ὀ]ϲṭοῦ ἢ μεταξύ | [ὀστοῦ καὶ μήνιγ-γος ἢ ἐγ]κεφάλου (vac.) 'How many are the types of hydrocephalus?' Four: either (1) between the scalp and the pericranium, or (2) [between the pericranium] and the skull, or (3) between the skull and the meninges, or (4) [between the meninges and the] brain.	235 *Quot differentiae sunt in hy⟨dro⟩cefalis? quattuor, enim inter cutem et omentum* […] *fit, et inter ipsum omentum* […] *fit, et inter omentum et testam, aut inter testam et miningam, aut inter miningam et cerebrum. fit autem huiusmodi collectio aut in parte aliqua capitis aut per totum.* 235 How many are the types of hydrocephalus? Four: it develops either between the scalp and the membrane (= pericranium) […], or into the same membrane […], or between this membrane and the skull, or between the skull and the meninx, or between the meninx and the brain. However, the accumulation occurs either in a part or in all the head.	*Int.* 19.3 (14.782.14–17 Kühn; 91.21–92.4 Petit) ὑδροκεφάλων δὲ εἴδη τέσσαρα. τὸ μὲν μεταξὺ ἐγκεφάλου καὶ μήνιγγος. τὸ δὲ μεταξὺ μήνιγγος καὶ ὀστοῦ. τὸ δὲ μεταξὺ ὀστοῦ καὶ περικρανίου. τὸ δὲ μεταξὺ ὀστοῦ καὶ δέρματος. There are four kinds of hydrocephalus: between the brain and the meninges, between the meninges and the skull, between the skull and the pericranium, between the skull and the skin.

The contents of these passages are quite similar and point to the definition of hydrocephalus as an accumulation of fluids in the head, but the phrasing and the level of detail are different. We see that:

- as to ll. 3–6 (definition):
  1) Ps.-Galen (ὑδροκέφαλον ἐστιν ὑδατώδους ὑγροῦ ἢ αἵματος τοῦ τρυγώδους συλλογή) is closer to Ps.-Soranus (*aquati humores collectio uel sanguinolentum uel fecilentum semper tamen humidum*) than the reconstructed text of the papyrus seems to be, even if the Galenic author includes some more details (κατά τι μέρος τῶν τὴν κεφαλὴν πλεκόντων σωμάτων);
  2) in ll. 3–4, the Latin question of the MS from Chartre (*Quid est hydrocefalon?*) does not help to restore the text of the papyrus since the presence of]α̣λης seems to conceal the plausible mention of the head at the end of l. 4. This makes the use of a more articulated question, such as the one proposed by the editors, more plausible than the simple one in Ps.-Soranus;
  3) in ll. 5–6 the editorial restoration reflects some passages of other medical authors, notably the two aforementioned versions of the account of hydrocephalus by Leonidas preserved in Aëtius.[29]

What is remarkable about the definition part is that the question-answer order is reversed in the papyrus when compared to Ps.-Soranus and Ps.-Galen. The papyrus departs from the sign/empirical fact, asking what is the water accumulation in the head, and then provides the technical terminology in the answer, declaring that the name of this condition is ὑδροκέφαλον. By contrast, Ps.-Soranus and Ps.-Galen depart from the technical terminology and then detail the sign/empirical fact. Such an inversion might give some insight into the different uses and purposes of these texts. The fact that the papyrus departs from what is instantly visible might perhaps mean that it had a more practical application, as a tool intended for doctors looking for a proper diagnosis 'on the spot', that would be perfectly compatible with the aforementioned hypothesis of a practical nature of the question-and-answer texts on papyrus.[30] Conversely, Ps.-Soranus and Ps.-Galen seem to have a more educational purpose serving as school manuals for memorising medical definitions.

---

29 For ll. 5–6 [τὸ πάθος προσαγορεύεται] ὑδροκέ[φαλον] | [διὰ τὸ ὑγρὸν ἐν κεφαλῇ συ]λλεγόμενον, cf. Aëtius 6.1 (2.123.2–3 Olivieri): τὸ ὑδροκέφαλον πάθος προσαγορεύεται ἀπὸ τοῦ ἐν τῇ κεφαλῇ ὑδατώδους ὑγροῦ συλλεγομένου, and also 15.12.1–2 (34.14–15 Zervos): ὑδροκέφαλον τὸ πάθος προσαγορεύεται ἀπὸ τοῦ ἐν τῇ κεφαλῇ ὑδατώδους ὑγροῦ συλλεγομένου ("the hydrocephalus condition is so called from the accumulation of watery fluid in the head").

30 On the practical nature of the catechisms on papyrus see also Andorlini (1999: 7–9). Thanks to Michiel Meeusen for this suggestion.

– as to ll. 7–10 (differentiation):

1) in l. 7 of the papyrus, the question ([πόσαι αἱ διαφοραὶ τῶν ὑδρ]ọκεφάλων;) is mainly modelled on the Latin of the MS from Chartre (*Quot differentiae sunt in hy⟨dro⟩cefalis?*) and Antyllus ap. Orib., *Coll. Med.* 46.28.2.1 (3.237.29 Raeder: διαφοραὶ δὲ τῶν ὑδροκεφάλων εἰσὶ κτλ.);

2) in ll. 9–10 (answer), the papyrus reflects the tradition of ancient medical writers to list the loci of fluid buildup from outermost scalp to innermost brain. Nevertheless, in Ps.-Galen, *Int.* 19.3 (14.782.14–17 Kühn; 91.21–92.4 Petit) the order is reversed, from innermost to outermost. Furthermore, in the papyrus catechism the loci are explicitly four, as is also the case in Ps.-Soranus and in the same Ps.-Galenic passage. By contrast, Antyllus ap. Orib., *Coll. Med.* 46.28.2.1–4 (3.237.29–32 Raeder) presents only three loci, but names four, for the one between the meninges and the brain is said to be "impossible", meaning deadly: διαφοραὶ δὲ τῶν ὑδροκεφάλων εἰσὶ τρεῖς· ἢ γὰρ μεταξὺ τοῦ δέρματος καὶ τοῦ περικρανίου ἢ μεταξὺ περικρανίου καὶ ὀστέου ἢ μεταξὺ ὀστέου καὶ μήνιγγος· μεταξὺ γὰρ μήνιγγος καὶ ἐγκεφάλου συστῆναι ὑγρὸν ἀδύνατον ("there are three different kinds of hydrocephalus: between the scalp and the pericranium, between the pericranium and the skull, between the skull and the meninges, for the formation of fluid between the meninges and the brain is impossible"). It is indeed specified that "the distension of the sutures is untreatable" (see 46.28.14.4–15.1 [3.239.1–2 Raeder]: διάστασις τῶν ῥαφῶν ἀθεράπευτός ἐστιν). Likewise, Aëtius 6.1.14–19 (2.123.15–20 Olivieri) focuses on three loci but mentions the fourth one saying that it is lethal: συνίσταται δὲ τὸ ὑγρὸν ἐπὶ τῶν ὑδροκεφάλων ἢ μεταξὺ τοῦ δέρματος καὶ τοῦ περικρανίου ὑμένος ἢ μυὸς τοῦ κροταφίτου ἢ ὑπὸ τὸν περικράνιον ὑμένα μεταξὺ αὐτοῦ καὶ τοῦ τῆς κεφαλῆς ὀστοῦ ἢ ὑπὸ τὸ κρανίον μεταξὺ τῆς μήνιγγος καὶ τοῦ ὀστέου. οἱ δὲ πρὸ ἡμῶν φασι καὶ μεταξὺ τῆς μήνιγγος καὶ αὐτοῦ τοῦ ἐγκεφάλου συνίστασθαι, ὅπερ ἐστὶν ὀλέθριον ("fluid associated with hydrocephalus collects either between the skin and the membrane round the skull [= pericranium] or the temporal muscle, or under the pericranium between the membrane and the bone of the head, or under the skull between the meninx and the bone. The ones before me also say that this fluid gathers between the meninx and the brain itself, which is lethal"). Also Paul of Aegina, *Medical Epitome* 6.3 (2.46.16–17 Heiberg), claims that there are three loci, omitting the innermost, perhaps because he considers it implicitly untreatable: ἢ γὰρ μεταξὺ περικρανίου καὶ δέρματος συνίσταται τὸ ὑγρὸν ἢ μεταξὺ περικρανίου καὶ ὀστέου ἢ μεταξὺ ὀστέου καὶ μήνιγγος ("fluid is formed either between the pericranium and the

skin, or between the pericranium and the skull, or between the skull and the meninx"). In this regard, it might be interesting to mention the appearance of the adjective ἀθεράπευτος (untreatable) in l. 18. It is the only readable word in that line since it occurs in the most scantly preserved part of the papyrus fragment. The immediate context is lost, but the adjective is perhaps referred to the most serious case of fluid accumulation (cf. ll. 13–14 συλλọọ|[γήν]), namely the one in the place most difficult to be treated (cf. l. 15]τατον τόπον, "the most … place").

To conclude, it seems that the compiler of the papyrus has selected sources close to what is excerpted by the late antique epitomists. These sources probably represented the best information on the topic in his time. Also the Ps.-Galenic author of the *Introductio* reflects the use of similar materials. Nevertheless, no one of these Greek authors seems to rely exactly and directly on the same source "of the excerptor as he was making the medical catechism, as we know it in Greek from the Yale papyrus and in Latin in the 'continental' version of the Pseudo-Soranian *Quaestiones medicinales*".[31] The conclusion is that, much in line with other compilers of papyrus *erôtapokriseis*, the compiler of this catechism is generally conservative and follows the traditional ordering of the entries, but he displays freedom in choosing what he offers as contents of his question-and-answer text.[32]

A2 *Affinities and Differences among Papyrus Catechisms on the Same Topic*

To further illustrate this point, it is particularly useful to compare the definitions provided by two ophthalmic catechisms from the II century CE: P.Ross.Georg. I 20 (MP3 2343, LDAB 4778, TM 63569) and P.Aberd. 11 (MP3 2342, LDAB 4539, TM 63332).[33] These papyri show how, despite their similarity in format, the organisation of the definition and the level of detail can vary on the same topic. P.Ross.Georg. I 20 contains remains of three columns discussing four eye diseases (col. II ll. 55–67 γλαύκωμα [glaucoma], ll. 68–93 σταφύλωμα [staphyloma], ll. 94–115 πτερύγιον [pterygium], col. III ll. 116–125 ῥευματισμός [discharge]), plus a question about ὑποσπαθισμός (a kind of operation for eye-affection, col. III l. 124), whereas P.Aberd. 11 preserves less than 20 readable lines

31 Hanson—Mattern (2001: 80).

32 Cf. Hanson (2003: 201 and 217).

33 The relationship between these two catechisms was first pointed out by Marganne (1978: 313–320), who republished them in Marganne (1994: 104–111 for P. Aberd. 11) and (112–132 for P.Ross.Georg. I 20). See also Hanson (2003: 205–207) and (2010: 192 n. 28).

on the eye condition called πτερύγιον[34] and overlaps with P.Ross.Georg. I 20 in its discussion of it. However, in spite of several textual affinities, neither of these papyri seems to be a copy of the other. Here follows the text of both as printed by Marganne,[35] divided into sets of question-answer:

P.Ross.Georg. I 20.94–115:

- τεί (*l.* τί) ἐστ[ι τὸ πτερύ]|γειον (*l.* πτερύγιον); | ἔκφυσεις (*l.* ἔκφυσις) ὑμενῴ[δης ἀπὸ τοῦ] | κανθοῦ ηὐξημέ[νη.]
- πῶ[ς γείνεται (*l.* γίνεται) τὸ] | π̣[τ]ε[ρύγειον (*l.* πτερύγιον);] | ἤτοι [σ]αρκὸς αὔ[ξησις τῆς] | ὑπὸ τοῦ κανθο[ῦ μὲν σωματο]|ποιουμένου, γε[ίνεται (*l.* γίνεται) δὲ καὶ] | ὑπὸ τοῦ κερ̣ατ̣[οειδοῦς χιτῶ]|νος.
- τ̣[είνει (*l.* τίνι) διαφέρουσι τὰ] | π̣[τερύγεια (*l.* πτερύγια); | διαφέρου̣[σειν (*l.* διαφέρουσιν) αὐτῶν μεγέ]|θει, σχήμα[τι, τόπῳ, χρώματει (*l.* χρώματι)] | ἢ φύσει.
- χ[ειρουργεία (*l.* χειρουργία) τοῦ | πτερυγείου (*l.* πτερυγίου)] | διαστείλα̣[ντες τὰ βλέφαρα, τὸ] | πτερύγει[ον (*l.* πτερύγιον) ἀγκίστρῳ ἐκ τοῦ] | ὀφθαλμοῦ [ἀναδεξάμενοι] | διεκφαν̣[οῦμεν.]

- What is pterygium? It is a membranous excrescence growing from the canthus.
- How does pterygium develop? It is a growth of flesh taking shape from under the canthus, but it also develops from the cornea.
- Which are the different kinds of pterygia? They differ among themselves in size, shape, location, color or nature.
- Surgery of pterygium. Having separated the eyelids, we/you[36] will raise and isolate the pterygium from the eye with a hook

34 For an in-depth study of this word and its sources, see *MedOn* s.v. πτερύγιον.

35 Marganne (1978: 313–320) and (1994: 104–132).

36 The previous editors, G. Zereteli and O. Krüger, integrate the verb as διεκφαν̣[εῖς, second person singular future, but διεκφαν̣[in l. 15 as well as in P.Aberd. 11.12, can also be reconstructed as a second person plural future, διεκφαν[εῖτε. In both cases it should be understood as an instruction, a direct address to the implied reader. This is speculative, since we do not have any parallel in the extant catechisms on papyrus preserving indications about therapy (cf., e.g., P.Mil.Vogl. I 15.21–32), but in medical literature, when describing the treatment and the operations to be performed, more often the first, other times the second person plural is found. A suitable example is represented by some passages of authors describing the (surgical or pharmaceutical) therapy of pterygium. For the second person, cf. Orib., *Eun.* 4.24.12–13 (6.3.448.2–3 Raeder): τὸ δὲ μικρὸν καὶ μαλακὸν (scil. πτερύγιον) θεραπεύσεις αἰγείρου ὀπῷ ("you will treat small and soft pterygium with juice of black poplar"). For the first person, cf. in particular Aëtius 7.62.1–15 (2.315.9–23 Olivieri): ἐγχειροῦμεν δὲ οὕτως πρὸς τὴν ἀφαίρεσιν τοῦ πτερυγίου· διαστέλλοντες τὰ βλέφαρα ἀπ' ἀλλήλων καὶ

P.Aberd. 11.2–20:

- τί̣ ἐστι ὦ̣ν̣ (*l.* οὖν) [τὸ πτερύγειον (*l.* πτερύγιον);] | ἔκφυσ̣ι̣ς̣ ὑμενώδης α[ὐξανομένη ἀπὸ τοῦ] | κα̣ν̣θοῦ ἢ σωματοποι̣[ουμένη] | ἀπὸ τοῦ κερατοειδοῦς [χιτῶνος.]
- τίνες [εἰσὶ διαφοραὶ πτερυγείων (*l.* πτερυγίων);] | διαφέρετε (*l.* διαφέρεται) αὐτῶν τ̣ό̣[πωι, μεγέθει,] | σχήματι, χρώματ[ι, φύσει ἢ ἀνα]|σκευῇ.
- χειρ[ουργεία (*l.* χειρουργία) τοῦ πτερυγείου (*l.* πτερυγίου).] | μετὰ τὸν καθέδρειο̣[ν (*l.* καθέδριον) ὄντα τὸν πάσχοντα, ἐκ] | τοῦ ὀφθαλμοῦ διφ[υῆ βλέφαρα διαστείλαντες] | τὸ πτερύγειον (*l.* πτερύγιον) δι̣[εκφανοῦμεν ἀγκι]|στρείοι (*l.* ἀγκιστρίῳ),

---

ἄγκιστρον καταπείροντες περὶ τὰ μέσα τοῦ πτερυγίου ἀνατείνομεν ἠρέμα, ἵνα μὴ ἡ ἐπιδερματὶς τοῦ κερατοειδοῦς μετεωρισθῇ [...]. εἶτα βελόνην λαμβάνομεν λίνον ἔχουσαν διῃρημένον καὶ τρίχα ἱππείαν, καὶ ταύτην ὑποβάλλομεν τῷ πτερυγίῳ ἀναταθέντι διὰ τοῦ ἀγκίστρου· εἶτα ἀποδήσαντες τῷ ὑποβληθέντι λίνῳ τὸ πτερύγιον ἀνατείνομεν [...], ἀμφοτέραις ταῖς χερσὶ κατέχοντες τὴν τρίχα διακινοῦμεν ἄνω τε καὶ κάτω, ὑποδέροντες τὸ πτερύγιον, ἀρχόμενοι ἀπὸ τοῦ μέλανος, μέχρι τοῦ κανθοῦ. εἶτα [...] ἀνατείνοντες τῷ λίνῳ ἀφαιροῦμεν πτερυγοτόμῳ ἐκ τῆς βάσεως τὸ πρὸς τὸν κανθὸν μέρος τοῦ πτερυγίου, φυλασσόμενοι τὰ βλέφαρα καὶ τὸν κανθόν ("we operate in this way for the removal of pterygium: having separated the eyelids one from the other and inserted a hook through the middle of the pterygium, we lift it up slightly, in order not to raise the skin of the cornea [...]. Then we take a needle armed with a flaxen thread and a horsehair and we insert it under the pterygium raised up with the hook. Next, bound the pterygium with the thread under it, we lift it up [...], and holding the horsehair with both hands we move it upwards and downwards, stripping off the pterygium from the black of the eye to the canthus. After that, [...] lifting it up with the thread, we separate with the instrument called the pterygotome the part of the pterygium on the side of the canthus from its base, taking care not to injure the eyelids and the canthus"). See also Paul. Aeg., *Medical Epitome* 6.18.1.5–18 (2.58.20–59.4 Heiberg): εὐιατότερα οὖν ὄντα τὰ λεπτομερῆ καὶ λευκανθίζοντα χειρουργοῦμεν οὕτως· διαστείλαντες τὰ βλέφαρα τὸ πτερύγιον ἀγκίστρῳ μικροκαμπεῖ ἀναδεξάμενοι ἀνατείνωμεν, βελόνην δὲ λαβόντες ἔχουσαν κατὰ τὸ οὖς ἱππείαν τρίχα καὶ λίνον ἰσχυρὸν ἐπικαμφθεῖσάν τε μικρὸν κατὰ τὸ ἄκρον ὑπὸ τὸ μέσον τοῦ πτερυγίου καταπείρωμεν καὶ τῷ μὲν λίνῳ τὸ πτερύγιον ἐκδήσαντες μετέωρον ἀνατείνωμεν, τῇ δὲ τριχὶ τὸ πρὸς τῇ κόρῃ μέρος αὐτοῦ ὥσπερ διαπρίζοντες ὑποδείρωμεν ἄχρι πέρατος, τὸ δὲ λοιπὸν αὐτοῦ τὸ πρὸς τῷ μεγάλῳ κανθῷ ἀναρραφικῷ σμιλίῳ ἐκτέμωμεν ἐκ βάσεως καταλιμπάνοντες τὸ φυσικὸν τοῦ κανθοῦ σαρκίον [...]. μετὰ δὲ τὴν χειρουργίαν ὀλίγους ἅλας λείους ἐμβαλόντες εἰς τὸν τόπον ᾠοβραχὲς ἔριον ἐπιδήσομεν. μετὰ δὲ τὴν ἐπίλυσιν ἐπὶ πολὺ τὴν ἅλμην αὐτοῖς ἐνστάξομεν ("we operate in the following way upon those which are thin and white, being easier to heal: having separated the eyelids and seised the pterygium with a hook with a small curve, we stretch it, and taking a needle having a horsehair and a strong flaxen thread in its ear [i.e., eye], a little bent on the edge, we transfix it through the middle of the pterygium and, binding the pterygium with the thread, we raise it upwards, whereas, with the horsehair, we strip off and saw as it were the part at the pupil up to its extremity, but the rest of it at the great canthus we cut out from the base with the scalpel used for the operation by suture, though leaving the natural flesh of the canthus [...]. After surgery, having applied some fine salt to the part, we will bind on it some wool soaked in an egg. After the removal of this we drop in the eye saltwater for a long time").

βελόνηṿ [δὲ λίνον καὶ τρίχα ἱππείαν] | ἔ̣χ̣ο̣ṳσ̣α̣[ν] |]σεως . [|]ματι . [|]μεν κα̣[|
]λ̣ε̣ιωṿ . [|] . ν ρει δ̣[ὲ] | [. .] . . ι̣ [

- What is pterygium? It is a membranous excrescence growing from the canthus or taking shape from the cornea.
- Which are the different kinds of pterygia? They differ among themselves in location, size, shape, color, nature or healing.
- Surgery of pterygium. After the patient is seated, having separated the two eyelids of the eye, we/you will isolate the pterygium from the eye with a hook, and a needle having a thread and a horsehair …

To outline some divergences, a first difference between the two texts is the number of their sections: P.Ross.Georg. I 20, immediately after the brief definition, continues with a question about aetiology (ll. 98–104 πῶ[ς γείνεται τὸ] | π̣[τ]ε[ρύγειον;] | ἤτοι [σ]αρκὸς αὔ[ξησις τῆς] | ὑπὸ τοῦ κανθο[ῦ μὲν σωματο]|ποιουμένου, γε[ίνεται δὲ καὶ] | ὑπὸ τοῦ κερ̣ατ̣[οειδοῦς χιτῶ]|νος), whereas P.Aberd. 11, instead of formulating a second question, has a longer definition including information that P.Ross.Georg. I 20 offers as aetiology in the second answer, namely the mention of the cornea as a part of the eye from which pterygium grows. So, whereas P.Aberd. 11 concentrates the mention of both the canthus and the cornea in a sort of 'double' or 'expanded' definition, P.Ross.Georg. I 20 repeats the mention of the canthus in the second answer and adds the cornea as the place of origin. The kind of definition in P.Aberd. 11 reflects a tendency highlighted by Leith: "the question-types are also tailored to a certain extent to the specific disease under discussion. Thus, for example, with the eye diseases especially, which are easily diagnosable, there is sometimes no separate question on signs, when the relevant details are tied up in the definition".[37]

These differential aspects in definition are clearly visible in the following table:

P.Ross.Georg. I 20.94–104	**P.Aberd. 11.2–5**
Definition: τεί ἐστ[ι τὸ πτερύ] γειον; ἔκφυσεις ὑμενῴ[δης ἀπὸ τοῦ] **κανθοῦ ηὔξημέ[νη.]**	Definition: τί̣ ἐστι ῷ̣ṿ [τὸ πτερύγειον;] ἔκφυσ̣ι̣ς ὑμενώδης **α[ὐξανομένη ἀπὸ τοῦ]** **κ̣α̣ṿθοῦ** ἢ σωματοποι̣[ουμένη] *ἀπὸ τοῦ κερατοειδοῦς [χιτῶνος.]*

37 Leith (2009a: 111).

(*cont.*)

P.Ross.Georg. I 20.94–104	**P.Aberd. 11.2–5**
Aetiology and location: πῶ[ς γείνεται τὸ] π̣[τ]ε[ρύγειον;] ἤτοι [σ]αρκὸς αὔ[ξησις τῆς] **ὑπὸ τοῦ κανθο**[ῦ μὲν σωματο-] ποιουμένου, γε[ίνεται δὲ καὶ] *ὑπὸ τοῦ κερ̣ατ̣[οειδοῦς χιτῶ-]* *νος.*	

It is hard to explain precisely why the description of the pathological condition named πτερύγιον is structured differently in the two papyri. It may be observed that its discussion in P.Ross.Georg. I 20 is more articulated and is set out systematically according to its definition, causes, differentiation and therapy, exactly like the discussion of the previous subject, σταφύλωμα, in ll. 68–93 of the same column. This is the only other fully preserved subject in the papyrus, whereas γλαύκωμα (col. II ll. 55–67) and ῥευματισμός (col. III ll. 116–125) are incomplete due to the fragmentary condition of the papyrus scrap. Thus, one might wonder whether the differences between these two catechisms on the same topic (πτερύγιον) depend, in general, on the mechanical repetition of a fixed set of topics for each disease, viz. definition, causes, differentiation and therapy in P.Ross.Georg. I 20, and definition, differentiation and therapy in P.Aberd. 11. But the comparison with what survives in the former shows that the other subjects were approached according to various sets of question-and-answers; for example, the last (and the only completely preserved) question-and-answer about γλαύκωμα (col. II ll. 57–67) does not deal with the therapy, like in the aforementioned cases of σταφύλωμα and πτερύγιον, but it inquires what differentiates the 'glaucoma' from another similar but distinct affection called ὑπόχυμα. This can be explained by the fact that—quoting again Leith's words—some 'topics' or 'attributes' (i.e., definition, cause, signs, differentiation and therapy) are "more relevant for some diseases than others (e.g., only certain diseases will have different species, or require distinctions to be drawn between them and similar affections; others will be untreatable, etc.)".[38]

38 Ibid.

In conclusion, the comparison between the discussion of πτερύγιον in P.Ross.Georg. I 20 and P.Aberd. 11 seems to point again to a certain freedom that the compilers of the catechisms had in choosing and arranging the contents of the sets of question-and-answers as a possible reason of the differences between these two papyri. This is particularly evident in the section devoted to surgery that in P.Ross.Georg. I 20 is differently expressed and noticeably shorter than in P.Aberd. 11. The corresponding portion of sheet is badly damaged in both papyri. Although the loss is extensive, restorations of lacunae can be made based upon the descriptions in Greek and Latin medical writers, mainly Celsus, Aëtius of Amida and Paul of Aegina.[39] According to the surgical procedure described by these authors, the eyelids are drawn aside certainly in P.Ross.Georg. I 20.112 (διαστείλα̣[ντες τὰ βλέφαρα), and likely in P.Aberd. 11.11 (τοῦ ὀφθαλμοῦ διφ[υῆ βλέφαρα διαστείλαντες]), since the adjective διφυής (double), albeit partially restored, seems to be applied to the two eyelids. Then, the pterygium is isolated from the eyeball with a hook, probably with a view toward removal, see P.Aberd. 11.12–13 (τὸ πτερύγειον δι̣[εκφανοῦμεν ἀγκι]|στρείοι), and P.Ross.Georg. I 20.112–115 (τὸ] | πτερύγει[ον ἀγκίστρῳ ἐκ τοῦ] | ὀφθαλμοῦ [ἀναδεξάμενοι] | διεκφαν̣[οῦμεν), where both the context and the word choice seem to assure the presence of ἄγκιστρον in the lacuna. What is perhaps more interesting is that P.Aberd. 11, although being increasingly damaged after l. 13, includes procedural information additional to that in the other papyrus: the patient is seated (l. 10 μετὰ τὸν καθέδρειο̣[ν ὄντα τὸν πάσχοντα),[40] as in Celsus, *Med.* 7.7.4.7 (313.11 Marx: *aduersus in sedili contra medicum is homo collocandus est*, "the patient is seated facing the surgeon"), and the usual needle threaded with a thread and a horsehair[41] is used in addition to the hook (ll. 13–14 ἀγκι]|στρείοι, βελόνην̣ [δὲ λίνον καὶ τρίχα ἱππείαν] | ἔχ̣ο̣υ̣σ̣α̣[ν]).

B *Technical Terminology in the* Erôtapokriseis *on Papyrus: a Lexical 'Particularisation'?*

The words employed to define the pterygium in P.Ross.Georg. I 20 and P. Aberd. 11 occasion some lexical observations. Particularly noteworthy is the juxtaposition of ἔκφυσις ὑμενώδης (membranous excrescence) mentioned in the defin-

39 For this aspect with references to the medical sources, see especially Olivieri (1928: 245–247), Marganne (1994: 111 and 129) and Hanson (2003: 207).

40 See *MedOn* s.v. καθέδριος.

41 Cf. notably Aëtius 7.62.5–6 (2.315.13–14 Olivieri: εἶτα βελόνην λαμβάνομεν λίνον ἔχουσαν διῃρημένον καὶ τρίχα ἱππείαν, "we take a needle armed with a flaxen thread and a horsehair"), and Paul. Aeg., *Medical Epitome* 6.18.1.7–8 (2.58.22–23 Heiberg: βελόνην δὲ λαβόντες ἔχουσαν κατὰ τὸ οὖς ἱππείαν τρίχα καὶ λίνον ἰσχυρόν, "taking a needle having a horsehair and a strong flaxen thread in its ear").

ition part of both papyri. Such an expression is never applied to πτερύγιον in medical authors, but its appearance in these catechisms might suggest that ἔκφυσις ὑμενώδης was perhaps the traditional definition of πτερύγιον in catechistic texts.

The noun ὑμήν (membrane) is often associated with πτερύγιον, but it is mostly qualified by νευρώδης (nervous), as in Paul of Aegina, *Medical Epitome* 6.18.1–2 (2.58.16–17 Heiberg: ὑμένος μὲν νευρώδους ἀπὸ τοῦ μεγάλου κανθοῦ τὸ ἐπίπαν τὴν ἀρχὴν δεξαμένου, "this disease [sc. pterygium] occurs by a nervous membrane having origin for the most part at the great canthus"), or it is found in the phrase νευρώδης τοῦ ἐπιπεφυκότος ὑμένος ὑπεροχή ("nervous excrescence of the conjunctiva"), as is the case in another passage from Paul of Aegina, *Medical Epitome* 3.22.25.1–2 (1.181.22–23 Heiberg: τὸ πτερύγιον νευρώδης ἐστὶν τοῦ ἐπιπεφυκότος ὑμένος ὑπεροχὴ ἐκφυομένη μὲν ἀπὸ τοῦ κανθοῦ, "pterygium is a nervous excrescence of the conjunctiva arising at the canthus"), and in Ps.-Galen, *Rem.* 2.5.1–2 (14.410.14–15 Kühn: τὸ πτερύγιον νευρώδης ἐστὶ τοῦ ἐπιπεφυκότος ὑμένος ὑπεροχή, "pterygium is a nervous excrescence of the conjunctiva arising at the canthus"), whereas the derivative adjective ὑμενώδης (membranaceous) is applied to πτερύγιον only once, in the *Hippiatrica* (*Hippiatr. Berol.* 11.39.8 [1.70.5 Oder—Hoppe]: πτερύγιον ὑμενῶδες). This parallel is intriguing, but it is not, of course, sufficient evidence to speculate about a possible hippiatric nature of these catechisms on papyrus.

Second, the meaning of 'excrescence' is expressed in these papyrus catechisms by the noun ἔκφυσις (outgrowth), which is the term used to define this eye condition only in Ps.-Galen's *Definitiones medicae*, entry 366 (19.439.5–6 Kühn: πτερύγιόν ἐστιν ἔκφυσις σώματος ἐπιφυομένη τῷ κερατοειδεῖ, "pterygium is an outgrowth of tissue growing upon the cornea"). The papyri indeed begin the discussion of pterygium in a manner resembling that of the Ps.-Galenic passage. This regards in particular P.Aberd. 11.3–5 since both this papyrus and the Ps.-Galenic text mention the cornea in the definition, whereas P.Ross.Georg. I 20 does not.

The example of this expression (ἔκφυσις ὑμενώδης), unparalleled in formal medical literature, raises the question as to whether there was a sort of 'particularisation' of medical technical language in the *erôtapokriseis* on papyrus. It is true that, in general, the catechisms on papyrus mirror the technical vocabulary employed by medical authors,[42] but some elements seem to suggest that there might also have been a further lexical specialisation or particular-

42 According to (Hanson 2003: 201), "medical language chosen by compilers for their teaching texts recycle back into formal medical literature via the students who become authors of medical treatises during their professional careers".

isation of the micro-language of medicine in this particular type of texts. Maybe the terminology of these texts was influenced by the already mentioned 'concrete' and practical nature of the catechisms on papyrus as teaching materials for apprentice physicians or as reference tools and succinct aides-mémoires for established practitioners. It might reflect specific aspects of the communication among doctors in the practice of their profession, at the very level of word-choice and phrasing. Therefore, my hypothesis is that, from a lexical viewpoint, the papyri in question-and-answer format might reveal features of the medical language as it was in the 'concrete' context in which the catechisms were copied, used and produced. So, by being situated at the linguistic intersection of both traditional (i.e., common to formal medical literature) and innovative (i.e., influenced by the practical communication current among physicians) medical situations, they might include lexical components of both sides.

This might also provide further support for the idea, originating from the close investigation of the technical vocabulary attested in the medical papyri, that it represents a 'missing link' for the reconstruction of the evolution of ancient Greek medical micro-language.[43] Its study enables us to supplement our picture of the Greek medical discourse as we know it from the more 'official' medical texts transmitted through the medieval manuscript tradition. Beside texts with a high level of technicality, medical papyri provide us with the opportunity to sketch the lexical situation of that part of medical language which best expresses the most concrete and everyday side of the medical practice. This includes the non-technical, but still 'medical', language and vocabulary used by lay people when writing about matters of health and disease, often characterised by elements of lexical simplification and intelligibility.[44] But it also includes the 'practical' communication among specialists in the exercise of their profession and the transmission of medical knowledge by way of written teaching materials, of which the *erôtapokriseis* on papyrus are a representative form.

Another example of this hypothesised lexical 'particularisation' in the catechistic genre may be found in an interesting, though quite problematic *addendum lexicis* recovered from a papyrus of the II–III century CE from Oxyrhynchus. This papyrus, P.Oxy. LXXIV 4972v (MP3 2354.01, LDAB 119317, TM 119317),

43 See Maravela (2018).

44 On this point, see Maravela (2018) and Hanson (2010: 187–202). Illuminating examples of utterances about health and disease by non-specialists in everyday situations are provided by private letters discussing medical matters. For a selection of *specimina*, see Bonati (2016a: 279–325, but also 251–276) and (2016b: 659–675).

contains a medical text in question-and-answer format offering a systematic exposition of the divisions of surgery: firstly discussing its 'forms' (σχήματα)—the categories of knowledge that surgery encompasses—, and secondly the different classes of surgical operations.[45] The term in question (ll. 16–17) is ἐγκατατομικός.[46] The compound adjective ἐγκατατομικός is referred to the noun σχῆμα (form), which is explicitly mentioned only in l. 7, even though it applies to all types of surgery outlined from that point onward. It belongs to the specialised language of obstetrics and is concerned with embryotomy,[47] an operation of last resort that was performed to save the mother's life in extreme cases of delivery complications; ἐγκατατομικός defines the most characteristic aspect of this operation, namely the technique used to dismember the fetus in the womb, as it is shown by its etymology. The structure of this derivative adjective is complex since it is formed by several lexical elements. The stem -τομ-, from τέμνω (to cut), constitutes the semantic core of the action. It is preceded by a double prepositional prefix (ἐν + κατά), which conveys specific shades of meaning detailing the action expressed by the verb 'to cut', and is followed by the suffix -ικός.

The first preverb ἐν- specifies that the action is carried out inside a confined inner space, viz. the uterus of a woman, while the preverb κατά might express a range of connotations, such as: a distributive sense, i.e., the division of a unit—the fetus—into segments; a sort of iterative value, i.e., the succession of actions required to complete the operation; the direction downwards, i.e., the movement of the surgical instrument, such as the knife called ἐμβρυοτόμος,[48] sinking down into the fetus to cut it up.

The suffix -ικός of Indo-European origin (< **-ikos*, formed by the i-stem suffix **-i-* + the adjectival suffix **-ko-*), usually expressing relationship and bearing the sense 'characteristic of', 'pertaining to', has been productive along the entire history of the ancient Greek language.[49] Widely used in the creation of scientific and technical terminology, it has become particularly common in Greek medical language.[50]

45 See Leith (2009b: 60).

46 For an in-depth discussion of this term, see *MedOn* s.v. ἐγκατατομικός.

47 The adjective is indeed concerned with a term that is undoubtedly a derivative noun from τέμνω (l. 18]οτομίας). The noun 'embryotomy' is itself a restoration, yet the fact that the word family to which ἐγκατατομικός belongs is semantically connected to that kind of surgical procedure makes both ἐνκατ̣α̣|[τομι]κ̣όν and [ἐμβρυ]οτομίας convincing.

48 For the ἐμβρυοτόμος, probably "a straight two-edged blade" for perforating the skull of the foetus, see Milne (1907: 43).

49 Cf. Budenz (1858: esp. 4–32); Debrunner (1917: 197–200); Chantraine (1933: 385–393).

50 Cf. Lipourlis (2010: 1110–1112) and Schironi (2010: 341).

In the papyrus catechism, the adjective is very plausibly restored by the *editor princeps* (ἐνκατ̣α̣|[τομι]κ̣όν). However, it must be noted that, on viewing the digital image of the papyrus,[51] it is possible to discern a trace at the end of l. 16 that, though very faded, might be compatible with the sloping vertical of a τ. This may imply that the actual word division was ἐνκατ̣α̣τ̣[ο|μι]κ̣όν, also because the letters το would seem to fit the space considering both the width of the right margin where it is preserved and the usual size of these letters in the papyrus.

The adjective appearing in this papyrus is a *hapax*, but it has a Hippocratic backdrop. It belongs to a family of medical terms that are scantily attested and quite challenging from a textual standpoint. Its cognates are the verb ἐγκατατέμνω (to cut up the fetus in the womb) and the noun ἐγκατατομή (cutting up of the fetus in the womb, cf. LSJ[9] 471 s.vv.). The main difficulty concerning these terms depends on the state of the manuscript tradition of the only medical source mentioning them, the title and the first line of the Hippocratic text *De exsectione foetus*, so printed in the Littré edition (*Foet. Exsect.* title and 1.1 [8.512.1–3 Littré; 368.0–2 Bourbon]): ΠΕΡΙ ΕΓΚΑΤΑΤΟΜΗΣ ΕΜΒΡΥΟΥ. περὶ δὲ τῶν μὴ κατὰ τρόπον κυϊσκομένων, ἀλλ' ἐγκατατεμνομένων οὕτως ("EXCISION OF THE FETUS. Regarding pregnancies that do not proceed in the normal way, but that are cut to pieces inside [sc. the uterus], the matter is as follows").[52] There is also another attestation of the verb ἐγκατατέμνω, albeit not in a medical but in an 'arithmetic' context, Pl., *R.* 565d9–e1 (ὁ γευσάμενος τοῦ ἀνθρωπίνου σπλάγχνου, ἐν ἄλλοις ἄλλων ἱερείων ἑνὸς ἐγκατατετμημένου, ἀνάγκη δὴ τούτῳ λύκῳ γενέσθαι: "he who tastes human entrails cut up among those of other victims inevitably becomes a wolf"). Here the meaning "to cut up among a number" (LSJ[9] 471 s.v. II) is not certainly technical, but it literally reflects the semantic components of the compound with the first preverb ἐν- specifying that the verb applies to an inner part of the body, the entrails, while κατά expresses the iterative sense of the action of cutting something up in small pieces.

It is important to stress again the word-formation of ἐγκατατομικός as an adjective ending in -ικός, in combination with the fact that all the adjectives defining the σχήματα, the 'forms' or 'categories' into which surgery is divided, end in this suffix. Another of these adjectives, viz. τομικός (ll. 7–8 το̣|[μικόν]), is also a *hapax*; it denotes the appropriate type of incision required by each sur-

---

51 See the image on the webpage: http://163.1.169.40/gsdl/collect/POxy/index/assoc/HASH0137/034fdc7f.dir/POxy.v0074.n4972.a.01.hires.jpg.

52 For a discussion of the topic, see *MedOn* s.v. ἐγκατατομικός C1. See also the most recent edition of the text by Bourbon (2017: *ad l.*).

gical procedure, i.e., "the incision-based form". In two other cases, already existing words acquire a more specific meaning that does not seem to be attested in any other source; as such, these adjectives represent two semantic neologisms: σχηματικόν (sc. σχῆμα, l. 3), "the position-based (sc. form)" concerned with appropriate patient positioning, and καιρικόν (sc. σχῆμα, l. 11), "the stage-based (sc. form)" regarding the post-operative measures to be taken. Furthermore, it is significant that the other unnamed forms, which are referred to at ll. 18–20 and were probably listed before each σχῆμα was individually explained in the surviving passage (ll. 1–18), are said "to be recognisable from the names" (τὰ δὲ ἄλλα ἀπ̣[| . . . . .]ν ὀνομάτων γνωριζό|[μενα] τυνχάνει [*l.* τυγχάνει]).[53] Therefore, it is reasonable to assume that these ὀνόματα were probably also terms ending in -ικός.

Also in the case of P.Oxy. LXXIV 4972v just treated, I suspect a lexical specialisation or particularisation of the micro-language of medicine. The presence of the *hapax* ἐγκατατομικός in this catechism, as well as the particular use of the other adjectives in -ικός defining the distinct σχήματα of surgery, suggest that the *erôtapokriseis* on papyrus reflect lexical features of the language influenced by the 'concrete' contexts in which these texts were used. Finally, the fact itself that adjectives like ἐγκατατομικός and τομικός seem to appear only in a papyrus catechism points at the significance of the vocabulary attested in the Greek medical papyri, making them important sources for reconstructing Greek medical micro-language.

3 Conclusions

The study of the *erôtapokriseis* on papyrus contributes to a more complete view of the catechistic genre as a whole, as it integrates what is already known about the more 'traditional' collections of medical question-and-answers that have come down to us via the medieval manuscript transmission. Indeed, the medical catechisms on papyrus help to illuminate the dynamic nature of these texts and their contexts of use, which would have remained undetected without the emergence of the medical papyri from the sands of Egypt. First, the number of papyrus copies to have survived attests to the popularity of catechistic texts in the Graeco-Roman world, with a peak in the II and III centuries CE. This is proof of the fact that the question-and-answer format was regarded as a methodologically effective way of approaching medical issues. Although

53 Transl. Leith (2009b: 63).

these texts are often extremely fragmentary, they enable us to identify some distinctive features. On the one side, their conservative tendency in the ordering of topics; on the other, their flexibility and the possibility of including or omitting some aspects of the subject according to the compiler's needs and probably the specific purpose of the particular catechism on papyrus (i.e., used by students learning the art or by practitioners in the exercise of their profession, as a tool for daily practice). At the same time, a certain freedom is displayed by the compiler in selecting and arranging the medical contents and their forms of expression. These aspects are confirmed (especially in the definition of the same topic) by comparison of the papyrus catechisms with medical literature and among the different catechisms on papyrus themselves.

A substantial part of my argument has focused on the innovative hypothesis of a lexical 'particularisation' of the micro-language of medicine in the *erôtapokriseis* on papyrus. The lexical observations drawn from the examination of *termini technici* and expressions referring to pathological conditions and surgical procedures in some catechisms on papyrus (but unparalleled in 'official' medical literature) have revealed features of the medical language and vocabulary that are presumably characteristic of this type of texts. The origin of these peculiar lexical aspects may be the concrete and practical contexts in and for which these texts were produced, copied, and used, thus reflecting particular features (at the very level of word-choice and phrasing) of the communication process among physicians when teaching the τέχνη to their students or when exercising their profession. This would imply a significant connection between the vocabulary and its contexts of use as well as the influence of these contexts on the texts themselves.

To conclude, this research emphasises, more generally, the significance of the study of technical terminology attested in the Greek medical papyri in order to refine and expand our acquaintance with the ancient Greek medical language as known from the 'official' medical tradition; more specifically, it points at the relevance of the analysis (hopefully more extensive in the future) of the language and vocabulary of the catechisms on papyrus in light of medical question-and-answer texts as a whole. Moreover, it can also contribute to shed new light on the purpose of the catechisms on papyrus—or, at least, some of these copies—compared to the traditional catechistic literature, which was intended primarily for memorising medical definitions. Some differences in expression and vocabulary, but also other elements, such as the inversion of the question-answer order (noted in GMP I 6), strengthen the hypothesis of a practical use of the papyri in question-and-answer format. This, of course, does not exclude their usefulness for didactic aims, but also suggests (in addition to their educational purposes) a more practical application as instruments used by established doctors for checking symptoms, identifying causes, making a diagnosis and looking for a therapy 'on the spot'.

Bibliography

Primary Sources

Bourbon, F. 2017. *Hippocrate 12.4. Femmes stériles. Maladies des jeunes filles. Superfétation. Excision du foetus*. Paris: Les Belles Lettres.

Heiberg, J.L. 1921–1924. *Paulus Aegineta*, 2 vols [CMG IX.1–2]. Leipzig—Berlin: Teubner.

Jouanna, J. 1983. *Hippocrate 10.2. Maladies II*. Paris: Les Belles Lettres.

Kühn, C.G. 1821–1833. *Claudii Galeni Opera Omnia*, 20 vols in 22. Leipzig: Car. Cnoblochii.

Littré, É. 1839–1861. *Oeuvres complètes d'Hippocrate: traduction nouvelle avec le texte grec en regard, collationné sur les manuscrits et toutes les éditions; accompagnée d'une introduction, de commentaires médicaux, de variantes et de notes philologiques; suivie d'une table générale des matières*, 10 vols. Paris: J.-B. Baillière.

Marx, F. 1915. *A. Cornelii Celsi quae supersunt* [CML I]. Leipzig—Berlin: Teubner.

Oder, E.—Hoppe, K. 1924–1927. *Corpus Hippiatricorum Graecorum*, 2 vols. Leipzig: Teubner (repr. Stuttgart 1971).

Olivieri, A. 1935–1950. *Aetii Amideni Libri medicinales*, 2 vols. [CMG VIII.1–2]. Leipzig—Berlin: Teubner.

Petit, C. 2009. *Galien 3. Le médecin. Introduction*. Paris: Les Belles Lettres.

Raeder, J. 1926. *Oribasii Synopsis ad Eustathium, Libri ad Eunapium* [CMG VI.3]. Leipzig—Berlin: Teubner.

Raeder, J. 1928–1933. *Oribasii Collectionum medicarum reliquiae*, 4 vols [CMG VI.1.1–2.2]. Leipzig—Berlin: Teubner.

Rose, V. 1870. *Anecdota graeca et graecolatina*, vol. 2. Berlin: Dümmler, 243–274.

Zervos, S.G. 1909. 'Aetius Amidenus. Logos dekatos pemptos', *Athena* 21: 7–138.

Secondary Sources

Andorlini, I. 1992. 'Papiri e medicina: P.Oxy. II 234 + P.Oxy. LII 3654', in A.H.S. El-Mosalamy (ed.), *Proceedings of the XIXth International Congress of Papyrology (Cairo, 2–9 September 1989)*, I. Cairo: Ain Shams University, Center of Papyrological Studies, 375–390.

Andorlini, I. 1997. 'Trattato o catechismo? La tecnica della flebotomia in PSI inv. CNR 85/86', in I. Andorlini (ed.), *"Specimina" per il Corpus dei Papiri Greci di Medicina. Atti dell'Incontro di studio (Firenze, 28–9 marzo 1996)*. Firenze: Istituto Papirologico G. Vitelli, 153–168.

Andorlini, I. 1999. 'Testi medici per la scuola: raccolte di definizioni e questionari nei papiri', in A. Garzya—J. Jouanna (eds.), *I testi medici greci. Tradizione e ecdotica. Atti del III Convegno internazionale (Napoli, 15–8 ottobre 1997)*. Napoli: M. D'Auria, 7–15.

Andorlini, I. 2017. 'Il corpus dei papiri medici online: la piattaforma editoriale', in A. Roselli (ed.), *Atti del VII Colloquio Internazionale sull'ecdotica dei testi medici greci (Procida, 11–3 giugno 2013)*. Napoli: M. D'Auria.

Bäckström, A. 1904. 'Fragment einer medizinischer Schrift', *APF* 3: 158–162.

Barns, J.W.B. 1949. 'Literary Texts from the Fayum', *CQ* 43: 1–8.

Bertonazzi, F. 2019. 'Digital Edition of P.Strasb. inv. 1187: between the Papyrus and the Indirect Tradition', in Nodar—Torallas Tovar (2019: 857–871).

Bonati, I. 2016a. *Il lessico dei vasi e dei contenitori greci nei papiri.* Specimina *per un repertorio lessicale degli angionimi greci*, APF-B 37. Berlin—Boston: De Gruyter.

Bonati, I. 2016b. 'Between Text and Context: P.Oslo II 54 Reconsidered', in T. Derda—A. Łajtar—J. Urbanik (eds.), *Proceedings of the 27th International Congress of Papyrology (Warsaw, 29 July–3 August), Vol. II: Subliterary Papyri, Documentary Papyri, Scribal Practices, Linguistic Matters*, JJP Suppl. 28. Warsaw: University of Warsaw, 659–675.

Bonati, I. 2018. 'Digital papyrological editions and the experience of a lexicographical database: Medicalia Online', in N. Reggiani (ed.), *Digital Papyrology II: Case Studies on the Digital Edition of Ancient Greek Papyri*. Berlin—Boston: De Gruyter, 149–173.

Bonati, I. 2019a. 'Medicalia Online: a lexical database of technical terms in medical papyri', in Nodar—Torallas Tovar (2019: 683–689).

Bonati, I. 2019b 'Medicalia Online: tecnicismi medici tra passato e presente', in N. Reggiani (ed.), *Greek Medical Papyri—Text, Context, Hypertext. Proceedings of the DIGMEDTEXT Final Conference held in Parma on November 2016, 2–4 (in memory of Isabella Andorlini)*, APF-B 40. Berlin—Boston: De Gruyter, 257–276.

Budenz, J. 1858. *Das Suffix kos (ikos, akos, ykos) im griechischen: ein Beitrag zur Wortbildungslehre*. Göttingen: Verlag der Dieterichschen Buchhandlung.

Chantraine, P. 1933. *La formation des noms en grec ancien*. Paris: Champion.

Cilliers, L. (ed.). 2008. *Asklepios. Studies on Ancient Medicine*. Acta Classica Supplementum II. Pretoria: V&R Printing Works.

Debrunner, A. 1917. *Griechische Wortbildungslehre*. Heidelberg: Carl Winters Universitätsbuchhandlung.

Fischer, K.D. 1998. 'Beiträge zu den pseudosoranischen Quaestiones Medicinales', in K.D. Fischer—D. Nickel—P. Potter (eds.), *Text and Tradition. Studies in Ancient Medicine and its Transmission presented to Jutta Kollesch*. Leiden: Brill, 1–54.

Hanson, A.E.—Mattern, S.P. 2001. 'Medical Catechism', in I. Andorlini (ed.), *Greek Medical Papyri I*. Firenze: Istituto Papirologico G. Vitelli, 71–83.

Hanson, A.E. 2003. 'Text and Context in Papyrus Catechisms on Afflictions of the Head', in A. Garzya—J. Jouanna (eds.), *Trasmissione e ecdotica dei testi medici greci. Atti del IV Convegno Internazionale (Parigi, 17–9 maggio 2001)*. Napoli: M. D'Auria, 199–217.

Hanson, A.E. 2010. 'Doctors' Literacy and Papyri of Medical Content', *Stud. Anc. Med.* 35: 187–202.

Ieraci Bio, A.M. 1995. 'L'ἐρωταπόκρισις nella letteratura medica', in C. Moreschini (ed.), *Esegesi, parafrasi e compilazione in età tardoantica. Atti del terzo Convegno dell'Associazione di Studi Tardoantichi*. Napoli: M. D'Auria, 187–207.

Jouanna, J. 2008. 'L'autre Hippocrate: un traité anonyme inédit "Sur les quatre humeurs" par questions et réponses (Vat.gr. 293, XIVe s., fol. 223r–225v)', in Cilliers (2008: 86–102).

Kollesch, J. 1973. *Untersuchungen zu den pseudogalenischen Definitiones Medicae*. Berlin: Akademie-Verlag.

Leith, D. 2007. 'A Medical Treatise "On Remedies"? P.Turner 14 Revised', *BASP* 44: 125–134.

Leith, D. 2009a. 'Question-Types in Medical Catechisms on Papyrus', in L.C. Taub—A. Doody (eds.), *Authorial Voices in Greco-Roman Technical Writing*. Trier: Wissenschaftlicher Verlag, 107–123.

Leith, D. 2009b. 'Medical and Related Texts. P.Oxy. 4972: Division of Surgery', in N. Gonis—D. Leith et al. (eds.), *The Oxyrhynchus Papyri. Vol. LXXIV. II*. London: Egypt Exploration Society with The Arts and Humanities Research Council and The British Academy, 60–66.

Leith, D. 2009c. 'A Note on the Greek Medical Fragment P.Golenischeff', in I. Andorlini (ed.), *Greek Medical Papyri II*. Firenze: Istituto Papirologico G. Vitelli, 211–218.

Lipourlis, D. 2010. 'Medical vocabulary', in A.F. Christidis (ed.), *A History of Ancient Greek from the Beginnings to Late Antiquity*. Cambridge—New York: Cambridge University Press, 1104–1115.

Magdelaine, C. 2004. 'Un nouveau questionnaire ophtalmologique (PStrasb gr. inv. 849)', in I. Andorlini (ed.), *Testi medici su papiro. Atti del Seminario di studio (Firenze, 3–4 giugno 2002)*. Firenze: Istituto Papirologico G. Vitelli, 63–77.

Maire, B. 2008. 'A Comparative Reading of Soranos and Mustio: an Example of ἐρωταπόκρισις', in Cilliers (2008: 103–115).

Manetti, D. 1973, 'P. Alex. inv. 614: testo medico', *SCO* 22: 46–49.

Manfredi, M. 1997. 'Modello di edizione di un testo letterario adespoto (PSI XV 1510: questionario sui παρίσθμια)', in I. Andorlini (ed.), *"Specimina" per il Corpus dei Papiri Greci di Medicina. Atti dell'Incontro di studio (Firenze, 28–9 marzo 1996)*. Firenze: Istituto Papirologico G. Vitelli, 73–79.

Maravela, A.—Leith, D. 1997. 'A Medical Catechism on Tumours from the Collection of the Oslo University Library', in J. Frösén—T. Purola—E. Salmenkivi (eds.), *Proceedings of the 24th International Congress of Papyrology (Helsinki, 1–7 2004)*, II. Helsinki: Societas Scientiarum Fennica, 637–650.

Maravela, A. 2018. 'Medical micro-language: The contribution of papyri to the study of medical Greek', in N. Reggiani—F. Bertonazzi (eds.), *Parlare la medicina: fra lingue e culture, nello spazio e nel tempo. Atti del Convegno Internazionale (Università di Parma, 5–7 settembre 2016)*. Firenze: Le Monnier, 12–29.

Marganne, M.-H. 1978. 'Deux questionnaires d'ophtalmologie: P. Aberdeen 11 et P. Ross. Georg. 1.20', *CE* 53: 313–320.

Marganne, M.-H. 1986. 'La "Cirurgia Eliodori" et le P. Genève inv. 111', *Etudes de Lettres*: 65–73.

Marganne, M.-H. 1987. 'Un questionnaire d'anatomie: P. Lund I 7. Réédition, traduction, commentaire', *CE* 62: 189–200.

Marganne, M.-H. 1994. *L'ophtalmologie dans l'Égypte gréco-romaine d'après les papyrus littéraires grecs*. Leiden—Köln—New York: Brill.

MedOn = Medicalia Online, see http://www.papirologia.unipr.it/CPGM/medicalia/vocab/index.php.

Milne, J.S. 1907. *Surgical Instruments in Greek and Roman Times*. Oxford: Clarendon Press.

Nicole, J. 1903. 'Un questionnaire de chirurgie', *APF* 2: 1–3.

Nodar, A.—Torallas Tovar, S. (eds.). 2019. *Proceedings of the 28th International Congress of Papyrology (Barcelona, 1–6 August 2016)*. Barcelona: Publicacions de l'Abadia de Montserrat—Universitat Pompeu Fabra.

Olivieri, A. 1928. 'Papiro medicinale', *Atti della Reale Accademia di Archeologia, Lettere e Belle Arti di Napoli* 10: 235–249.

Papadoyannakis, Y. 2006. 'Instruction by Question and Answer: the case of Late Antique and Byzantine Erotapokriseis', in S.F. Johnson (ed.), *Greek Literature in Late Antiquity: dynamism, didacticism, classicism*. Aldershot: Ashgate, 91–106.

Reggiani, N. 2015. 'A Corpus of Literary Papyri Online: the Pilot Project of the Medical Texts via SoSOL', in R. Lafer—K. Strobel (eds.), *Antike Lebenswelten Althistorische und papyrologische Studien*. Berlin—New York: De Gruyter, 341–352.

Reggiani, N. 2017. *Digital Papyrology I. Methods, Tools and Trends*. Berlin—Boston: De Gruyter.

Reggiani, N. 2019. 'The Corpus of Greek Medical Papyri Online and the digital edition of ancient documents', in Nodar—Torallas Tovar (2019: 843–856).

Schironi, F. 2010. *Technical Languages: Science and Medicine*, in E.J. Bakker (ed.), *A Companion to the Ancient Greek Language*. Malden—Oxford: Wiley Blackwell, 338–353.

Zalateo, G. 1961. 'Papiri scolastici', *Aegyptus* 41: 160–235.

Zalateo, G. 1964. 'Papiri di argomento medico redatti in forma di domanda e risposta', *Aegyptus* 44: 52–57.

CHAPTER 8

Digitizing Medical Papyri in Question-and-Answer Format

Nicola Reggiani

Abstract

This chapter presents a general overview of the Greek medical papyri in question-and-answer format, focusing in particular on their layout and on the graphical strategies deployed by the ancient scribes in highlighting the main articulations of the texts. Discussion will then move from the ancient sources to their modern digital representation, where the current strategies to encode such ancient layout and graphical devices will be presented and analysed, pinpointing their fundamental relevance in our comprehension of this peculiar textual typology.

1 Introduction: Medical Catechisms on Papyrus as a Technical Genre*

The term 'catechism' usually defines a technical genre of writing that, by its typical question-and-answer format (ἐρωταπόκρισις, with a Middle Byzantine word),[1] was particularly useful for teaching, learning, and referencing purposes. The papyrological evidence of such catechisms is not limited to the field of ancient medicine alone,[2] but the relatively large amount of medical papyri that

---

* This contribution stems from the project DIGMEDTEXT ("Online Humanities Scholarship: A Digital Medical Library Based on Ancient Texts", Principal Investigator Prof. Isabella Andorlini) funded by the European Research Council (Advanced Grant no. 339828) at the University of Parma. See http://www.papirologia.unipr.it/ERC for further details.

1 In general, on erotapocritic literature in Antiquity, see Ieraci Bio (1995).

2 The fields of poetry, philosophy, rhetoric, mythology, law, and religion are represented as well. Poetry: P.Lond.Lit. 160 (on Homer's *Odyssey*); philosophy: P.Heid. inv. G 1716 = LDAB 4699 (on ethics; cf. Bilabel [1925: 339–340]; Körte [1927: 266]; Ingenkamp [1969]); rhetoric: PSI I 85 (definitions of *chreia*; cf. Bastianini [2004]; Hock-O'Neil [2002: II, 94–98]) and P.Vindob. inv. G 754 = LDAB 6396 (cf. Oellacher [1937]); mythology: P.Oxy. XXXIV 2688v (cf. Fernandez-Delgado [2013: 133 n. 3]) and 2689; law: P.Berol. inv. 11866a/b = LDAB 6078 (commentary on Roman law; cf. Schönbauer [1933a and 1933b]; McNamee [2007: 503–504]); religion: BKT IX

 | DOI:10.1163/9789004442672_010

came down to us in this format (22 published fragments, and one unpublished) seems to underline the importance of this type of discourse for knowledge transmission specifically in the ancient medical sector.[3] Such questionnaires provide key medical notions in a dialogue format, where a question about theoretical definitions or practical procedures is typically followed by a more or less detailed answer.[4] All the interpretations that have been advanced to explain this peculiar textual typology focus on its Q&A structure.[5] This in itself pinpoints the central role played by the erotapocritic format, which arguably stems from the very origins of medicine as an orally transmitted type of knowledge[6] as well as from its scientific nature as an enquiring, empirical discipline (cf., e.g., Hipp., *Ant. Med.* 13.1–2 [1.598.3–4 Littré; 133.7–8 Jouanna]: "those who pursue their researches in the art").[7] Medical questionnaires as technical reference manuals are indeed flanked by a proper 'literary' genre of 'definitions', i.e., broader and more detailed treatises connected with the research and teaching practice of Graeco-Roman medicine as attested, for instance, in Ps.-Galen's *Definitiones medicae* and in Ps.-Soranus' *Quaestiones medicinales*,[8] but also in papyrus fragments. Both textual typologies, catechisms and definitions, testify to a well-rooted medical tradition in the practical and theoretical use of questions and answers as schemes of cognition, the difference being between more schematic and practical texts and more articulated and theoretical discourses respectively (see also below).

It speaks for itself that ancient doctors required the necessary technical skills to exercise their profession properly; but there were also situations where they could undergo some sort of 'examination', either by private clients[9] or by

100 (Mithraic liturgy; cf. Brashear [1992]; Turcan [1992 and 1993: 152–156]: possibly not Mithraic, possibly not a catechism).

3 Cf. Ieraci Bio (1995). It was recently brought to my attention that students of medicine take advantage of a very similar learning methodology still today, making use of 'flash cards' with questions on one side and answers on the other: see, e.g., Drake—Vogl—Mitchell (2015), in the *Preface* of which we read: "The question-and-answer format stimulates learning, and pertinent clinical information on most cards provides relevance".

4 For a detailed overview, see Bonati's chapter in this volume.

5 Teaching manuals for students of medicine: Andorlini (1999); Hanson (2003). An Aristotelian way of systematizing medical knowledge: Leith (2009a). Zalateo (1964) gave a very peculiar interpretation by relating these texts to the official examination of the δημόσιοι ἰατροί (public physicians) of Roman Egypt, but his hypothesis is now outdated. See Ricciardetto in this volume.

6 Cf., e.g., Andorlini (2006), *passim*, with further bibliography.

7 τῶν [...] τὴν τέχνην [...] ζητεόντων. Translation from Schiefsky (2005: 89).

8 On which, cf. Kollesch (1963) and Fischer (1998) respectively.

9 Galen gives instructions to the patients that they should choose the best doctor after an

public authorities,[10] in which they had to demonstrate their acquired knowledge in practice. The transmission of this knowledge was carefully carried out through a specialised education, initially based on oral teachings and subsequently entrusted to written supports. The relevance of written texts for medical education is stressed already in the Hippocratic corpus,[11] while Galen explains how written records of his oral lectures passed from hand to hand (these are the notes, or ὑπομνήματα, of which he says that they were not actually destined for wide publication).[12] These writings, compiled within a didactic framework, aimed at preserving, condensing and disseminating the medical knowledge and practice taught: they were the 'study textbooks' on which medical education—in terms of both learning and training—was built, and of which brief excerpts survive in the fragmentary papyri that came down to us—including the medical catechisms. Extremely significant is the introductory section of one of such writings, preserved as an *adespoton* in PSI XII 1275v (II century AD): "For those among the young people who approach medicine with a theoretical attitude, Demosthenes, since it is a primary and essential requirement for an introductory learning to master the names of internal and external body parts, we believe that it is best to first write each of such names in the form of a definition, and once a certain experience relating to these things has been acquired [...]".[13] The text is unfortunately incomplete, but either its writer or its

---

enquiry: cf. Nutton (1990), describing Galen's lost treatise *On Examining the Physician*, preserved thanks to an Arabic version. At 5.4 (70.13–15 Iskandar) it is said that "[a] man who is well trained in demonstrative logic can find out the truth simply by questioning the would-be healer on his learning" (tr. Nutton [1990: 245]).

10 Even though the official request for scientific proofs of a physician's actual medical capacity as recorded in P.Oxy. I 40 + BL I 312, V 74, VI 95 (copy of court proceedings from Oxyrhynchus, II cent. AD, in which a public doctor claims for immunity from some public obligations, and the judge asks for proofs) can be interpreted in different ways due to the fragmentary state of the papyrus, the practice of the δοκιμασία, i.e., the official examination by which a physician became a 'public doctor', is well attested (cf. Reggiani [2018c]).

11 "I consider the ability to evaluate correctly what has been written as an important part of the art", says the author of the *Epidemics* adding that: "He who has knowledge of it and knows how to use it will not commit, in my opinion, serious errors in the professional practice" (*Epid.* 3.3.16.1–4 [3.100.7–102.2 Littré; 113.5–8 Jouanna—Guardasole—Anastassiou]: μέγα δὲ μέρος ἡγεῦμαι τῆς τέχνης εἶναι τὸ δύνασθαι κατασκοπέεσθαι περὶ τῶν γεγραμμένων ὀρθῶς. ὁ γὰρ γνοὺς καὶ χρεόμενος τούτοισιν, οὐκ ἄν μοι δοκέῃ μέγα σφάλλεσθαι ἐν τῇ τέχνῃ).

12 *Libr. Propr.*, *Pref.* (19.8–11 Kühn; 1.131–135 Boudon-Millot); cf. Nutton (1972); Nieddu (1992: 555–567); Andorlini (2003: 14). On the topic of ancient medical education (and literacy) cf. also Hanson (2010).

13 τῶν νέων τοῖς κατὰ λόγοις εἰς | τὸ ἰατρεύειν προσάγουσιν, ὦ Δημό|σθενες, πρώτ[ο]ụ καὶ ἀναγκαιοτάτο[υ] | πρὸς [εἰ]σαγωγὴ̣ν ὑπάρχοντος τοῦ δι|ακατασχεῖν τῷ̣ν ἐπὶ τοῖς ἐντός τε | καὶ ἐκτὸς

user seems to have put such a recommendation into practice by transcribing a definition of the parts of the head on the other side of the papyrus. Similarly, the anonymous introduction to surgery preserved in BKT III, pp. 22–26 (I century AD) claims that beginners should learn an adequate basic terminology, of which the author provides some examples, structured, not inappropriately, in a sequence of questions.[14]

2 Digitizing the Medical Questionnaires on Papyrus

In the questionnaires on papyrus, utilised as handbooks and as reference tools for the doctors' preparation and practice, the importance of the erotapocritic structure is stressed by a complex set of graphic and paratextual devices deployed to highlight the articulation of the text.[15] As we already saw, this Q&A format is probably inspired by some sort of oral teaching, later entrusted to writing, at which point the articulation becomes a distinct discursive technique. This explains why the scribes took specific care to highlight the articulation of the text by means of a wide range of devices affecting the overall layout.[16] The questions are very often indented in *eisthesis* and further marked with diacritical and lectional marks (see below), which introduce the answers as well. This *mise en page* reflects the central role played by the Q&A structure of the didactical tool, and is therefore a constitutive part of the text, of its composition and transmission. For this reason it ought to be preserved carefully when the texts are moved to a modern medium. This is not only a matter of formal reproduction, but also of detailed analysis and interpretation. Due to the often-fragmentary state of the scattered sources on papyrus and the related difficulty in recognizing their textual genre,[17] scholars have to rely on any possible textual

τόποις τοῦ σώματος κε[ι]|μένων ὀνομάτων, βέλτιον οἰό|μεθα εἶναι τ[ο]ύτων πρότερον ἕκα|στ[ο]ν ὁρ[ικ]ῶς ὑπογράψαι καὶ πε|πρ[αγ]ματευμένοις περὶ τούτω[ν] […].

14 Cf. Andorlini (1992: 375–378).

15 In such technical and practical writings as medical textbooks, traces of different stages of transmission and use are preserved on the written support (cf. Andorlini [2003]; Reggiani [2019a and 2019d]), so that the very textual data interweave with a broad range of paratextual devices (see details below). These contribute to the articulation of an expressive discursive network that is essential to the formulation of the medical writing itself, to its transmission, to its learning, and to its practical use. According to Gérard Genette's textual theory, paratextuality is the relation between one text and what surrounds the main body of the text itself, e.g., titles, headings, and—so one may add—any graphical devices. Cf. Genette (1992: 83–84), as later developed in Genette (1997: 1–7).

16 Cf. Andorlini (1999: 8).

17 Cf. Andorlini (1997b: 159).

feature to ensure a proper understanding of the kind of text they are dealing with. As a matter of fact, some very fragmentary texts have been identified as questionnaires on the basis of the presence of blank spaces exclusively, as is the case with P.Oxford Sackler s.n., a small papyrus scrap from the II century BC dealing with apoplexy,[18] and more recently with GMP I 6 and P.Strasb. inv. 489, to which we will turn further on.[19] It is fundamental, therefore, to consider such texts with the necessary attention to their paratextual garment.

The following observations contextualise what precedes in the framework of the ERC-funded DIGMEDTEXT project, conducted by Isabella Andorlini at the University of Parma between 2014 and 2016, which was aimed at the creation of a digital textual database of the Greek papyri dealing with medicine. Encoding Greek medical papyri raises a very peculiar set of editorial issues, due to their special status as technical (para)literary texts,[20] for which reason they have been excluded from the extant databases so far. They express a specialised type of knowledge (namely, medicine) that mirrors itself in a particular "graphic and expressive jargon",[21] which ought to be properly represented in the digital editions, since it is an essential part of the texts themselves and of their interpretation. The Q&A catechisms are particularly challenging from this point of view, because of their structural complexity, and deserve further consideration, in view of which I will first provide a very short overview of how texts are digitally encoded in the current papyrological databases.

Papyrologists use a particular markup language called Leiden+ after the 'Leiden conventions' established for the critical editions of ancient texts;[22] this language represents papyrological features in a way that can be easily managed by any scholar, enabling him/her to encode texts according to the collaborative method deployed by the 'Son of Suda online' (SoSOL) platform on the Papyri.info website (http://papyri.info). In the so-called *Papyrological Editor* (the editing environment of SoSOL), this markup is converted into both an HTML display output resembling a print edition and an XML layer, where each papyrological feature of the text is represented by a specific label or "tag" according to the TEI EpiDoc standards.[23] This type of annotation is not

18 Cf. Barns (1949: 4–5).
19 Cf. Hanson—Mattern (2001: 72) and Magdelaine (2004: 63).
20 For the peculiar category of paraliterary texts and their difficult digital treatment, see Reggiani (2017: 78).
21 Andorlini (2006).
22 Cf. Reggiani (2017: 234 ff.).
23 On the TEI/EpiDoc markup, see Bodard (2010). In general, on digital editions of papyri, see Sosin (2010); Andorlini—Reggiani (2012); Reggiani (2017: 232 ff.); Reggiani (2018a); Reggiani (2018b).

descriptive but semantic: this means that when we, for instance, underdot an *alpha* in the Leiden+ editor (α̣), which renders the XML string <unclear>α </unclear>, we do not just want to *draw* an *alpha* with a dot below, but to *represent* an unclear character that may be read as *alpha*. The final user will see an underdotted *alpha* as usual, and s/he will understand it as an unclear letter as usual, but the system stores the semantic information rather than its visual rendering. Due to historical and technical reasons, the currently available set of Leiden+ marks was designed to encode documentary papyri only and did not take into consideration many features of literary and paraliterary papyri: critical, diacritical, lectional signs but also layout features that are deeply interconnected with the text itself. For this reason, the Parma DIGMEDTEXT project acted as a partner of the ongoing *Digital Corpus of Literary Papyrology* (DCLP), which is aimed at creating a complete online database of papyrus texts of literary and paraliterary content. Digitizing medical papyri raised several methodological and technical issues that proved useful to enhance both digital and traditional scholarship.[24]

The case of *eisthesis* (line indention) is the most meaningful in the present context. This layout device is perhaps the most evident way of highlighting a section in a text—in our case the question headings.[25] P.Ross.Georg. I 20 (Fig. 8.1)—an ophthalmological catechism on papyrus roll dated to the II century AD[26]—illustrates the use of *eisthesis* best, but we do find the same feature in several other papyri, among which, for instance, P.Aberd. 125v, dealing with trichological questions (III cent. AD, second half[27]) (Fig. 8.2).[28]

24 More detailed discussion of this can be found in Reggiani (2019b). On the digitisation of medical papyri and the Parma project, see also Reggiani (2015, 2016, and 2017: *passim*). On the DCLP, see now Ast—Essler (2018).

25 Its use is not, however, limited to medical questionnaires only: e.g., in poetry, *eisthesis* marks a change in metre. On the mechanics of *eisthesis* in ancient texts more generally, cf. Savignago (2008) and Agosti (2010).

26 Isabella Bonati deals with this text (ll. 94–115, regarding pterygium) in her contribution to the present volume.

27 Cf. Andorlini (1999: 9–10).

28 Other instances are: P.Strasb. inv. 489 (ophthalmological questionnaire, IV AD: cf. Magdelaine [2004]); P.Gen. inv. 111v (surgical definitions, II–III AD: cf. Nicole [1903]; Marganne [1998: 85–95]); GMP II 15; PSI XV 1510; P.Oxy. LXXIV 4972v (see below for these three papyri); possibly also P.Oxy. LXXX 5241v (ophthalmological definitions, II–III AD), although its left-hand side is lost and the answers cannot be supplemented entirely (see *ed.pr.*). Transcriptions of the papyri studied here can be found online via the links provided in the Appendix below. When pictures were not available, but the description of the papyrus layout required an image to be appended here for the sake of clarity, the transcription of the main edition was provided instead, if the treatment of graphical devices was sufficiently clear.

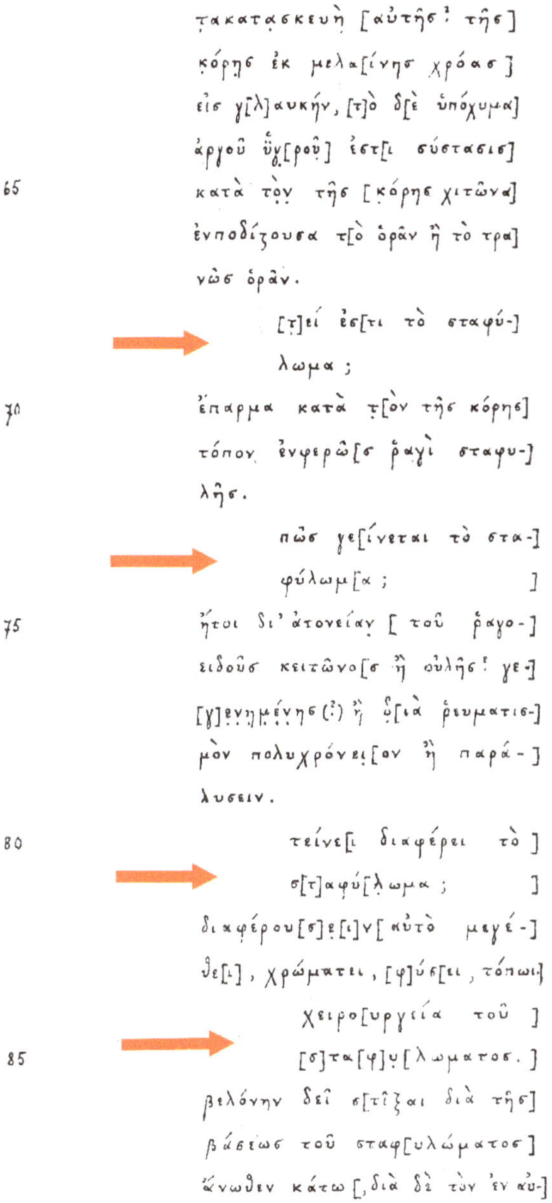

τακατασκευὴ [αὐτῆς; τῆς]
κόρης ἐκ μελα[ίνης χρόας]
εἰς γ[λ]αυκήν, [τ]ὸ δ[ὲ ὑπόχυμα]
ἀργοῦ ὑγ[ροῦ] ἐστ[ι σύστασις]
κατὰ τὸν τῆς [κόρης χιτῶνα]
ἐνποδίζουσα τ[ὸ ὁρᾶν ἢ τὸ τρα]
νῶς ὁρᾶν.

[τ]ί ἐσ[τι τὸ σταφύ-]
λωμα;

ἔπαρμα κατὰ τ[ὸν τῆς κόρης]
τόπον ἐνφερῶ[ς ῥαγὶ σταφυ-]
λῆς.

πῶς γε[ίνεται τὸ στα-]
φύλωμ[α;]

ἤτοι δι' ἀτονείαν [τοῦ ῥαγο-]
ειδοῦς κειτῶνο[ς ἢ οὐλῆς; γε-]
[γ]ενημένης (?) ἢ ὑ[ιὰ ῥευματισ-]
μὸν πολυχρόνει[ον ἢ παρά-]
λυσειν.

τείνε[ι διαφέρει τὸ]
σ[τ]αφύ[λωμα;]

διαφέρου[σ]ε[ι]ν[αὐτὸ μεγέ-]
θε[ι], χρώματει, [φ]ύσ[ει, τόπωι]

χειρο[υργεία τοῦ]
[σ]τα[φ]υ[λώματος.]

βελόνην δεῖ σ[τῖξαι διὰ τῆς]
βάσεως τοῦ σταφ[υλώματος]
ἄνωθεν κάτω [, διὰ δὲ τὸν ἐν αὐ-]

FIGURE 8.1 P.Ross.Georg. I 20

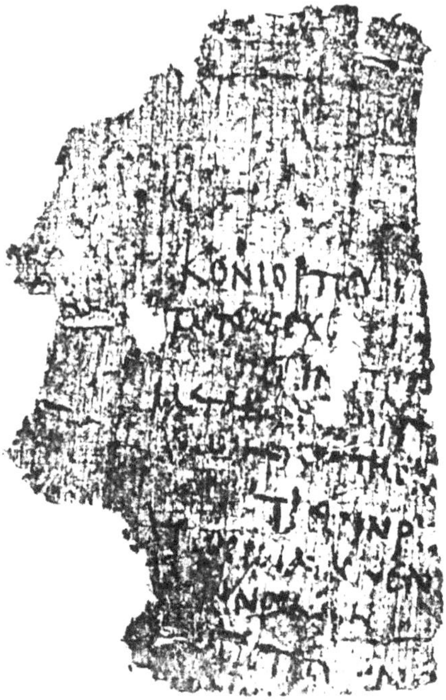

<margine ca. cm 3>
κονιορτοῦ ἢ .[τρίχας μολυνο-
μένας ἔχο[υ]σ̣ι̣ν̣[
  τί ἐστιν πολ̣ί̣[ωσις;
μεταβολὴ [τ]ῶ̣ν τ̣ρ[ιχῶν ἐπὶ τὸ λευκὸν
χρῶμα πρὸ τῆς κ̣α̣[θη- κούσης ἡλικίας.
  τί ἐστιν ῥύ[ις;
ἀπόρροια τῶν ε̣γ̣[
..ινομ... [

FIGURE 8.2 P.Aberd. 125v

Since a specific way of encoding *eisthesis* was lacking, we were tempted, at first, to equate it to a *vacat* (a space intentionally left blank by the ancient scribe) and therefore to encode it as such according to the well-established Leiden+ custom (i.e., vac.? = XML <space extent="unknown" unit="character"/>).[29] However, as noted above, when we encode a text digitally we aim not only at creating a pleasant display output, but above all at annotating the text with the necessary semantic information. In this case, we are not dealing with a mere space that was left blank by the scribe, but with a graphical displacement of the line beginning that flags the start of a new question and thus puts particular emphasis on it. The use of *ekthesis* in the papyri (i.e., an extension of the line out of the left-hand margin)[30] makes the point more clear: surely, it would be inappropriate to indicate this layout device with a virtual *vacat* at the beginning of each of the surrounding lines. This is the case, for instance, with P.Oxy. LII 3654 (Fig. 8.3), a fragmentary catechistic section of a wider roll

29 Cf. the EpiDoc guidelines at http://www.stoa.org/epidoc/gl/latest/trans-vacatchar.html. A more compact description and discussion of Leiden+ and XML strategies for the encoding of the Greek papyri can now be found in Reggiani (2019c: Appendix after p. 400).

30 Cf. again Savignago (2008).

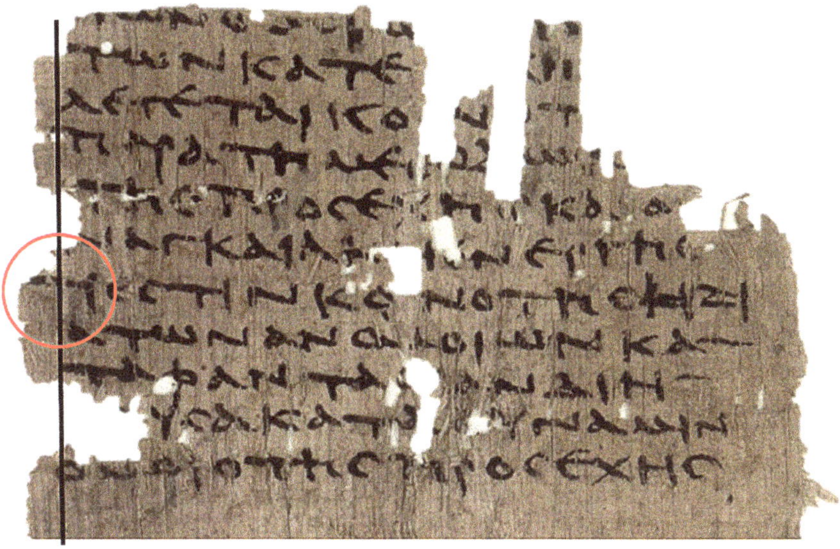

FIGURE 8.3 P.Oxy. LII 3654
COURTESY OF THE EGYPT EXPLORATION SOCIETY AND IMAGING PAPYRI PROJECT, OXFORD

containing a therapeutic work of Methodist provenance,[31] dated between the last quarter of the II century AD and the first quarter of the III. The *ekthesis* is slightly perceivable only in fr. 8, line 7 (τί ἐστιν κο[ι]νότης; "what is pathologic generality?") but was likely employed throughout.[32]

A peculiar case is GMP II 15 (Fig. 8.4) (III cent. AD, questionnaire of gynaecology/pathology), where (at least in the extant fragments and according to Albert Bäckström's drawings) questions in *eisthesis* seem to be followed by answers with the first line in *ekthesis* (col. ii, ll. 25–27), which makes it evident that the *vacat*-system is not refined enough to be applicable to such circumstances.[33]

We therefore suggested that *eisthesis* should be encoded, according to the EpiDoc guidelines, as an attribute describing a special rendering of the line:

31 Andorlini (1992). The fragments belong to the same roll as P.Oxy. II 234.

32 See probably fr. 1+5+2, l. 12, and the supplements to fr. 7, ll. 3–5, according to Andorlini (1992).

33 From Bäckström's transcription in the Russian *editio princeps* of the text (Bäckström [1904a]) it seems that the second line of the question in *eisthesis* is more indented than the first one, but his drawing does not support this rendering, which indeed disappears from his German edition (Bäckström [1904b]). The *ekthesis* is not noted in either of the editions but is quite evident in the drawing. I am very grateful to David Leith, latest editor of the papyrus (Leith [2009b]), who kindly provided me with his scans of Bäckström's material.

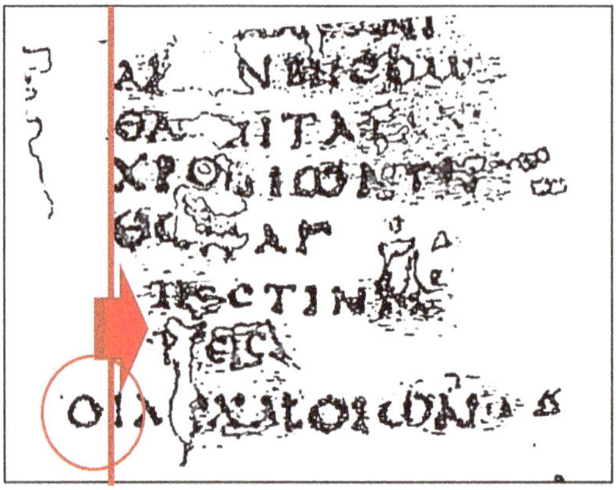

FIGURE 8.4 GMP II 15

<lb n="1" rend="indent"/>,[34] which in Leiden+ appears as (1, indent)—the same way marginal annotations are tagged.[35] This seems to work fine: it is recognised by the system and is now fully supported also by the HTML display output, which displaces the line accordingly. Thus, each indented line can be marked as *eisthesis*, and this feature may be searched for in the database. When the last question line does not fit the line entirely, the scribe leaves it blank: this is a proper *vacat* and can be encoded accordingly (see above for the markup of blank spaces) within the "eisthesis" tag, because it is part of the *eisthesis* scheme. Note that in the Oxyrhynchus fragments, on the contrary, the answers seem to follow the questions without any break.[36]

A further problem arises when, in some catechisms, the question does not start on a new line, but on the same line as the end of the previous answer, following a blank space. This feature occurs, e.g., in P.Oxy. LXXX 5239 (II–III century AD), a catechism dealing with pathology (tumour-like diseases, as far as the surviving fragment goes), the text of which is partly overlapped by P.Oslo inv. 1576v (III AD),[37] which deploys the very same device to highlight the questions (Fig. 8.5A/B). Such blank spaces cannot be considered as true *vacat*'s for the

34 On line tagging and its attributes, see the online documentation at http://www.stoa.org/epidoc/gl/latest/trans-linebreak.html and http://www.stoa.org/epidoc/gl/latest/trans-linebreakdirection.html.

35 See documentation at http://papyri.info/docs/leiden_plus. For *ekthesis*, one should of course just replace the "rend" attribute with the appropriate indication (i.e., "outdent" instead of "indent").

36 Papyrus catechisms show a wide variety of graphical and layout indications for questions and answers and it is almost always hard to find any rationale, if any. Likely it depended on the scribe's own sensibility.

37 Maravela—Leith (2007). The papyrus will be republished with substantial updates

same reasons as explained above. Moreover, if we were to tag the entire line as "eisthesis" we would not represent the situation correctly. A possible solution would be to tag the question phrase with the XML <hi> label, which is used to mark "highlighted characters or words", "with a rend attribute specifying the kind of highlighting".[38] In our case, the attribute would be "eisthesis", and would account for this special 'inline indention'. At the moment, this code is not supported by SoSOL, but it seems meaningful to implement a proper way of displaying this peculiar type of layout.

P.PisaLit. 6 (an ophthalmological catechism, II–III AD)[39] (Fig. 8.6) shows a different, yet comparable situation: questions start in *eisthesis* on new lines (the indention is visible at l. 15, cf. also ll. 8 and 12, in the transcription by Isabella Andorlini), but answers start on the very same line as the preceding questions. This is clearly a case in which it may prove more helpful to tag the question-phrase, rather than the entire line. A somewhat opposite case is found in P.Oxy. LXXX 5238 (II–III AD) (Fig. 8.7), where therapeutical questions are highlighted by means of 'inline' *eisthesis* (ll. 4, 12),[40] but are indented if they run over more than one line (ll. 6–7, 13), staying aligned with the starting point of the question phrase itself. This rather peculiar case proves difficult to be treated and may well lead to further distinctions in *eisthesis* types in the encoding markup ('inline', 'indented', 'mixed' *eisthesis*?).

In P.Aberd. 11 (another questionnaire on ophthalmology, dating back to the II century AD)[41] (Fig. 8.8) the two kinds of *eisthesis* (the proper and the inline type) seem to occur together, though it is not unlikely that the rationale followed here is actually that of the proper *eisthesis* (ll. 2 and 6), while the apparent inline type at l. 9 is likely due to the practical need of placing the last letters of the preceding section, which did not fit line 8, on the same line as the new section heading (which is not, however, phrased in question form but concerns "surgery of pterygium", χειρ[ουργεία τοῦ πτερυγείου]).[42] It is indeed clear that

and enhancements in the forthcoming fourth volume of the *Papyri Osloenses*. I am most grateful to Anastasia Maravela for sharing her drafts of the new edition and for discussing with me some textual and linguistic details.

38 http://www.stoa.org/epidoc/gl/latest/trans-charactershighlighted.html.

39 Cf. P.Alex. 614 *descr.*; Manetti (1973); Andorlini (1999: 13–15).

40 At some points these resemble an indention, viz. when they occur at line beginnings (ll. 2, 17), as noted by the editor, David Leith, and paralleled in P.Oxy. LXXX 5235 (see below); l. 36 is uncertain because no text survives to the left.

41 Cf. Winstedt (1907: 266); Körte (1941: 145); Marganne (1978); Marganne (1994: 104–111). Isabella Bonati discusses ll. 2–20 of this papyrus (about pterygium) in her chapter in the present volume.

42 Nevertheless, this is still implicitly interrogative: "surgery of the *pterygion*", i.e., "which is the ...?".

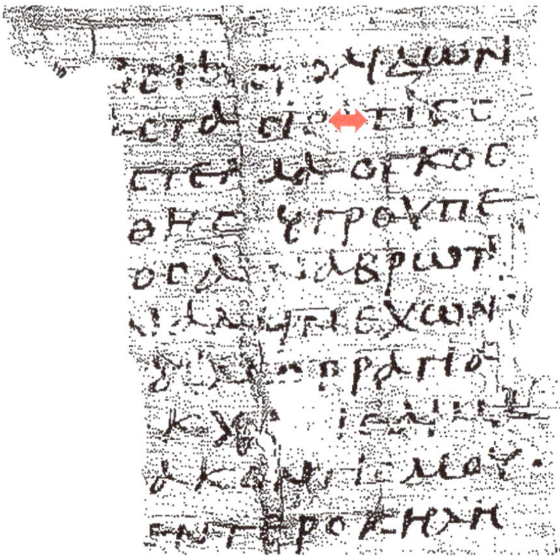

FIGURE 8.5A P.Oxy. LXXX 5239
COURTESY OF THE EGYPT EXPLORATION SOCIETY AND IMAGING PAPYRI PROJECT, OXFORD

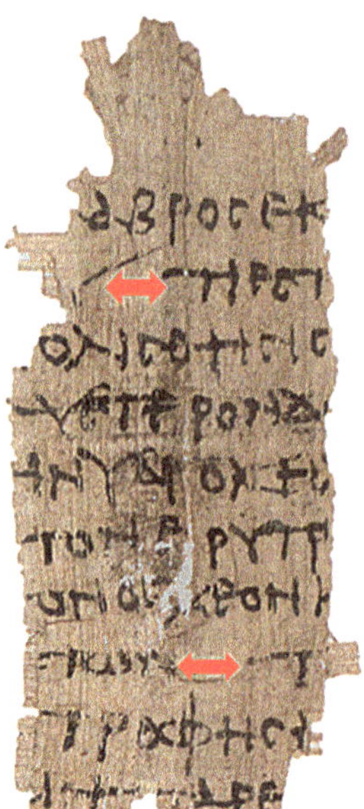

FIGURE 8.5B
P.Oslo inv. 1576v
COURTESY OF THE PAPYRUS COLLECTION, UNIVERSITY OF OSLO LIBRARY

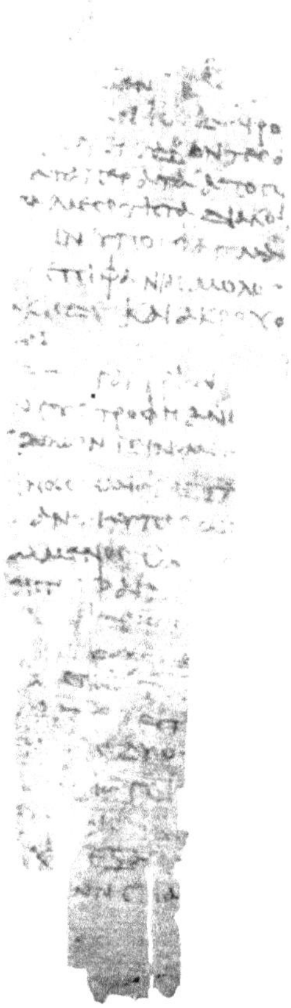

— — — —
].[ ].[ ]. . . κ̣. [
]μεν .[ ]. . [
]. ν η̣.. δ̣ιαιρο[
]κ̣α̣ι ἐκ̣λαβόντες ἀ[γκίστρῳ ἀμ-
φότερ]α τὰ πέρατα ἀποσφ[ίγγομεν καὶ
διὰ τ]ὴν μεσότητα διακόπ̣[τομεν.
τί ἐσ]τ̣ιν ὑπόσφαγμα; [γίνεται ἐξω-
θεν τῆς] ἐπιφαν<ε>ίας μόλω̣π̣[ι παραπλήσιον:
πολλ]άκις δὲ καὶ ἀκροχο[ρδων-
] α̣ν.
τί ἐ]στ[ιν] γαγγρίον; [ἐστὶ νεύρου παρὰ
φύσι]ν̣ συστροφὴ ἀνα̣[λγὴς ἐπὶ τῶν
ὀρθοκ]ύ̣λλων γεινομέν[ων μορίων
] τ̣ίνα σημ<ε>ῖα γαγγλ[ίου;
ὄγκο]ς̣ ἀντίτυπος ὡ̣ς [ἐπὶ τὸ πολὺ συν-
εστρ]α̣μμένος ὁμ[ό]χ̣[ρους

FIGURE 8.6 P.PisaLit. 6

the section heading on line 9 is aligned to the previous ones. This looks like another plausible reason to prefer the second way of encoding the *eisthesis* as described above (rather than simply using *vacat* or line attribute). A third reason is that when the question is spread over multiple lines, the *eisthesis* is sometimes repeated (as is the case in the diplomatic transcription of the P.Ross.Georg., above); by using the proper encoding we can avoid that the "eisthesis" phenomenon is connected to specific lines, and thus allows for tagging an appropriate semantic unity in the interrogative phrase as a whole.

Aberdeen papyrus 11 further deploys horizontal rules (*paragraphoi*)[43] to clearly distinguish separate definition sections (consisting of question and

43 On the typology of *paragraphos*, see Barbis Lupi (1994) and Schironi (2010: 16 and *passim*).

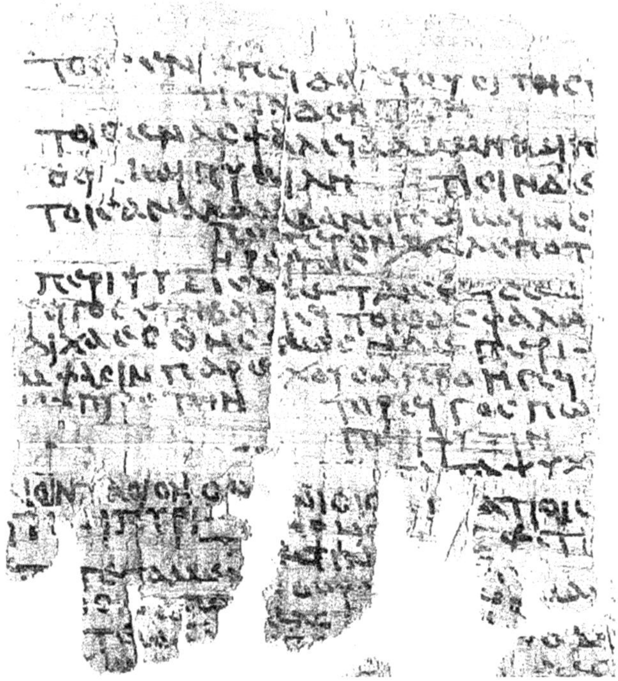

FIGURE 8.7 P.Oxy. LXXX 5238
COURTESY OF THE EGYPT EXPLORATION SOCIETY AND IMAGING PAPYRI PROJECT, OXFORD

answer). This does not cause any problem with the digital encoding, since *paragraphoi* are widespread in documentary papyri too, and are already supported by the SoSOL editing platform: they are encoded as "milestones", i.e., markers of non-structural text parts (XML: <milestone rend="paragraphos" unit="undefined"/>; Leiden+: ----).[44] A similar mark, very recently introduced into the platform, is the *diple obelismene* or forked *paragraphos*, i.e., a horizontal rule preceded by a closing angle bracket (*diple*).[45] It is used, e.g., in GMP II 14, a surgical (?) catechism dealing with anatomy dated to II–III century AD,[46] to mark the end of an answer section and the beginning of a new question section (col. ii, ll. 7–8) (Fig. 8.9). The new proposed "milestone" tag (not yet working) for the forked *paragraphos* is <milestone rend="diple-obelismene" unit="undefined"/> (Leiden+: >->->->-). This distinction is not superfluous:

44 Cf. http://www.stoa.org/epidoc/gl/latest/trans-nonstructural.html.
45 On the typology of *diple obelismene*, see Barbis Lupi (1988); cf. Schironi (2010: 19).
46 Formerly PSI III 252r; cf. Fausti (1980); Mavroudis (1986).

[. . . .] . ντο καὶ τ.οει[ ]
· τί ἐστι ὧν [τὸ πτερύγειον ;]
ἔκφυσις ὑμενώδης α[ὐξανομένη ἀπὸ τοῦ]
κανθοῦ ἢ σωματοποι[ουμένη]
ἀπὸ τοῦ κερατοειδοῦς [χιτῶνος.]
τίνες [εἰσὶ διαφοραὶ πτερυγείων ;]
διαφέρετε αὐτῶν τό[πωι, μεγέθει,]
σχήματι, χρώματ[ι, φύσει ἢ ἀνα-]
σκευῇ. χειρ[ουργεία τοῦ πτερυγείου.]
μετὰ τὸν καθέδρειο[ν ὄντα τὸν πάσχοντα, ἐκ]
τοῦ ὀφθαλμοῦ διφ[υῆ βλέφαρα διαστείλαντες]
τὸ πτερύγειον δι[εκφανοῦμεν ἀγκι-]
στρείοι, βελόνην [δὲ λίνον καὶ τρίχα ἱππείαν]
ἔχουσα[ν]
σεωσ . [ ]
ματι . [ ]
μεν κα[ ]
λειων . [ ]
. ν ρει δ[ὲ]
[. .] . . ι [ ]

FIGURE 8.8 P.Aberd. 11

compared to a 'simple' *paragraphos*, the *diple obelismene*, in its more elegant look, seems to show a certain 'bookish' or 'literary' flavour that might attest to a greater concern for accuracy towards the copying of the medical text. As Leith distinguishes two types of medical Q&A texts, namely, on the one hand, the proper catechisms, or questionnaires, which are introductory manuals for the student of medicine, and, on the other, more general treatises on remedies (see below), we may ask whether careful attention to the paratextual architecture of the text could help us in distinguishing different levels of this textual typology.[47] At any rate, a careful digital annotation of these peculiarities proves very helpful for research. Other stylistic trends are found in GMP II 14, for example, in the underlines and overlines that highlight the first and last letters of the question sentences, which is a feature usually to be found in association with book titles.[48] Encoding such marks is not a problem, since the current Leiden+ syntax supports both underlined and overlined characters—with few insignificant display issues. The real problem is to overcome any possible shortcom-

47 Leith (2007).
48 Cf., e.g., Caroli (2007: 55).

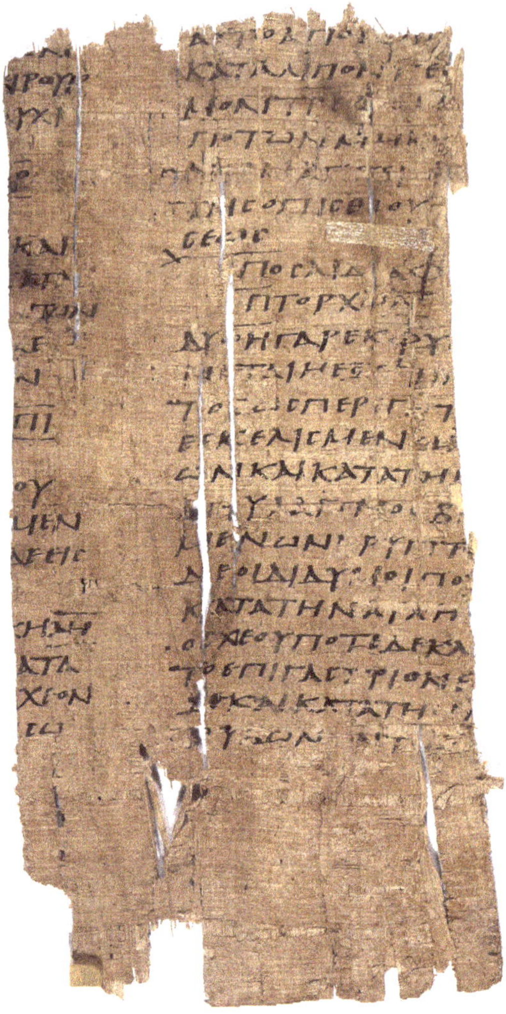

FIGURE 8.9 GMP II 14
COURTESY OF THE ISTITUTO PAPIROLOGICO "G. VITELLI", UNIVERSITY OF FLORENCE

ings of previous printed editions in order to represent correctly and accurately the ancient texts. The case of GMP II 14 is relevant here. While the picture patently exhibits a forked *paragraphos* as the marker of the new Q&A section, both the *editio princeps* (PSI III 252) and the *editio altera* print a simple *paragraphos*.[49] This is a clear example of how digital encoding becomes a critical

49 Fausti (1980). The partial re-edition in the second volume of *Greek Medical Papyri* (Leith—Maravela [2009]) does not take this section into consideration.

edition not only of the text itself, but also of the previous printed editions, if we want to represent the ancient document in its entirety.[50] PSI XV 1510 (catechism on anatomy, III AD)[51] likely shows a case comparable to GMP II 14: questions are in *eisthesis*, while a slight enlargement of the initial letters of the answer (ll. 4 ἐξ, 11 εἵ̈να with *trema* for ἵ̈να) seems intended to have the same use as *paragraphoi* or over/underlines (Fig. 8.10).[52]

Line fillers represent another paratextual typology that raises some interesting theoretical and technical issues. They are not absent from documentary papyri, where they are commonly used to fill the final blank in the event that the text is not long enough to complete the entire line, thus allowing to keep the alignment on the right (justification).[53] The SoSOL platform developed a way to encode them as non-alphabetical "glyphs" (e.g., *filler* = XML <g type="filler"/>),[54] and indeed they usually do not bear any other meaning than being filling symbols. In medical catechisms they can be used when questions and answers are articulated as separated sections, and therefore final blanks may occur if the text does not fill out the last line of a section (see the cases above, where the remaining blank space is left empty). Yet sometimes they can become a further mark to highlight the Q&A structure. This is the case in MPER XIII 19, a fragment of a questionnaire of likely medical content in codex format (II cent. AD) (Fig. 8.11), where questions seem to be introduced by short *paragraphoi* (side A, ll. 5–6). On side B, a sentence (likely belonging to an answer section) ends much before the right-hand margin, and a small hyphen is added (l. 5). This is not enough to cover the entire blank space, and therefore is clearly not acting as a line filler.[55] This kind of situation is even more evident in PSI inv. 3783, a questionnaire about surgery (phlebotomy, in the surviving fragments; I–II AD)[56] (Fig. 8.12) where the questions are pinpointed by blanks ('inline' *eistheseis*) before and after the sentence, and further highlighted by groups of elaborate S-shaped 'fillers' at the line ends (fr. A, col. I, l. 43; col. ii, *passim*; a *paragraphos* is used at ll. 44–45 of the second column of fr. A, but it looks isolated), which according to Isabella Andorlini's interpretation act as

50 For digital criticism, cf. the observations in Reggiani (2017: 264 ff.).

51 Cf. Manfredi (1997); Andorlini (2007: 414).

52 For the lack of uniformity in such phenomena, see above.

53 On the typology of filling marks in literary papyri, see Barbis Lupi (1992). See also Di Matteo (2007), with a particular focus on the Herculaneum papyri.

54 See http://147.142.225.252/paptrac/wiki/gtypes and http://papyri.info/docs/leiden_plus.

55 It must be noted that while the *editio princeps* (MPER I 32) does transcribe the hyphen, the re-edition in the thirteenth volume of MPER omits it.

56 Cf. Andorlini (1997b). A full edition is being published in the forthcoming third volume of the *Greek Medical Papyri*.

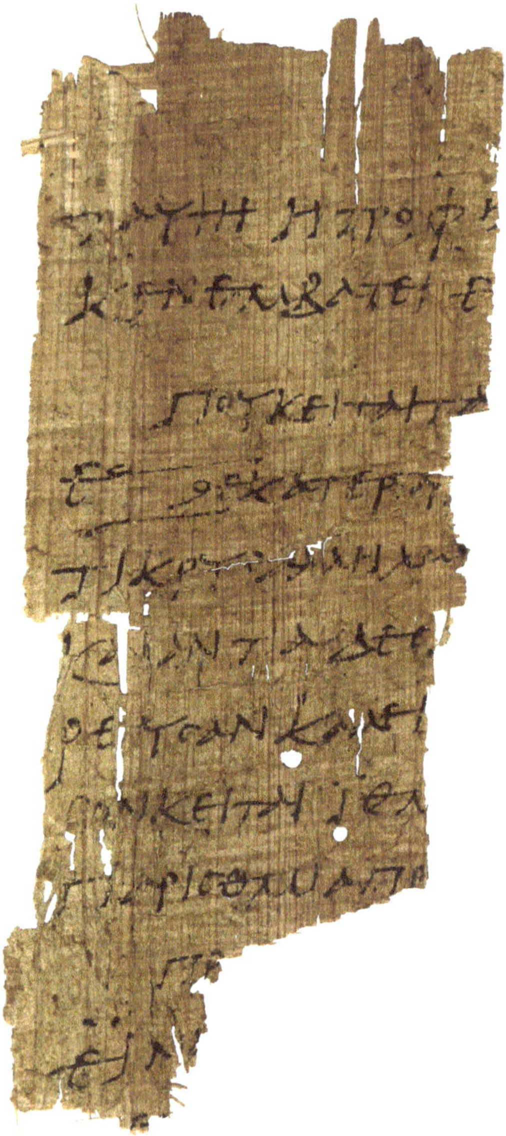

FIGURE 8.10 PSI XV 1510
COURTESY OF THE ISTITUTO PAPIROLOGICO "G. VITELLI", UNIVERSITY OF FLORENCE

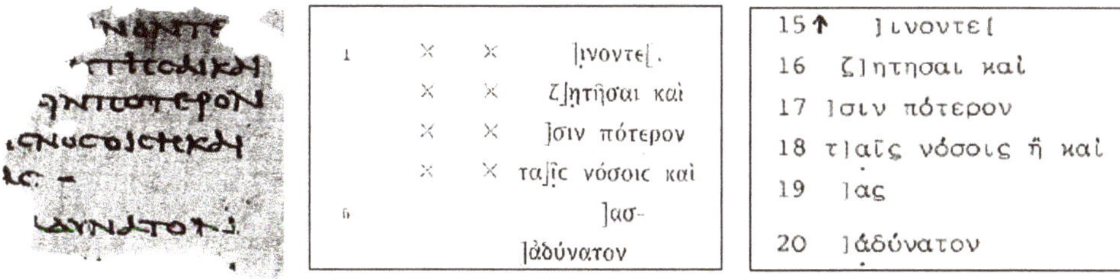

FIGURE 8.11 MPER XIII 19
© AUSTRIAN NATIONAL LIBRARY

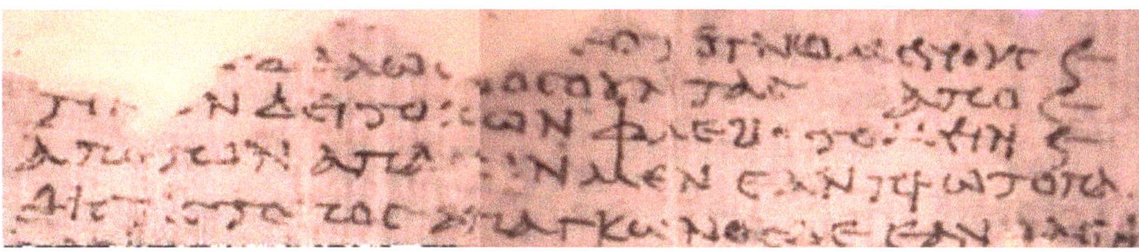

FIGURE 8.12 PSI inv. 3783
COURTESY OF THE ISTITUTO PAPIROLOGICO "G. VITELLI", UNIVERSITY OF FLORENCE

highlighters of key questions, which resemble common line fillers but carry out a different function, namely to mark the occurrence of a question phrase.[57]

The same practice, in fact, does appear in SB XXVI 16458, a parchment sheet dated to the first half of the IV cent. AD (possibly from a notebook in codex format?),[58] containing a series of medical recipes separated by means of *paragraphoi*. Each text section ends with peculiar 'filling marks' (ll. 2, 5, 12) that are very similar to the ones in the Florentine catechism. The first editor of the sheet (A. Olivieri, PSI VI 718) considered them as indications of weight measures (abbreviation for drachmas + number, overlined in one case: ll. 2 and 12) and tachygraphic marks (l. 5).[59] The second editor correctly read them as graphical devices aimed at separating different recipes, and described them as shaped in the same way: an S-like sign followed by a horizontal line, ending in a curl,

57 Andorlini (1997b: 160 with n. 13).
58 Cf. Reggiani (2019a) with further bibliography. Digital edition at http://papyri.info/dclp/64564. I was unable to publish a picture of this text because of restrictions applied by the holding institution (Biblioteca Mediceo-Laurenziana, Florence); an online image can be found at http://www.psi-online.it/documents/psi;6;718.
59 Cf. also McNamee (1981: 82), where it is transcribed as part of the preceding abbreviation.

the length of which depends on the blank space to be filled.[60] However, from the photo of the sheet it appears that at the end of l. 5 we have three signs: the S-shaped one; a curled one, which closely resembles the first one; and the horizontal line. The combination of the first two is the same as ll. 2 and 12, without horizontal line. We may infer that we are dealing with two different sets of signs: (1) a double 'curl', for which the old definition of "Koronis",[61] advanced by Wilcken, seems appropriate;[62] (2) a horizontal line acting as a filler mark. That the alleged *koronis* acts as more than a filling mark may be inferred from l. 12, where it is used to mark the end of a recipe, while the following one starts on the very same line.

Coming back to the Florentine catechism, it seems therefore that encoding those symbols as simple 'line fillers' might be rather inadequate with respect to their original meaning (namely indicators of the question sections). They do not even act as proper *koronides* as in GMP II 15, at the end of the fourth column (not indicated in Bäckström's transcriptions, see above) (Fig. 8.13). They are much more similar to the forked *paragraphoi* which in P.Lund I 7 (anatomical catechism, III–IV cent. AD)[63] (Fig. 8.14A/B) are located at the end of each definition block (i.e., at the end of the answers, and before the questions in *eisthesis*). Also in this case, this is not a 'line filler', since in some cases it simply does not fill the line entirely. P.Mil.Vogl. I 15 (therapeutic questionnaire, IV AD)[64] (Fig. 8.15) is even more clear in this use: here, the forked *paragraphoi* at the end of each answer are followed by blank spaces acting as 'inline' *eistheseis* before each question.[65] These are layout devices aimed at marking definition blocks, not mere filling marks. The same should apply to P.Oxy. LXXIV 4972v (surgical text, II–III AD) (Fig. 8.16), though here the 'answer-marks' seem to reach the line ends.

The distinction mentioned earlier between proper catechisms (i.e., introductory manuals for the student of medicine) and more general treatises on remedies (for study and reference use by physicians and learned laymen), also in Q&A form,[66] seems to be further stressed by the present reconsideration

---

60 Ronconi (2000).

61 On the *koronis*, the bird-like symbol that was commonly used in literary copies to mark the end of a book or a text section, cf., e.g., Schironi (2010: 16–18 and *passim*).

62 Wilcken (1924: 86).

63 Cf. Körte (1939: 127); Marganne (1987).

64 Cf. Körte (1939: 126–127); Snell (1939: 532); Leith (2014).

65 Cf. Moretti (1995: 22). P.Oxy. LXXX 5235, identified as belonging to the same work as the Milan fragment, seems to feature an indented question (col. ii, l. 5), but this may be due to the fact that the preceding answer exactly fits line 4, so that the 'inline' *eisthesis* coincides with the subsequent line beginning.

66 Suggested by David Leith in 2007, but already envisaged by Andorlini (1997b: 160).

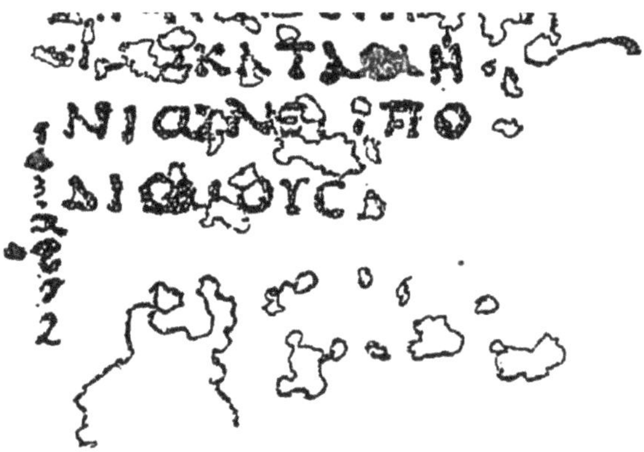

FIGURE 8.13 GMP II 15

of paratextual marks as favoured by the digital edition of the medical papyri. Leith's suggestion derives from the similarities detected between *erotapokriseis* on papyrus such as P.Turner 14 (see below) and PSI inv. 3783 and the excerpts from the physicians Herodotus and Antyllus as preserved in Oribasius' *Collectiones medicae*, but is not limited to those cases only: as Isabella Andorlini wrote apropos of PSI inv. 3783, the papyrus samples attest to the diffusion of medical catechisms in various formats and contents. Beside the simple articulation in question-like ὅροι, serving as a practical teaching system (cf. P.PisaLit. 6), there are more articulated and theoretical discourses, structured in the didactic catechistic model (cf. P.Mil.Vogl. I 15).[67]

We noted above that both PSI inv. 3783 and P.Mil.Vogl. I 15 exhibit the feature of the 'inline' *eisthesis*, accompanied by a special use of forked *paragraphoi* (or similar signs) to mark the Q&A structure; the same does indeed occur in P.Turner 14 (pharmacological/therapeutical questionnaire, II AD)[68] (Fig. 8.17), which deploys 'inline' *eisthesis* and *diple obelismene*—now in its 'standard' interlinear place—along with a double dot (*dikolon*) at the end of both the question sentence and the answer section. Conversely, it is understandable that more practical manuals needed to display the relevant information in a more usable format than inline marks, such as an emphasised indention. High dots are deployed by GMP I 6 (II–III AD)[69] (Fig. 8.18), apparently at the end of each question, though it is not clear how the *eisthesis* system works in this case, since all the beginnings of the questions are lost, and the blanks, clearly recognisable on the right (they led the editors to identify the papyrus as a questionnaire, see

67 Andorlini (1997b: 160).

68 Cf. Leith (2007).

69 This papyrus is discussed by Isabella Bonati in her chapter in the present volume.

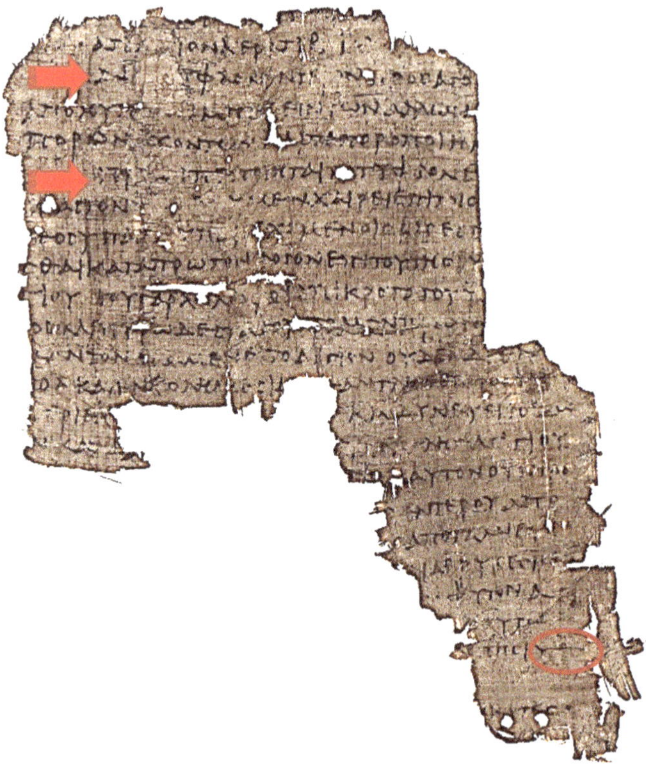

FIGURE 8.14A P.Lund I 7 recto
© LUND UNIVERSITY LIBRARY (I WAS UNABLE TO REACH ANY COPYRIGHT HOLDER)

above), may well point either to *vacat*'s before and after indented *eisthesis* or to the blanks of an 'inline' *eisthesis* (line 7, in particular, is supplemented by the editors as if it was not in *eisthesis*).

It does not seem unlikely to conceive of a differentiation in paratextual use according to different textual subgenres, but this requires further investigation and discussion: unfortunately, the fragmentary state of the available documentation makes things more complicated. What I want to stress here is the new series of observations that may arise from a deep and accurate reconsideration of papyrus texts as favoured by their digital encoding, which can—in turn—lead to new possibilities of research and comparison with other known texts. Medical papyri show how important it is to account for any paratextual feature deployed by the ancient scribes in the phases of text transmission, as this provides valuable information which 'traditional' printed editions often do not take into consideration, because it is not regarded as particularly relevant for the reconstruction of the texts.

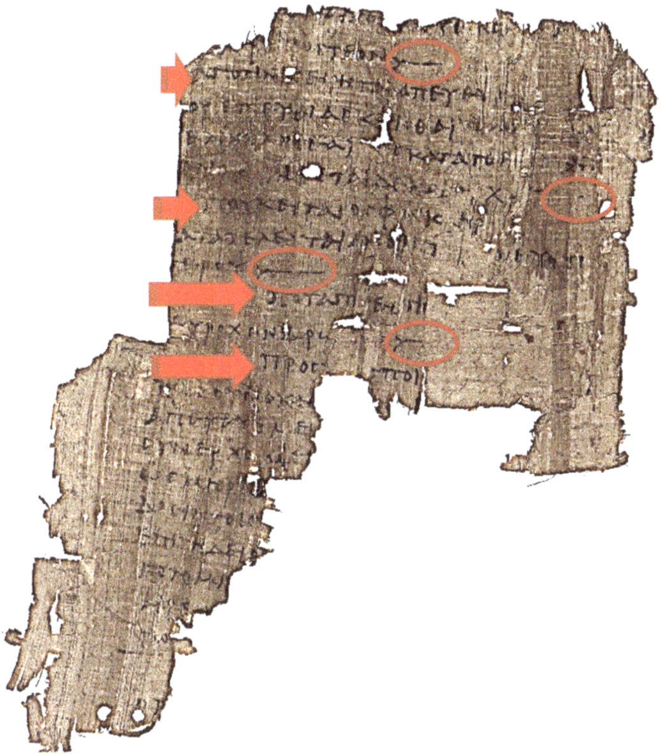

FIGURE 8.14B P.Lund I 7 verso

3 Concluding Remarks

Thanks to their peculiar textual structure, the medical catechisms on papyrus in Q&A prove extremely useful as *specimina* of the theoretical and practical issues raised by the digital encoding of ancient papyri in general, and more in specific of those belonging to a very technical corpus of medical texts. We have seen how the layout strategies and the paratextual framework deployed to enhance the peculiar articulation in questions and answers are strictly related to the educational and functional uses of this textual typology, fundamental in ancient medical learning and training. In turn, their technical use produced textual phenomena, the description and transmission of which go far beyond a traditional, 'static' philological model. Digital encoding provides a momentous opportunity to produce an accurate reproduction of the ancient texts presenting all their constitutive parts in an enhanced way: not just a mere graphical representation—often even lacking from printed editions—but a wider and

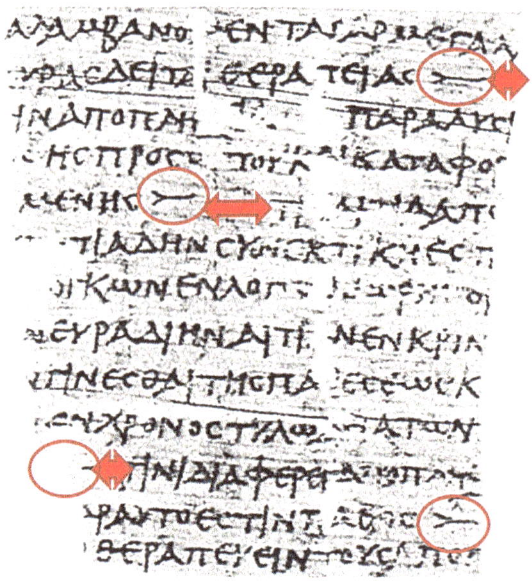

FIGURE 8.15 P.Mil.Vogl. I 15

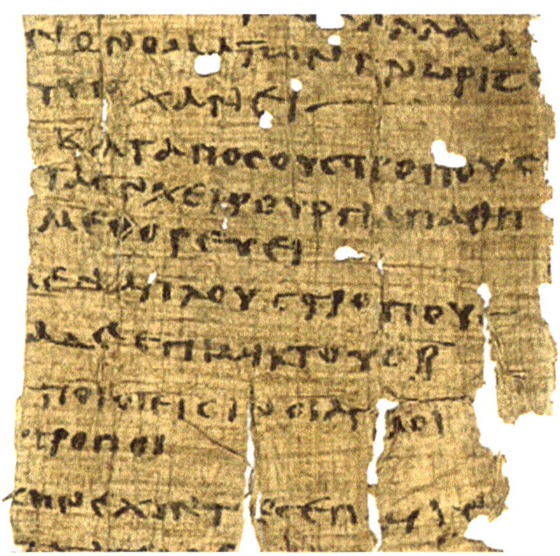

FIGURE 8.16 P.Oxy. LXXIV 4972v

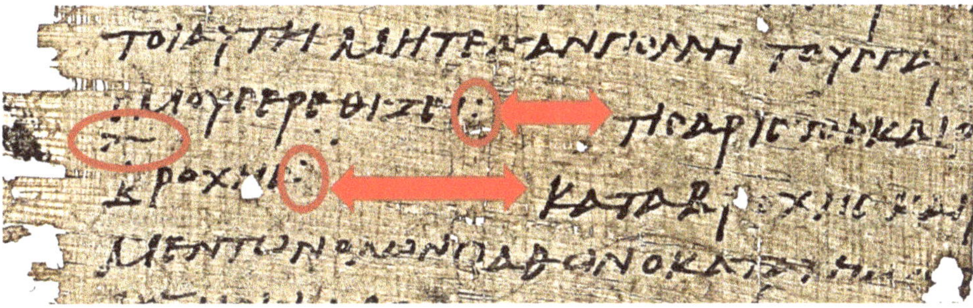

FIGURE 8.17 P.Turner 14
COURTESY OF THE UNIVERSITY OF MICHIGAN PAPYROLOGY COLLECTION

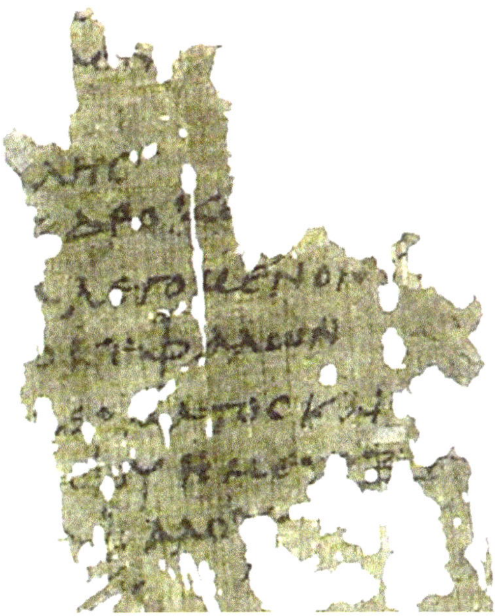

↓

— — — — — —
]̣ [
]δ̣ε̣ν̣ (*vac.*)
τι εϲτι το υγρον ον] (*vac.*)
(*vac.*) εν τινι μερει τηϲ κεφ]α̣ληϲ (*vac.*)
το παθοϲ προϲαγορευεται] υδροκε[φαλον]
δια το υγρον εν κεφαλη ϲυ]λλεγομενον·
ποϲαι αι διαφοραι των υδρ]ο̣κεφαλων (*vac.*)
τεϲϲαρεϲ η γαρ μεταξὺ του] δερματοϲ και
περικρανιου η ? και ο]ϲ̣τ̣ου η μεταξυ
οϲτου και μηνιγγοϲ η ? εγ]κεφαλου· (*vac.*)
(*vac.*) ποϲαι ειϲι] α̣ι̣ [αιτι]α̣[ι]̣ (*vac.*)

FIGURE 8.18 GMP I 6
COURTESY OF THE BEINECKE RARE BOOK AND MANUSCRIPT LIBRARY, YALE UNIVERSITY

deeper semantic comprehension. Moreover, it is an occasion to rethink and reread these texts, and to pay specific attention to peculiar features sometimes neglected or misunderstood by printed editions (devoted as they were—and still are—to the reconstruction of an archetypical, 'ideal' text, sometimes far from the actual document at our disposal). It is, to sum up, fundamental to understand (and further transmit)[70] the objects of our study.

70 I have argued that digital critical editions may act as a further step in the textual transmission in Reggiani (2020).

Appendix: Overview of Digital Editions of Medical Questionnaires on Papyrus

Text	Link to the digital edition
P.Oxford Sackler s.n. (II BC), fragment on apoplexy	http://www.papyri.info/dclp/65633
PSI inv. 3783 (I–II AD), treatise on phlebotomy	http://www.papyri.info/dclp/63244
MPER XIII 19 (II AD), on physiology (anatomy?)	http://www.papyri.info/dclp/63723
P.Aberd. 11 (II AD), on ophthalmology	http://www.papyri.info/dclp/63332
P.Ross.Georg. I 20r (II AD), on ophthalmology	http://www.papyri.info/dclp/63569
P.Turner 14r (II AD), on therapy	http://www.papyri.info/dclp/63560
P.Oxy. LII 3654v (+ II 234) (II–III AD), composite roll, definitions on therapy followed by prescriptions	http://www.papyri.info/dclp/59150
P.Gen. inv. 111v (II–III AD), on surgery	http://www.papyri.info/dclp/63819
P.PisaLit. 6r (II–III AD), on ophthalmic surgery	http://www.papyri.info/dclp/63748
GMP II 14 (II–III AD), fragment dealing with diseases	http://www.papyri.info/dclp/63804
GMP I 6 (II–III AD), on afflictions of the head	http://www.papyri.info/dclp/69007
P.Oxy. LXXIV 4972v (II–III AD), on surgery	http://www.papyri.info/dclp/119317
P.Oxy. LXXX 5238 (II–III AD), on therapy	Forthcoming
P.Oxy. LXXX 5239 (II–III AD), on pathology	Forthcoming
P.Oxy. LXXX 5241v (II–III AD), on ophthalmology	Forthcoming
P.Oxford Ashmolean inv. 28 (Petrie Box A3) (II–IV AD)	Unpublished
GMP II 15 (III AD), on gynaecology	http://www.papyri.info/dclp/64216
P.Aberd. 125v (III AD), on trichology	http://www.papyri.info/dclp/64262
PSI XV 1510 (III AD), on anatomy	http://www.papyri.info/dclp/64024
P.Oslo inv. 1576v (III AD), on pathology	Forthcoming
P.Lund I 7 (III–IV AD), on anatomy	http://www.papyri.info/dclp/64316
P.Mil.Vogl. I 15 + P.Oxy. LXXX 5235 (IV AD), on pathology	http://www.papyri.info/dclp/64473
P.Strasb. inv. 489 (IV AD), on ophthalmology	http://www.papyri.info/dclp/69028

Bibliography

Primary Sources[71]

Bekker, I. 1846. *Iulii Pollucis Onomasticon*. Berolini: Nicolai.

Boudon-Millot, V. 2007. *Galien 1. Introduction générale. Sur l'ordre de ses propres livres. Sur ses propres livres. Que l'excellent médecin est aussi philosophe*. Paris: Les Belles Lettres.

Duffy, J.M. 1983. *Stephani Philosophi In Hippocratis Prognosticum commentaria III* [CMG XI.1.2]. Berlin: Teubner.

Iskandar, A.Z. 1988. *Galeni De optimo medico cognoscendo libelli* [CMG Suppl. Or. IV]. Berlin: Akademie-Verlag.

Jouanna, J. 1990. *Hippocrate 2.1. De l'ancienne médecine*. Paris: Les Belles Lettres.

Jouanna, J.—Guardasole, A.—Anastassiou, A. 2016. *Hippocrate 4.1. Épidémies I et III*. Paris: Les Belles Lettres.

Kühn, C.G. 1821–1833. *Claudii Galeni Opera Omnia*. 20 vols in 22. Lipsiae: Car. Cnoblochii.

Littré, É. 1839–1861. *Hippocrate, Œuvres complètes*. 10 vols. Paris: Baillière.

Petit, C. 2009. *Galien 3. Le médecin. Introduction*. Paris: Les Belles Lettres.

Secondary Sources

Agosti, G. 2010. '*Eisthesis*, divisione dei versi, percezione dei *cola* negli epigrammi epigrafici in età tardoantica', *Segno & Testo* 8: 67–98.

Andorlini, I. 1992. 'Papiri e medicina: P.Oxy. II 234 + P.Oxy. LII 3654', in El-Mosalamy (1992: 1.375–390).

Andorlini, I. (ed.). 1997a. *"Specimina" per il Corpus dei Papiri Greci di Medicina. Atti dell'Incontro di studio (Firenze 1996)*. Firenze: Istituto Papirologico Vitelli

Andorlini, I. 1997b. 'Trattato o catechismo? La tecnica della flebotomia in PSI inv. CNR 85/86', in Andorlini (1997a: 153–168).

Andorlini, I. 1999. 'Testi medici per la scuola: raccolte di definizioni e questionari nei papiri', in A. Garzya—J. Jouanna (eds.), *I testi medici greci. Tradizione e ecdotica. Atti del III Convegno internazionale (Napoli 1997)*. Napoli: D'Auria, 7–15.

Andorlini, I. 2003. 'L'esegesi del libro tecnico: papiri di medicina con scolî e commento', in *Studi e Testi per il Corpus dei Papiri Filosofici Greci e Latini 11: Papiri filosofici. Miscellanea di studi IV*. Firenze: Olschki, 9–29.

71 Papyri are cited according to the abbreviations listed in the *Checklist of Editions of Greek, Latin, Demotic, and Coptic Papyri, Ostraca, and Tablets*, online at http://papyri.info/docs/checklist. LDAB numbers refer to the *Leuven Database of Ancient Books* catalogue (http://www.trismegistos.org/ldab).

Andorlini, I. (ed.). 2004. *Testi medici su papiro. Atti del Seminario di studio (Firenze 2002)*. Firenze: Istituto Papirologico Vitelli.
Andorlini, I. 2006. 'Il 'gergo' grafico ed espressivo della ricettazione medica antica', in A. Marcone (ed.), *Medicina e società nel mondo antico: Atti del convegno di Udine (4–5 ottobre 2005)*. Firenze: Le Monnier, 142–167.
Andorlini, I. 2007. 'Teaching Medicine in Late Antiquity: Methods, Texts and Contexts', in P. Lendinara—L. Lazzari—M.A. D'Aronco (eds.), *Form and Content of Instruction in Anglo-Saxon England in the Light of Contemporary Manuscript Evidence. Papers presented at the International Conference (Udine, 6–8 April 2006)*. Turnhout: Brepols, 385–398.
Andorlini, I. (ed.). 2009. *Greek Medical Papyri II*. Firenze: Istituto Papirologico Vitelli.
Andorlini, I.—Reggiani, N. 2012. 'Edizione e ricostruzione digitale dei testi papiracei', in N. Palazzolo (ed.), *Diritto romano e scienze antichistiche nell'era digitale. Convegno di studio (Firenze 2011)*. Torino: Giappichelli, 131–146.
Ast, R.—Essler, H. 2018. '*Anagnosis*, Herculaneum, and the *Digital Corpus of Literary Papyri*', in Reggiani (2018a: 63–73).
Bäckström, A. 1904a. 'Demetrius of Apamea and His Fragments', *Journal of the Ministry of People Education* 356: 547–555 [in Russian].
Bäckström, A. 1904b. 'Fragment einer medizinischer Schrift', *Archiv für Papyrusforschung* 3: 158–162.
Barbis Lupi, R. 1988. 'La diplè obelismene: precisazioni terminologiche e formali', in B.G. Mandilaras (ed.), *Proceedings of the XVIII Inernational Congress of Papyrology (Athens, 25–31 May 1986)*. Athens: Greek Papyrological Society, II, 473–476.
Barbis Lupi, R. 1992. 'Uso e forma dei segni di riempimento nei papiri letterari greci', in El-Mosalamy (1992: 1.503–510).
Barbis Lupi, R. 1994. 'La Paragraphos: analisi di un segno di lettura', in A. Bülow-Jacobsen (ed.), *Proceedings of the 20th International Congress of Papyrologists (Copenhagen, 23–29 August 1992)*. Copenhagen: Museum Tusculanum Press, 414–417.
Barns, J.W.B. 1949. 'Literary Texts from the Fayum', *Classical Quarterly* 43: 1–8.
Bastianini, G. 2004. 'PSI 85 e la definizione di "chreia"', in M.S. Funghi (ed.), *Aspetti di letteratura gnomica nel mondo antico*, II, Firenze: Olschki, 249–263.
Bilabel, F. 1925. 'Fragmente aus der Heidelberger Papyrussammlung', *Philologus* 80: 331–341.
Bodard, G. 2010. 'EpiDoc: Epigraphic Documents in XML for Publication and Interchange', in F. Feraudi-Gruénais (ed.), *Latin On Stone: Epigraphic Research and Electronic Archives*. Lanham (MD): Lexington Books, 101–118.
Bonati, I. 2014. 'ὑδροκέφαλον', in I. Andorlini (ed.), *Medicalia Online*. Parma: http://www.papirologia.unipr.it/CPGM/medicalia/vocab/index.php?tema=44.
Brashear, W.M. 1992. *A Mithraic Catechism from Egypt (P. Berol. 21196)*. Wien: Holzhausen.

Caroli, M. 2007. *Il titolo iniziale nel rotolo librario greco-egizio*. Bari: Levante.

Di Matteo, T. 2007. 'Segni di riempimento nei papiri ercolanesi', in Frösén—Purola—Salmenkivi (2007: 1.259–265).

Drake, R.L.—Vogl, A.W.—Mitchell, A.W.M. 2015[3]. *Gray's Anatomy for Students Flash Cards*. Philadelphia (PA): Churchill Livingstone.

El-Mosalamy, A.H.S. (ed.). *Proceedings of the XIXth International Congress of Papyrology (Cairo 1989)*. Cairo: Center for Papyrological Studies.

Fausti, D. 1980. 'PSI III 252: manuale di medicina redatto in forma di questionario', in R. Pintaudi (ed.), *Miscellanea Papyrologica*. Firenze: Gonnelli, 61–65.

Fernandez-Delgado, J.A. 2013. 'Nuove testimonianze dell'opera di Plutarco', in G. Pace—V. Cacciatore (eds.), *Gli scritti di Plutarco: tradizione, traduzione, ricezione, commento. Atti del IX Convegno della International Plutarch Society (Ravello, 29 settembre–1 ottobre 2011)*. Napoli: D'Auria, 133–142.

Fischer, K.-D. 1998. 'Beiträge zu den pseudosoranischen Quaestiones Medicinales', in K.-D. Fischer—D. Nickel—P. Potter (eds.), *Text and Tradition. Studies in Ancient Medicine and its Transmission presented to Jutta Kollesch*. Leiden-Boston-Köln: Brill, 1–41.

Fournet, J.-L. 2004. 'La bibliothèque d'un médecin ou d'un apothicaire de Lycopolis?', in Andorlini (2004: 175–197).

Frösén, J.—Purola, T.—Salmenkivi, E. (eds.). 2007. *Proceedings of the 24th International Congress of Papyrology (Helsinki, 1–7 August 2004)*. Helsinki: Societas Scientiarum Fennica.

Genette, G. 1992. *The Architext: An Introduction*. Berkeley (CA): Quantum Books [1979. *Introduction à l'architexte*. Paris: Seuil].

Genette, G. 1997. *Palimpsests. Literature in the Second Degree*. Lincoln (NE): University of Nebraska Press [1982. *Palimpsestes: la littérature au second degré*. Paris: Seuil].

Gignac, F.T. 1976. *A Grammar of the Greek Papyri of the Roman and Byzantine Periods, I: Phonology*. Milano: Cisalpino-Goliardica.

Hanson, A.E. 1997. 'Fragmentation and the Greek Medical Writers', in G.W. Most (ed.), *Collecting Fragments / Fragmente Sammeln*. Göttingen: Vandenhoeck & Ruprecht, 289–314.

Hanson, A.E. 2003. 'Text and Context in Papyrus Catechisms on Afflictions of the Head', in A. Garzya—J. Jouanna (eds.), *Trasmissione e ecdotica dei testi medici greci. Atti del IV Convegno Internazionale (Napoli 2001)*. Napoli: D'Auria, 199–217.

Hanson, A.E. 2010. 'Doctors' Literacy and Papyri of Medical Content', in M. Horstmanshoff (ed.), *Hippocrates and Medical Education*. Leiden—Boston: Brill, 187–204.

Hanson, A.E.—Mattern, S.P. 2001. 'Medical Catechism', in I. Andorlini (ed.), *Greek Medical Papyri I*. Firenze: Istituto Papirologico Vitelli, 71–83.

Hock, R.F.—O'Neil, E.N. 2002. *The Chreia and Ancient Rhetoric: Classroom Exercises*. Atlanta (GA): Society of Biblical Literature.

Ieraci Bio, A.M. 1995. 'L'ἐρωταπόκρισις nella letteratura medica', in *Esegesi, parafrasi e compilazione in età tardoantica*. Napoli: D'Auria, 187–207.

Ingenkamp, H.G. 1969. 'τὸ ἅμα? Zu einem Papyrus mit Fragen und Antworten', *Rheinisches Museum* 112: 48–53.

Körte, A. 1927. 'Referate: Literarische Texte mit Ausschluß der christlichen', *Archiv für Papyrusforschung* 8: 251–272.

Körte, A. 1939. 'Referate: Literarische Texte mit Ausschluß der christlichen', *Archiv für Papyrusforschung* 13: 78–132.

Körte, A. 1941. 'Referate: Literarische Texte mit Ausschluß der christlichen', *Archiv für Papyrusforschung* 14: 103–150.

Kollesch, J. 1963. *Untersuchungen zu den pseudogalenischen* Definitiones Medicae. Berlin: Akademie-Verlag.

Leith, D. 2007. 'A Medical Treatise "On Remedies"? P.Turner 14 Revised', *Bulletin of the American Society of Papyrologists* 44: 125–135.

Leith, D. 2009a. 'Question-Types in Medical Catechisms on Papyrus', in L.C. Taub—A. Doody (eds.), *Authorial Voices in Greco-Roman Technical Writing*. Trier: Wissenschaftlicher Verlag, 107–123.

Leith, D. 2009b. 'A Note on the Greek Medical Fragment PGolenischeff', in Andorlini (2009: 211–218).

Leith, D. 2014. 'Medical Doxography in P. Mil. Vogl. I 15', *Zeitschrift für Papyrologie* 189: 225–232.

Leith, D.—Maravela, A. 2009. 'Notes on PSI III 252', in Andorlini (2009: 201–209).

Magdelaine, C. 2004. 'Un nouveau questionnaire ophtalmologique (PStrasb gr. inv. 849)', in Andorlini (2004: 63–77).

Manetti, D. 1973. 'P. Alex. inv. 614: testo medico', *Studi Classici e Orientali* 22: 46–49.

Manfredi, M. 1997. 'Modello di edizione di un testo letterario adespoto (PSI XV 1510: questionario sui παρίσθμια)', in Andorlini (1997a: 73–79).

Maravela, A.—Leith, D. 2007. 'A Medical Catechism on Tumours from the Collection of the Oslo University Library', in Frösén—Purola—Salmenkivi (2007: 2.637–650).

Marganne, M.-H. 1978. 'Deux questionnaires d'ophtalmologie: P. Aberdeen 11 et P. Ross. Georg. 1.20', *Chronique d'Egypte* 53: 313–320.

Marganne, M.-H. 1986. 'La « Cirurgia Eliodori » et le P. Genève inv. 111', *Etudes de Lettres*: 65–73.

Marganne, M.-H. 1987. 'Un questionnaire d'anatomie: P. Lund I 7. Réedition, traduction, commentaire', *Chronique d'Egypte* 62: 189–200.

Marganne, M.-H. 1994. *L'ophtalmologie dans l'Egypte gréco-romaine d'après les papyrus littéraires grecs*. Leiden—Boston: Brill.

Marganne, M.-H. 1998. *La chirurgie dans l'Egypte gréco-romaine d'après les papyrus littéraires grecs*. Leiden—Boston: Brill.

Mavroudis, A.D. 1986. 'Critical Notes on a Medical Papyrus (PSI III 252)', *Annual of the Faculty of Medicine, Aristotelian University of Thessaloniki* 16: 187–209.

McNamee, K. 2007. *Annotations in Greek and Latin Texts from Egypt*. s.l.: American Society of Papyrologists.

McNamee, K. 1981. *Abbreviations in Greek Literary Papyri and Ostraca*. Chico (CA): American Society of Papyrologists.

Moretti, A.F. 1995. 'Revisione di alcuni papiri greci letterari editi tra i P.Mil.Vogl.', *Analecta Papyrologica* 7: 19–30.

Nicole, J. 1903. 'Un questionnaire de chirurgie', *Archiv für Papyrusforschung* 2: 1–3.

Nieddu, G.F. 1992. 'Il ginnasio e la scuola: scrittura e mimesi del parlato', in G. Cambiano—L. Canfora—D. Lanza (ed.) *Lo spazio letterario della Grecia antica, I.1: La produzione e la circolazione del testo—La* polis. Roma: Salerno, 555–585.

Nutton, V. 1972. 'Galen and Medical Autobiography', *Proceedings of the Cambridge Philological Society* 198: 50–62.

Nutton, V. 1990. 'The Patient's Choice: A New Treatise by Galen', *Classical Quarterly* 40: 236–257.

Oellacher, H. 1937. 'Rhetorischer Katechismus in einem Wiener Papyrus', *Wiener Studien* 55: 63–78.

Petit, C. 2009. *Galien: Le médicin. Introduction*. Paris: Les Belles Lettres.

Reggiani, N. 2015. 'A Corpus of Literary Papyri Online: The Pilot Project of the Medical Texts via SoSOL', in R. Lafer—K. Strobel (eds.), *Antike Lebenswelten. Althistorische und papyrologische Studien*. Berlin—Boston: De Gruyter, 341–352.

Reggiani, N. 2016. 'The Corpus of Greek Medical Papyri and Digital Papyrology: New Perspectives from an Ongoing Project', in M. Berti—F. Naether (eds.), *Altertumswissenschaften in a Digital Age—Egyptology, Papyrology and Beyond. Proceedings of a Conference and Workshop in Leipzig (November 4–6, 2015)*. Leipzig: Universität Leipzig, ch. 1.9: http://nbn-resolving.de/urn:nbn:de:bsz:15-qucosa-201726.

Reggiani, N. 2017. *Digital Papyrology I: Methods, Tools and Trends*. Berlin—Boston: De Gruyter.

Reggiani, N. (ed.). 2018a. *Digital Papyrology II: New Methods and Tools for the Digital Edition of Ancient Greek Papyri*. Berlin—Boston: De Gruyter.

Reggiani, N. 2018b. 'The Corpus of the Greek Medical Papyri and a New Concept of Digital Critical Edition', in Reggiani (2018a: 1–59).

Reggiani, N. 2018c. 'I papiri greci di medicina come fonti storiche: il caso dei rapporti dei medici pubblici nell'Egitto greco-romano', *Aegyptus* 98: 107–130.

Reggiani, N. 2019a. 'Transmission of Recipes and Receptaria in Greek Medical Writings on Papyrus Between Ancient Text Production and Modern Digital Representation', in R. Berardi—N. Bruno—L. Fizzarotti (eds.), *On the Track of the Books: Scribes, Libraries and Textual Transmission*. Berlin—Boston: De Gruyter, 167–188.

Reggiani, N. 2019b. *The Corpus of Greek Medical Papyri Online and the Digital Edition of Ancient Documents*, in A. Nodar—S. Torallas Tovar (eds.), *Proceedings of the 28th International Congress of Papyrology (Barcelona 2016)*. Barcelona: Universitat Pompeu Fabra, 843–856.

Reggiani, N. 2019c. *La papirologia digitale. Prospettiva storico-critica e sviluppi metodologici*, Parma: Athenaeum.

Reggiani, N. 2019d. 'Ancient Doctors' Literacies and the Digital Edition of Papyri of Medical Content', *Classics@* 17: http://nrs.harvard.edu/urn-3:hlnc.essay:ReggianiN.Ancient_Doctors_Literacies.2019.

Reggiani, N. 2020. 'The Digital Edition of Ancient Sources as a Further Step in the Textual Transmission', forthcoming in the proceedings of the workshop "Digital Classics III: Re-Thinking Text Analysis" (Heidelberg, 12–13 May 2017).

Ronconi, F. 2000. 'Riedizione di PSI VI 718: ricette mediche e geoponiche', *Analecta Papyrologica* 12: 143–149.

Savignago, L. 2008. Eisthesis. *Il sistema dei margini nei papiri dei poeti tragici*. Alessandria: Edizioni dell'Orso.

Schiefsky, M.J. 2005. *Hippocrates On Ancient Medicine*. Leiden—Boston: Brill.

Schironi, F. 2010. *ΤΟ ΜΕΓΑ ΒΙΒΛΙΟΝ. Book-ends, End-titles, and* Coronides *in Papyri with Hexametric Poetry*. Durham (NC): American Society of Papyrologists.

Schönbauer, E. 1933. 'Ein neues vorjustinianisches Werk (P. Festheft Wilcken)', *Zeitschrift der Savigny-Stiftung für Rechtsgeschichte / Romanistische Abteilung* 53: 451–464.

Schönbauer, E. 1933. 'Ein neuer juristischer Papyrus', *Aegyptus* 13: 621–643.

Snell, B. 1939. Review to P.Mil.Vogl. I, *Gnomon* 15: 529–543.

Sosin, J.D. 2010. 'Digital Papyrology', *The Stoa Consortium* 26 October 2010: http://www.stoa.org/archives/1263.

Turcan, R. 1992. 'Un 'catéchisme' mithriaque?', *Comptes Rendus de l'Académie des Inscriptions* 136.3: 549–564.

Turcan, R. 1993. *Mithras et le mithriacisme*. Paris: Les Belles Lettres.

Wilcken, U. 1924. 'Referate: Papyrus-Urkunden', *Archiv für Papyrusforschung* 7: 67–114.

Winstedt, E.O. 1907. 'Some Greek and Latin Papyri in Aberdeen Museum', *Classical Quarterly* 1: 257–267.

Zalateo, G. 1964. 'Papiri di argomento medico redatti in forma di domanda e risposta', *Aegyptus* 44: 52–57.

CHAPTER 9

Questions on the Unseen: Alexander of Tralles' Patient Interaction

Laura Mareri

Abstract

The aim of this contribution is to explore, for the very first time, the ways in which the Byzantine physician Alexander of Tralles (4th century AD) interacts with his patients, and so to extend contemporary scholarship into hitherto unexplored terrain. More concretely, I will examine the role which Alexander ascribes to questions and answers in diagnosing his patients. Alexander generally relies on direct observation and past experience in the treatment of internal diseases, yet some exceptions show that this is not the only kind of approach he employs in the diagnostic process, as in some cases he resorts to various questions in order to obtain information about what is not immediately visible to his eyes. This is the case primarily when no help is provided by what becomes manifest through his observation of the patient's body or symptoms at the moment of the medical examination (e.g., the patient's own sensation and perception of heat/cold, heaviness, pain). At the same time, Alexander's discussion of cases of melancholy and phrenitis demonstrate that the interaction with the patient also relates to mental disorders, as Alexander relies on the patient's behaviour in determining whether s/he is in the process of healing or not. By focusing on Alexander's use of questions and answers in his patient communication, the present contribution aims to demonstrate that this specific mode of interaction is unavoidable in some cases and is even employed by a physician who generally prefers diagnosing diseases mainly through direct observation than through human communication.

1 Alexander of Tralles' Life, Work and Therapeutic Approach

Little is known about Alexander of Tralles' life (ca. 525–605 AD), except from the fact that he was born in a wealthy family. The historian Agathias tells us that Alexander's father, Stephanus, was a famous doctor in Tralles, and that his brother Anthemius was one of the architects of the Hagia Sophia in Constantinople. He also had other brothers, namely Metrodorus, a mathematician and a grammarian, Olympius, a famous jurist, and Dioscorus, who was a doc-

 | DOI:10.1163/9789004442672_011

tor but exercised the medical profession in his hometown and did not travel, unlike Alexander. Agathias was so impressed by the eminence of Alexander of Tralles' family that he even congratulated his mother for having given birth to such a great offspring, abounding with a variegated culture (ποικίλης παιδείας: 171.3–6 Keydell).

As to his professional life, Alexander of Tralles largely based his medicine on a critical re-use of the Hippocratic and Galenic medical systems in combination with his own professional experience, which he gained through a long career as a practicing physician. He drew up his main work, the *Therapeutica*, at a late age.[1] In this work, the diagnosis of internal illnesses, which is essential for the prescription of a proper therapy, is generally conducted on the basis of patient observation and supported by the knowledge of Hippocratic and Galenic medicine.

The aim of this paper is to examine the use which Alexander ascribes to questions and answers for medical diagnosis. Although an initial investigation shows that he only rarely engages in a dialogue with his patients in order to gain information about their symptoms and underlying medical conditions, there are some specific cases in which he cannot but rely on the patients' answers in order to establish a proper diagnosis. As such, the focus of this study will be on those situations in which Alexander changes his usual diagnostic method (usually based on Hippocratic and Galenic advice and on his own personal experience), and instead relies on his patients' words. The reason why he sometimes breaks away from his usual approach is key to our better understanding of Alexander's medicine.

2 Alexander's Communication with His Readers

In diagnosing his patients, Alexander generally prefers to rely on his own eyes and only rarely asks questions, let alone establish a dialogue concerning his patients' health conditions. Yet, questions and answers are not completely absent from his work. In fact, the *Therapeutica* come in the very form of the author's response to the request of one Cosmas to publish the methods of treatment of internal diseases that Alexander as a physician was able to collect

1 For a number of recent studies on (the Greek) Alexander of Tralles, his life, time, style, ideas and manuscript tradition, see: Scarborough (1997) on Alexander's life and time; Guardasole (2004a) on his *editio princeps*; Guardasole (2004b) on his use of natural remedies; Guardasole (2004c) on his relationship to Galen; Guardasole (2006) on his life, style and ideas; Zipser (2005) on the manuscript tradition; and Bouras-Vallianatos (2014) on his therapy of epilepsy.

thanks to his sound experience gained while exercising his profession.[2] Similarly, his treatise on intestinal worms (*De lumbricis*) is directed at a certain Theodorus in response to his request for an effective remedy to cure his son, who was facing death due to the infection under discussion.[3]

Of course, in both cases, the physician uses dedication as a literary device, aimed at defining the work's context and specifying its purpose and usefulness to the reader. Nonetheless, it is significant that there is a will to establish a dialogue with the dedicatee, a dialogue that can be real or fictitious, but in either case is the answer to a precise health-related request by an individual. As such, these passages show that Alexander was considered a great authority by his dedicatees, who consulted him for his medical expertise. Being asked for his therapeutic advice, he is more than happy to share his knowledge with them.

Both in the *Therapeutica* and in the treatise on intestinal worms we thus find a response to a personal request for help. But at a more general level, this response is of use to any reader looking for practical advice on internal diseases and intestinal worms respectively, including the doctors involved in the treatment of such ailments. Eventually, it is the patients—and not only Cosmas or Theodorus—who are the final 'recipients' of the texts, and more precisely of the therapies prescribed therein. They are the ones that Alexander—so he explicitly declares elsewhere—intends to cure by *any* means possible (πάσῃ μηχανῇ)—even if this involves using 'natural', that is magical, remedies.[4] So

2 Next to nothing is known about this Cosmas, except from the fact that he was particularly dear to the author. 1.289.1–4 Puschmann: "I promptly listened to your request, my dearest Cosmas, to publish the methods of treatment of the various diseases I collected thanks to my long-standing experience, in order to express my gratitude to you and your father—thus responding to your will—for your constant good disposition towards me." (Αἰτήσαντί σοι, Κοσμᾶ φίλτατε, τὰς ἐκ πείρας ἡμῖν πολλάκις ἀνυσθείσας ἐπὶ διαφόρων νοσημάτων ἐκθέσθαι θεραπείας ἑτοίμως ὑπήκουσα χάριτας ἀμφοτέροις εἰκότως ὁμολογῶν σοί τε καὶ τῷ σῷ πατρὶ τῆς εἰς ἐμὲ παρ' ὑμῶν φιλοφρόνως ἑκάστοτε γενομένης εὐνοίας.) All the translations of Alexander's text are mine.

3 2.587.1–3 Puschmann: "My dearest Theodorus, you wrote to me about your son in danger of death, so that I could give you some remedy for eliminating worms and help him." (Γέγραφάς μοι, φίλτατε Θεόδωρε, περὶ τοῦ σοῦ παιδὸς ἀπολέσθαι κινδυνεύοντος, ὅπως ἄν τι τῶν ἕλμινθας ἀναιρεῖν δυναμένων ὑμῖν ἀποστείλαντες φάρμακον οἷοί τε γενοίμεθα βοηθεῖν αὐτῷ.)

4 See LSJ, s.v. φῠσικός, iii: "later, belonging to occult laws of nature, magical, φ. φάρμακα spells or amulets" (with an indication of its use in Alexander of Tralles; cf. Meeusen in this volume, n. 12). The aim of Alexander of Tralles' work is mostly therapeutic. He uses the metaphor of victory in war (νικῆσαι) in order to describe the saving (σῶσαι) of a patient from an illness, which, so he generalises, should be implemented to any patient by any means (πάσῃ μηχανῇ). 2.475.2–4 Puschmann: "I deemed it necessary to expose also some of these [sc. natural/magical] remedies—especially in view of the people who love virtue—in order to save the man and win the fight against the illness; in fact, it is good to overcome it and help a

apparently, as far as this last point is concerned, even the prescription of natural/magical remedies is entrusted to the doctor, whose therapeutic method is not solely based on 'rational' medicine but also involves 'alternative' (i.e., non-rational/popular) elements. As a matter of fact, the doctor's authoritative advice is not strictly required in each and every case: at some point we read that when a popular remedy is available, it is not needed to ask for a doctor (μηδὲ ἐρωτῶντες ἰατρούς) but that self-medication suffices. This is in the chapter on colic, where Alexander writes that everyone knows by experience that in case of stomach ache it is advisable to consume tops of celery and boiled leek and, along with caucalis, wild asparagus and garlic, and that for this reason it is unnecessary to ask for a doctor; especially farmers use such a diet instead of taking powerful drugs.[5]

3 Questions on the Unseen

Apart from the two apostrophes just mentioned, which show Alexander's willingness to engage in direct communication with his patient (or with the patient's close relatives) by responding to a specific request for help, he seems to avoid the use of questions and answers in diagnosing his patient's condition almost completely. Alexander thus only relies on the knowledge from the medical sources he draws on and above all on his own personal experience. Health conditions, including the perception of pain, are usually not diagnosed by formulating questions and obtaining corresponding answers, as the cause of pain is often manifested by the patient's body (e.g., in the case of wounds) and so perceptible to the physician's observation. Nevertheless, even if direct obser-

person in every possible way" (ἀναγκαῖον ἐνόμισα καὶ τούτων [sc. φυσικῶν] ἐκθέσθαι τινὰ καὶ μάλιστα διὰ τοὺς φιλαρέτους ἕνεκα τοῦ σῶσαι ἄνθρωπον καὶ δυνηθῆναι νικῆσαι πάθος· καλὸν γὰρ νικᾶν καὶ πάσῃ μηχανῇ βοηθεῖν). On Alexander of Tralles' use of natural/magical remedies, see Guardasole (2004b).

5 2.339.11–19 Puschmann: "It is useful for those [affected by colic] to eat, among the vegetables, the tops of celery and boiled leek; and it is also good for them to eat caucalis, wild asparagus and, above all, garlic; everybody knows, by experience, that it produces a considerable benefit, and for this reason, when a person feels some pain in the stomach, without calling the doctor, he immediately takes these vegetables; and especially the farmers use this food instead of some other very powerful drug." (Τῶν δὲ λαχάνων ἐσθίειν αὐτοὺς συμφέρει τῶν τε σελίνων καὶ τῶν πράσων ἑφθῶν τὰς κεφαλάς· καλὴ δέ ἐστιν ἐπὶ τούτων καὶ ἡ καυκαλὶς καὶ ὁ ἕλειος ἀσπάραγος καὶ τὰ σκόρδα πλείονα πάντων. ἴσασι δὲ τοῦτο πάντες ἐξ αὐτῆς μεμαθηκότες τῆς πείρας, ὅτιπερ οὐ μικρὸν τὸ ἐξ αὐτῶν ὄφελός ἐστι, καὶ διὰ τοῦτο, ἐπειδὰν αἴσθωνταί τινος ὀδύνης οἱ πολλοὶ περὶ τὴν γαστέρα, μηδὲ ἐρωτῶντες ἰατροὺς εὐθὺς ταῦτα προσφέρονται καὶ μάλιστα οἱ γεωργοὶ ἀντὶ μεγίστου τινὸς φαρμάκου ταύτῃ κέχρηνται τῇ τροφῇ.)

vation and knowledge of Hippocratic and Galenic antecedents form the basis of the diagnosis of diseases, in some specific cases these are not sufficiently adequate as diagnostic tools. This is the case when no help is provided by what becomes manifest to the doctor through the observation of the patient's body or symptoms at the moment of the medical examination.

For instance, in the case of the first type of melancholy, due to an overabundance of blood (Alexander's classification of the other types of melancholy is discussed below), we read that an excess of fluid is shown by the patient's temperament and complexion (κρᾶσις), such as increased facial blushing and tense and dilated veins, the tangibility of which makes it unnecessary to question the patient. But the fact that the body contains an excess of blood also implies a previous accumulation of it, which is not exclusively shown through clearly recognisable signs, precisely because it relates to a past condition. It follows that the interruption of its normal outflow, which in the case of men occurs through the blockage of the hemorrhoidal flow and, in the case of women, of the menstrual flux, makes it unavoidable to question (ἐρωτᾶν) the patient, as this phenomenon has already happened, and therefore cannot be subjected to medical observation.[6]

Bearing this passage in mind, there is much reason to assume—although this remain implicit—that in another paragraph concerning a phlebotomy that should be performed on a patient with angina, the doctor who learns (μάθῃς) that the patient usually loses blood through hemorrhoids did so by questioning him in order to obtain the desired information about these bleedings. We are dealing here with a phenomenon only known to the patient, who is accustomed to it (εἰωθότα) because he has previous experience, whereas the physician probably only found out by asking.[7]

Besides the behaviour of bodily fluids and the physiological processes that regulate them, certain sensations and sensory perceptions can also be subject to medical questioning. Thus, one of the ways to find out which part is affected is to ask if the patient feels a sensation of heat (θέρμη) or perceives heaviness (βάρος) in that area. This is the case, for instance, if a patient has a lung inflammation: in order to find out if the inflammation has produced pus,

6 1.593.7–9 Puschmann: "and it is also necessary to ask whether there was an interruption of the usual bleeding through the hemorrhoid—in the case of men—or through the monthly menstruation—in the case of women" (ἐρωτᾶν δὲ δεῖ πρὸς τούτοις, μὴ ἄρα τις ἐπίσχεσις γένοιτο συνήθους κενώσεως, ἐπὶ μὲν ἀνδρῶν, αἱμορροίας, ἐπὶ δὲ γυναικῶν, ἐμμήνου καθάρσεως).

7 2.143.15–16 Puschmann: "this [i.e., bloodletting] should also be performed on a man, if you find out that he usually evacuates blood through hemorrhoids" (τοῦτο δὲ καὶ ἐπ' ἀνθρώπου δεῖ ποιεῖν, ἐὰν μάθῃς αὐτὸν δι' αἱμορροΐδων εἰωθότα αἷμα κενοῦν).

the physician should ask (ἐρωτώμενον) the patient whether the right part of the chest is particularly hot and if he is feeling a sense of heaviness.[8] The same type of sensation is the subject of a direct interaction between the doctor and the patient in the paragraph dedicated to kidney inflammation, again as a way to discover the presence of pus. In this case, the emphasis is also put on two precise actions, namely the perception of heaviness (βάρους αἰσθάνεσθαι) and the action to report (λέγειν) it to the doctor.[9]

The perception of heat and heaviness concern the inner part of the patient's body which is not observable by the doctor's eye or touch. So since relying on his own sensation is impossible, the doctor is obliged to ask the patient how s/he is feeling, just as in the case of the interruption of hemorrhoids and menstrual flow, albeit for different reasons. In the latter case, the blockage is unknowable because it concerns the patient's state of health in the past, while in the former case health conditions are examined at the time of diagnosis. In either case, the patient's words convey important information to the doctor which is vital for a proper diagnosis. As such, questioning the patient serves as a useful tool for diagnosing physical ailments.

4 Diagnosing Mental Health

While the examples mentioned above are connected with the body's physiology, the use of questions and answers is also an important method to exclude or confirm the presence of mental illness, which in ancient medicine was believed to have well-defined physiological origins, but of which the behavioural consequences are equally well-identifiable.

8 2.211.24–27 Puschmann: "it is necessary to diagnose the affected area also on the basis of what the questioned patient says, if by chance even the right part of the chest is warmer and he feels a sense of heaviness, as if something is pending when he bends over to the other side" (διαγνωστέον δὲ τὸν πεπονθότα τόπον καὶ ἐκ τοῦ ἐρωτώμενον τὸν κάμνοντα λέγειν, εἰ τύχοι καὶ τὸ δεξιὸν μέρος τοῦ θώρακος εἶναι θερμότερον μᾶλλον καὶ βάρους συναίσθησιν ἔχειν, ὡς κρεμαμένου τινὸς ἐξ αὐτοῦ, ὁπηνίκα περὶ τὸ ἕτερον μέρος ἀνακλιθείη).

9 2.481.5–11 Puschmann: "Recognise that the phlegmon is turning into pus [...] also from the fact that the patient, when bending over to the healthy side, says that he feels a great weight in the affected part, heavier than before the phlegmon turned into a suppurative inflammation." (Τὴν δὲ φλεγμονὴν μέλλουσαν εἰς πῦον μεταβάλλεσθαι διαγίνωσκε [...] πρὸς τοῦτο ἀνακλινόμενον αὐτὸν εἰς τὸ ὑγιαῖνον μέρος ἐκ τοῦ πεπονθότος βάρους πολλοῦ μᾶλλον αὐτὸν αἰσθάνεσθαι λέγειν ἢ πρὸ τοῦ εἰς ἀπόστασιν ἄρχεσθαι τὴν φλεγμονήν.) The imperative (διαγίνωσκε) is directed at the recipients of the text, namely doctors or, more generally, people engaged in taking care of patients suffering from kidney inflammation.

Alexander devotes a specific chapter (the seventeenth of the first book of the *Therapeutica*) to melancholy, where he draws a distinction between four different types: melancholy due to the abundance of blood (discussed above), melancholy due to excessively acrid and bilious blood, melancholy due to melancholic blood, and chronic melancholy. The paragraph dedicated to melancholy caused by melancholic blood is largely aimed at identifying the typical behaviours of patients affected by this type of melancholy. Here, Alexander describes the case of a woman who suffered from this pathological condition because of the absence of her husband, who had left for a long journey, and, for that reason, replied angrily to everyone (ὀργίλως [...] ἀποκρινομένην).[10] Unlike the cases discussed above, we are not dealing here with a reply to a question concerning a specific physiological matter, nor is the woman necessarily addressed by the physician: the reference is rather to the external observation of her irritable behaviour in answering to a probably more generic type of question asked by any bystander trying to interact with her. Nevertheless, such type of interacton is still useful to the doctor who is observing the dialogue to probe the patient's mental condition.

Likewise, in the chapter on phrenitis (the thirteenth of the first book of the *Therapeutica*), when discussing the first signs of the illness, Alexander reports that one of the typical behavioural changes is that the patients reply (ἀποκρινόμενοι) in a more insolent and irascible manner than before (other signs include insomnia and tormented sleep, the will to predict the future and forgetting what one wants to say or do).[11] This kind of behaviour has to be seen in the broader context of the inability of those affected by phrenitis to use articulate language, as is clear from the paragraph dealing with false phrenitis, which immediately follows. People suffering from this illness behave similarly to those suffering from real phrenitis (they suffer from insomnia, with short moments of delirium, followed by a deep and comatose sleep and then by loud awakening), and also reply (ἀποκρίνονται) with incoherent and mad expressions to those who address them.[12]

While answering angrily, incoherently, impudently and madly falls within the behaviours indicating the presence of a mental illness (as is shown by the

---

10 1.607.10–11 Puschmann: "and I saw another woman experiencing melancholy because her husband had left for a long journey, and she replied wrathfully to everyone" (καὶ ἄλλην δέ τινα μελαγχολίᾳ περιπεσοῦσαν ἐπὶ μακρᾷ τοῦ ἀνδρὸς ἀποδημίᾳ καὶ ὀργίλως πρὸς ἅπαντας ἀποκρινομένην).

11 1.511.30–31 Puschmann: "and, when replying, they appear more insolent and irascible than in the past" (καὶ ἀποκρινόμενοι δὲ θρασύτεροι καὶ ὀργιλώτεροι φαίνονται τοῦ πρόσθεν).

12 1.513.14–15 Puschmann: "and they reply to those who address them with incoherent and mad expressions" (καὶ ἀποκρίνονται πρὸς τοὺς λαλοῦντας ἄτακτα καὶ μανίας ἐχόμενα ῥήματα).

above passages on melancholy and phrenitis), the path to healing can also be diagnosed on the basis of the answers given by the patients. At least in the case of recovery from melancholy, we read that the answers are consistently expressed (ἀποκρινόμενον ἀκολούθως), and the patient's reasoning appears sensible, while his behaviour in general is no longer barbaric, indicating that the doctor should administer a specific diet in view of the definitive remission of the disease.[13]

5 Conclusion

In the cases previously considered, the medical use of questions and answers regards the area of diagnostic analysis. We have seen that it is useful for diagnosing not only physical but also mental pathologies. Interaction by means of questions and answers gives the physician a proper understanding of humoural excess in the patient's body (in particular, that of the blood) but also of the patient's own sensory perception, which are both essentially inaccessible to the doctor. Also in the case of mental illness, the patient's answers (although not necessarily to questions asked by the doctor) serve as useful signs in the diagnostic process. This is the case specifically when patients suffer from phrenitis or melancholy. In the latter case, the patient's answers can also serve as a useful tool to understand whether the healing process has commenced or not.

As such, questions and answers serve as a fundamental diagnostic tool for the practicing physician: their presence in Alexander's medicine demonstrates the inevitability of the use of the spoken word in medical practice. Therefore, it would be an oversimplification to reduce Alexander's work to a mere encyclopaedic compilation by a voiceless Byzantine doctor. It is true that the theories Alexander learned from his predecessors are fundamental to his own art (esp. Hippocrates and Galen), but he also relies on the medical experience that he gained during his long activity as a practicing physician. As part of this practice, we have seen that, in some cases, the doctor has to rely on verbal

13 1.615.10–15 Puschmann: "and when you notice that he (i.e., the melancholic) answers in a coherent way, his reasoning is sensible and his behaviour is no longer barbaric, you have to give to the patient more food, including partridges, birds and pheasants—the parts without fat—and even sparrows, avoiding all the animals raised in the marshes and, among the types of fish, cetaceans, with the exception of rock fish" (καὶ ἐπειδὰν εὕρῃς αὐτὸν ἀποκρινόμενον ἀκολούθως καὶ τοὺς λογισμοὺς ἐρρωμένους ἔχοντα καὶ τὸ βαρβαρικὸν ἦθος ἀποθέμενον, ἔτι τε καὶ μᾶλλον ἐπιδίδου πλείονα τῷ κάμνοντι τροφὴν περδίκων τε καὶ ὀρνίθων καὶ φασιανῶν τὰ μὴ λιπαρὰ καὶ στρουθίων ὁμοίως, παραιτούμενος δὲ τὰ ἐν τοῖς ἕλεσι τρόφιμα πάντα καὶ τῶν ἰχθύων τοὺς κητώδεις πλὴν τῶν πετραίων).

communication in order to establish a proper diagnosis, where the patient's answers to specific questions, as well as the way in which those answers are formulated, have a seminal role to play.

Bibliography

Primary Sources

Keydell, R. 1967. *Agathiae Myrinaei historiarum libri quinque*. Berlin: De Gruyter.

Puschmann, T. 1963. *Alexander von Tralles: original-Text und Übersetzung nebst einer einleitenden Abhandlung*. 2nd ed. Amsterdam: Hakkert.

Secondary Sources

Bouras-Vallianatos, P. 2014. 'Clinical Experience in Late Antiquity: Alexander of Tralles and the Therapy of Epilepsy', *Medical History* 58.3: 337–353.

Guardasole, A. 2004a. 'Sur l'*editio princeps* d'Alexandre de Tralles', in V. Boudon-Millot—G. Cobolet (eds.), *Lire les médecins grecs à la Renaissance*. Paris: De Boccard, 323–337.

Guardasole, A. 2004b. 'Alexandre de Tralles et les remèdes naturels', in F. Collard—E. Samama (eds.), *Mires, physiciens, barbiers et charlatans*. Langres: D. Gueniot, 81–99.

Guardasole, A. 2004c. 'L'héritage de Galien dans l'œuvre d'Alexandre de Tralles', in J. Jouanna—J. Leclant (eds.), 'La médecine grecque antique', *Cahiers de la Villa Kérylos* 15.1: 219–234.

Guardasole, A. 2006. 'Alessandro di Tralle', in A. Garzya (ed.), *Medici bizantini*. Torino: UTET, 555–679.

Scarborough, J. 1997. 'The Life and Times of Alexander of Tralles', *Expedition* 39.2: 51–60.

Zipser, B. 2005. 'Die *Therapeutica* des Alexander Trallianus: ein medizinisches Handbuch und seine Überlieferung', in R.M. Piccione—M. Perkams (eds.), *Selecta Colligere II*. Alessandria: Edizioni Dell'Orso, 211–234.

Index Locorum

Index Rerum Nominumque

www.ingramcontent.com/pod-product-compliance
Ingram Content Group UK Ltd.
Pitfield, Milton Keynes, MK11 3LW, UK
UKHW022224051026
15624UKWH00002B/335

9 789004 437654